a LANGE medical book

Endocrine Physiology

fourth edition

Patricia E. Molina, MD, PhD
Richard Ashman, PhD Professor
Head, Department of Physiology
Louisiana State University Health Sciences Center
New Orleans, Louisiana

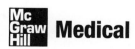 **Medical**

New York Chicago San Francisco Lisbon London Madrid Mexico City
Milan New Delhi San Juan Seoul Singapore Sydney Toronto

The McGraw·Hill Companies

Endocrine Physiology, Fourth Edition

Copyright © 2013, 2010, 2006, 2004 by the McGraw-Hill Companies, Inc. All rights reserved. Printed in the United States of America. Except as permitted under the United States Copyright Act of 1976, no part of this publication may be reproduced or distributed in any form or by any means, or stored in a data base or retrieval system, without the prior written permission of the publisher.

3 4 5 6 7 8 9 0 DOC/DOC 18 17 16 15

ISBN 978-0-07-179677-4
MHID 0-07-179677-0
ISSN 1545-2344

This book was set in Adobe Garamond Pro by Thomson Digital.
The editors were Michael Weitz and Christie Naglieri.
The production supervisor was Catherine Saggese.
Cover Image: The thyroid gland. Credit: Anatomical Travelogue / Photo Researchers, Inc.
RR Donnelly was printer and binder.

This book is printed on acid-free paper.

McGraw-Hill books are available at special quantity discounts to use as premiums and sales promotions, or for use in corporate training programs. To contact a representative please e-mail us at bulksales@mcgraw-hill.com.

*To my friend, colleague, and husband,
Miguel F. Molina, MD, for his
unconditional support and constant
reminder of what is really
important in life.*

Contents

Preface

This fourth edition of *Endocrine Physiology* provides comprehensive coverage of the fundamental concepts of hormone biological action. The content has been revised and edited to enhance clarity and understanding, and illustrations have been added and annotated to highlight the principal concepts in each chapter. In addition, the answers to the test questions at the end of the chapter have been expanded to include explanations for the correct answers.

The concepts herein provide the basis by which first- and second-year medical students will better grasp the physiologic mechanisms involved in neuroendocrine regulation of organ function. The information presented is also meant to serve as a reference for residents and fellows. The objectives listed at the beginning of each chapter follow those established and revised in 2012 by the American Physiological Society for each hormone system and are the topics tested in Step I of the United States Medical Licensing Examination (USMLE).

As with any discipline in science and medicine, our understanding of endocrine molecular physiology has changed and continues to evolve to encompass neural, immune, and metabolic regulation and interaction. The suggested readings have been updated to provide guidance for more in-depth understanding of the concepts presented. They are by no means all inclusive, but were found by the author to be of great help in putting the information together.

The first chapter describes the organization of the endocrine system, as well as general concepts of hormone production and release, transport and metabolic fate, and cellular mechanisms of action. Chapters 2–9 discuss specific endocrine systems and describe the specific hormone produced by each system in the context of the regulation of its production and release, the target physiologic actions, and the clinical implications of either its excess or deficiency. Each chapter starts with a short description of the functional anatomy of the organ, highlighting important features pertaining to circulation, location, or cellular composition that have a direct effect on its endocrine function. Understanding the mechanisms underlying normal endocrine physiology is essential in order to understand the transition from health to disease and the rationale involved in pharmacological, surgical, or genetic interventions. Thus, the salient features involved in determination of abnormal hormone production, regulation or function are also described. Each chapter includes simple diagrams illustrating some of the key concepts presented and concludes with sample questions designed to test the overall assimilation of the information given. The key concepts provided in each chapter correspond to the particular section of the chapter that describes them. Chapter 10 illustrates how the individual endocrine systems described throughout the book dynamically interact in maintaining homeostasis.

As with the previous editions of this book; the modifications are driven by the questions raised by my students during lecture or when studying for an examination. Those questions have been the best way of gauging the clarity of the writing and they have also alerted me when unnecessary description complicated or obscured the understanding of a basic concept. Improved learning and understanding of the concepts by our students continues to be my inspiration. I would like to thank them, as well as all the faculty of the Department of Physiology at LSUHSC for their dedication to the teaching of this discipline.

General Principles of Endocrine Physiology

1

OBJECTIVES

▶ *Contrast the terms endocrine, paracrine, and autocrine.*
▶ *Define the terms hormone, target cell, and receptor.*
▶ *Understand the major differences in mechanisms of action of peptides, steroids, and thyroid hormones.*
▶ *Compare and contrast hormone actions exerted via plasma membrane receptors with those mediated via intracellular receptors.*
▶ *Understand the role of hormone-binding proteins.*
▶ *Understand the feedback control mechanisms of hormone secretion.*
▶ *Explain the effects of secretion, degradation, and excretion on plasma hormone concentrations.*
▶ *Understand the basis of hormone measurements and their interpretation.*

The function of the endocrine system is to coordinate and integrate cellular activity within the whole body by regulating cellular and organ function throughout life and maintaining **homeostasis**. Homeostasis, or the maintenance of a constant internal environment, is critical to ensuring appropriate cellular function.

THE ENDOCRINE SYSTEM: PHYSIOLOGIC FUNCTIONS AND COMPONENTS

Some of the key functions of the endocrine system include:

- Regulation of sodium and water balance and control of blood volume and pressure
- Regulation of calcium and phosphate balance to preserve extracellular fluid concentrations required for cell membrane integrity and intracellular signaling
- Regulation of energy balance and control of fuel mobilization, utilization, and storage to ensure that cellular metabolic demands are met

1

- Coordination of the host hemodynamic and metabolic counterregulatory responses to stress
- Regulation of reproduction, development, growth, and senescence

In the classic description of the endocrine system, a chemical messenger or **hormone** produced by an organ is released into the circulation to produce

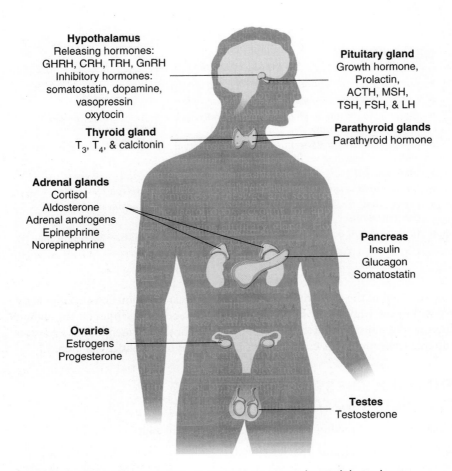

Figure 1–1. The endocrine system. Endocrine organs are located throughout the body, and their function is controlled by hormones delivered through the circulation or produced locally or by direct neuroendocrine stimulation. Integration of hormone production from endocrine organs is regulated by the hypothalamus. ACTH, adrenocorticotropic hormone; CRH, corticotropin-releasing hormone; FSH, follicle-stimulating hormone; GHRH, growth hormone-releasing hormone; GnRH, gonadotropin-releasing hormone; LH, luteinizing hormone; MSH, melanocyte-stimulating hormone; TRH, thyrotropin-releasing hormone; TSH, thyroid-stimulating hormone; T_3, triiodothyronine; T_4, thyroxine.

an effect on a distant target organ. Currently, the definition of the endocrine system is that of an integrated network of multiple organs derived from different embryologic origins that release hormones ranging from small peptides to glycoproteins, which exert their effects either in neighboring or distant target cells. This endocrine network of organs and mediators does not work in isolation and is closely integrated with the central and peripheral nervous systems as well as with the immune systems, leading to currently used terminology such as "neuroendocrine" or "neuroendocrine-immune" systems for describing their interactions. Three basic components make up the core of the endocrine system.

Endocrine glands—The classic endocrine glands are ductless and secrete their chemical products (hormones) into the interstitial space from where they reach the circulation. Unlike the cardiovascular, renal, and digestive systems, the endocrine glands are not anatomically connected and are scattered throughout the body (Figure 1–1). Communication among the different organs is ensured through the release of hormones or neurotransmitters.

Hormones—Hormones are chemical products, released in very small amounts from the cell, that exert a biologic action on a target cell. Hormones can be released from the endocrine glands (ie, insulin, cortisol); the brain (ie, corticotropin-releasing hormone, oxytocin, and antidiuretic hormone); and other organs such as the heart (atrial natriuretic peptide), liver (insulin-like growth factor 1), and adipose tissue (leptin).

Target organ—The target organ contains cells that express hormone-specific receptors and that respond to hormone binding by a demonstrable biologic response.

HORMONE CHEMISTRY AND MECHANISMS OF ACTION

Based on their chemical structure, hormones can be classified into proteins (or peptides), steroids, and amino acid derivatives (amines). Hormone structure, to a great extent, dictates the location of the hormone receptor, with amines and peptide hormones binding to receptors in the cell surface and steroid hormones being able to cross plasma membranes and bind to intracellular receptors. An exception to this generalization is thyroid hormone, an amino acid–derived hormone that is transported into the cell in order to bind to its nuclear receptor. Hormone structure influences the half-life of the hormone as well. Amines have the shortest half-life (2–3 minutes), followed by polypeptides (4–40 minutes), steroids and proteins (4–170 minutes), and thyroid hormones (0.75–6.7 days).

Protein or Peptide Hormones

Protein or peptide hormones constitute the majority of hormones. These are molecules ranging from 3 to 200 amino acid residues. They are synthesized as preprohormones and undergo post-translational processing. They are stored in secretory granules before being released by exocytosis (Figure 1–2), in a

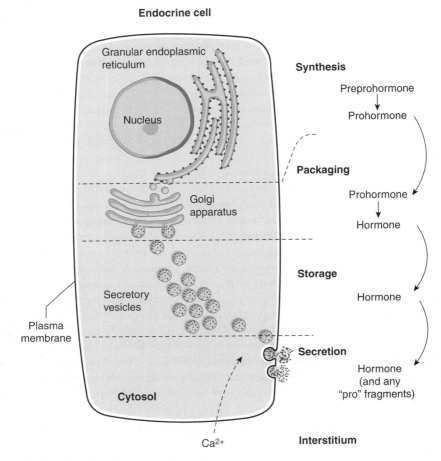

Figure 1–2. Peptide hormone synthesis. Peptide hormones are synthesized as preprohormones in the ribosomes and processed to prohormones in the endoplasmic reticulum (ER). In the Golgi apparatus, the hormone or prohormone is packaged in secretory vesicles, which are released from the cell in response to an influx of Ca^{2+}. The increase in cytoplasmic Ca^{2+} is required for docking of the secretory vesicles in the plasma membrane and for exocytosis of the vesicular contents. The hormone and the products of the post-translational processing that occurs inside the secretory vesicles are released into the extracellular space. Examples of peptide hormones are adrenocorticotropic hormone (ACTH), insulin, growth hormone, and glucagon.

manner reminiscent of how neurotransmitters are released from nerve terminals. Examples of peptide hormones include insulin, glucagon, and adrenocorticotropic hormone (ACTH). Some hormones in this category, such as the gonadotropic hormone, luteinizing hormone, and follicle-stimulating hormone, together with thyroid-stimulating hormone (TSH) and human chorionic gonadotropin, contain carbohydrate moieties, leading to their designation as glycoproteins. The carbohydrate moieties play important roles in determining the biologic activities and circulating clearance rates of glycoprotein hormones.

Steroid Hormones

Steroid hormones are derived from cholesterol and are synthesized in the adrenal cortex, gonads, and placenta. They are lipid soluble, circulate bound to binding proteins in plasma, and cross the plasma membrane to bind to intracellular cytosolic or nuclear receptors. Vitamin D and its metabolites are also considered steroid hormones. Steroid hormone synthesis is described in Chapters 5 and 6.

Amino Acid–Derived Hormones

Amino acid–derived hormones are those hormones that are synthesized from the amino acid tyrosine and include the catecholamines norepinephrine, epinephrine, and dopamine; as well as the thyroid hormones, derived from the combination of 2 iodinated tyrosine amino acid residues. The synthesis of thyroid hormone and catecholamines is described in Chapters 4 and 6, respectively.

Hormone Effects

Depending on where the biologic effect of a hormone is elicited in relation to where the hormone was released, its effects can be classified in 1 of 3 ways (Figure 1–3). The effect is **endocrine** when a hormone is released into the circulation and then travels in the blood to produce a biologic effect on distant target cells. The effect is **paracrine** when a hormone released from 1 cell produces a biologic effect on a neighboring cell, which is frequently a cell in the same organ or tissue. The effect is **autocrine** when a hormone produces a biologic effect on the same cell that released it.

Recently, an additional mechanism of hormone action has been proposed in which a hormone is synthesized and acts intracellularly in the same cell. This mechanism has been termed **intracrine** and has been identified to be involved in the effects of parathyroid hormone–related peptide in malignant cells and in some of the effects of androgen-derived estrogen (see Chapter 9).

Hormone Transport

Hormones released into the circulation can circulate either freely or bound to carrier proteins, also known as *binding proteins*. The binding proteins serve as a reservoir for the hormone and prolong the hormone's **half-life**, the time during which the concentration of a hormone decreases to 50% of its initial concentration. The free or unbound hormone is the active form of the hormone, which binds to the specific hormone receptor. Thus, hormone binding to its carrier protein serves to regulate the activity of the hormone by determining how much hormone is free to exert a biologic action. Most carrier proteins are globulins and are synthesized in the liver. Some of the binding proteins are specific for a given protein, such as cortisol-binding proteins. However, proteins such as

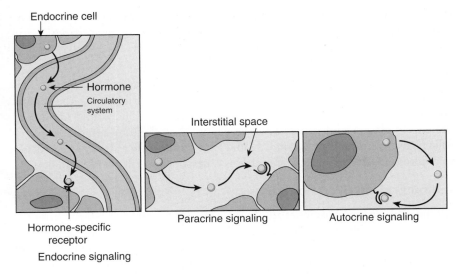

Figure 1–3. Mechanisms of hormone action. Depending on where hormones exert their effects, they can be classified into endocrine, paracrine, and autocrine mediators. Hormones that enter the bloodstream and bind to hormone receptors in target cells in distant organs mediate endocrine effects. Hormones that bind to cells near the cell that released them mediate paracrine effects. Hormones that produce their physiologic effects by binding to receptors on the same cell that produced them mediate autocrine effects.

globulins and albumin are known to bind hormones as well. Because for the most part these proteins are synthesized in the liver, alterations in hepatic function may result in abnormalities in binding-protein levels and may indirectly affect total hormone levels. In general, the majority of amines, peptides, and protein (hydrophilic) hormones circulate in their free form. However, a notable exception to this rule is the binding of the insulin-like growth factors to 1 of 6 different high-affinity binding proteins. Steroid and thyroid (lipophilic) hormones circulate bound to specific transport proteins.

The interaction between a given hormone and its carrier protein is in a **dynamic equilibrium** and allows adjustments that prevent clinical manifestations of hormone deficiency or excess. Secretion of the hormone is adjusted rapidly following changes in the levels of carrier proteins. For example, plasma levels of cortisol-binding protein increase during pregnancy. Cortisol is a steroid hormone produced by the adrenal cortex (see Chapter 6). The increase in circulating levels of cortisol-binding protein leads to an increased binding capacity for cortisol and a resulting decrease in free cortisol levels. This decrease in free cortisol stimulates the hypothalamic release of corticotropin-releasing hormone, which stimulates ACTH release from the anterior pituitary and consequently cortisol synthesis and release from the adrenal glands. The cortisol, released in greater amounts, restores free cortisol levels and prevents manifestation of cortisol deficiency.

As already mentioned, the binding of a hormone to a binding protein prolongs its half-life. The half-life of a hormone is inversely related to its removal from the circulation. Removal of hormones from the circulation is also known as the **metabolic clearance rate**: the volume of plasma cleared of the hormone per unit of time. Once hormones are released into the circulation, they can bind to their specific receptor in a target organ, they can undergo metabolic transformation by the liver, or they can undergo urinary excretion (Figure 1–4). In the liver, hormones can be inactivated through phase I (hydroxylation or oxidation) and/or phase II (glucuronidation, sulfation, or reduction with glutathione) reactions, and then excreted by the liver through the bile or by the kidney. In some instances, the liver can actually activate a hormone precursor, as is the case for vitamin D synthesis, discussed in Chapter 5. Hormones can be degraded at their

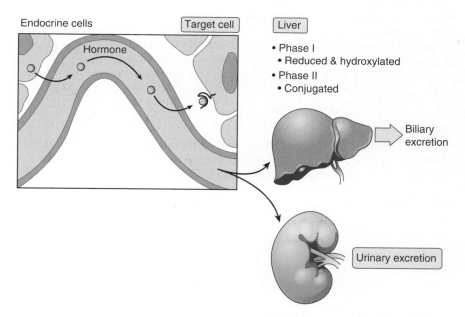

Figure 1–4. Hormone metabolic fate. The removal of hormones from the organism is the result of metabolic degradation, which occurs mainly in the liver through enzymatic processes that include proteolysis, oxidation, reduction, hydroxylation, decarboxylation (phase I), and methylation or glucuronidation (phase II) among others. Excretion can be achieved by bile or urinary excretion following glucuronidation and sulfation (phase II). In addition, the target cell may internalize the hormone and degrade it. The role of the kidney in eliminating hormone and its degradation products from the body is important. In some cases urinary determinations of a hormone or its metabolite are used to assess function of a particular endocrine organ based on the assumption that renal function and handling of the hormone are normal.

target cell through internalization of the hormone-receptor complex followed by lysosomal degradation of the hormone. Only a very small fraction of total hormone production is excreted intact in the urine and feces.

HORMONE CELLULAR EFFECTS

The biologic response to hormones is elicited through binding to hormone-specific receptors at the target organ. Hormones circulate in very low concentrations (10^{-7} – 10^{-12} M), so the receptor must have high affinity and specificity for the hormone to produce a biologic response.

Affinity is determined by the rates of dissociation and association for the hormone-receptor complex under equilibrium conditions. The equilibrium dissociation constant (K_d) is defined as the hormone concentration required for binding 50% of the receptor sites. The lower the K_d, the higher the affinity of binding. Basically, affinity is a reflection of how tight the hormone-receptor interaction is. **Specificity** is the ability of a hormone receptor to discriminate among hormones with related structures. This is a key concept that has clinical relevance as will be discussed in Chapter 6 as it pertains to cortisol and aldosterone receptors.

The binding of hormones to their receptors is saturable, with a finite number of hormone receptors to which a hormone can bind. In most target cells, the maximal biologic response to a hormone can be achieved without reaching 100% hormone-receptor occupancy. The receptors that are not occupied are called *spare receptors*. Frequently, the hormone-receptor occupancy needed to produce a biologic response in a given target cell is very low; therefore, a decrease in the number of receptors in target tissues may not necessarily lead to an immediate impairment in hormone action. For example, insulin-mediated cellular effects occur when less than 3% of the total number of receptors in adipocytes is occupied.

Abnormal endocrine function is the result of either excess or deficiency in hormone action. This can result from abnormal production of a given hormone (either in excess or in insufficient amounts) or from decreased receptor number or function. Hormone-receptor agonists and antagonists are widely used clinically to restore endocrine function in patients with hormone deficiency or excess. Hormone-receptor agonists are molecules that bind the hormone receptor and produce a biologic effect similar to that elicited by the hormone. Hormone-receptor antagonists are molecules that bind to the hormone receptor and inhibit the biologic effects of a particular hormone.

HORMONE RECEPTORS AND SIGNAL TRANSDUCTION

As mentioned previously, hormones produce their biologic effects by binding to specific hormone receptors in target cells, and the type of receptor to which they bind is largely determined by the hormone's chemical structure. Hormone receptors are classified depending on their cellular localization, as **cell membrane** or **intracellular receptors**. Peptides and catecholamines are unable to cross the cell membrane lipid bilayer and in general bind to cell membrane receptors, with the exception of thyroid hormones as mentioned above. Thyroid hormones are transported into the cell and bind to nuclear receptors. Steroid hormones are lipid soluble, cross the plasma membrane, and bind to intracellular receptors.

Cell Membrane Receptors

These receptor proteins are located within the phospholipid bilayer of the cell membrane of target cells (Figure 1–5). Binding of hormones (ie, catecholamines, peptide and protein hormones) to cell membrane receptors and formation of the

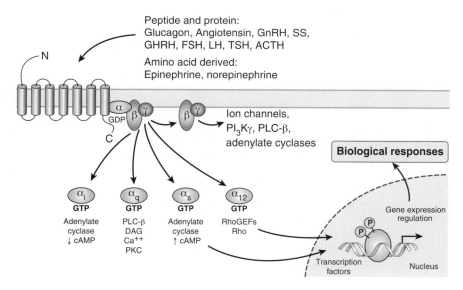

Figure 1–5. G protein–coupled receptors. Peptide and protein hormones bind to cell surface receptors coupled to G proteins. Binding of the hormone to the receptor produces a conformational change that allows the receptor to interact with the G proteins. This results in the exchange of guanosine diphosphate (GDP) for guanosine triphosphate (GTP) and activation of the G protein. The second-messenger systems that are activated vary depending on the specific receptor, the α-subunit of the G protein associated with the receptor, and the ligand it binds. Examples of hormones that bind to G protein–coupled receptors are thyroid hormone, arginine vasopressin, parathyroid hormone, epinephrine, and glucagon. ACTH, adrenocorticotropic hormone; ADP, adenosine diphosphate; cAMP, cyclic 3′,5′-adenosine monophosphate; DAG, diacylglycerol; FSH, follicle-stimulating hormone; GHRH, growth hormone-releasing hormone; GnRh, gonadotropin-releasing hormone; IP_3, inositol trisphosphate; LH, luteinizing hormone; $PI_3K\gamma$, phosphatidyl-3-kinase; PIP_2, phosphatidylinositol bisphosphate; PKC, protein kinase C; PLC-β, phospholipase C; RhoGEFs, Rho guanine-nucleotide exchange factors; SS, somatostatin; TSH, thyroid-stimulating hormone.

hormone-receptor complex initiates a signaling cascade of intracellular events, resulting in a specific biologic response. Functionally, cell membrane receptors can be divided into ligand-gated ion channels and receptors that regulate activity of intracellular proteins.

LIGAND-GATED ION CHANNELS

These receptors are functionally coupled to ion channels. Hormone binding to this receptor produces a conformational change that opens ion channels on the cell membrane, producing ion fluxes in the target cell. The cellular effects occur within seconds of hormone binding.

RECEPTORS THAT REGULATE ACTIVITY OF INTRACELLULAR PROTEINS

These receptors are transmembrane proteins that transmit signals to intracellular targets when activated. Ligand binding to the receptor on the cell surface and activation of the associated protein initiate a signaling cascade of events that activates intracellular proteins and enzymes and that can include effects on gene transcription and expression. The main types of cell membrane hormone receptors in this category are the **G protein–coupled receptors** and the **receptor protein tyrosine kinases**. An additional type of receptor, the receptor-linked kinase receptor, activates intracellular kinase activity following binding of the hormone to the plasma membrane receptor. This type of receptor is used in producing the physiologic effects of growth hormone (see Figure 1–5).

G protein–coupled receptors—G protein–coupled receptors are single polypeptide chains that have 7 transmembrane domains and are coupled to heterotrimeric guanine-binding proteins (G proteins) consisting of 3 subunits: α, β, and γ. Hormone binding to the G protein–coupled receptor produces a conformational change that induces interaction of the receptor with the regulatory G protein, stimulating the release of guanosine diphosphate (GDP) in exchange for guanosine triphosphate **(GTP)**, resulting in activation of the G protein (see Figure 1–5). The activated G protein (bound to GTP) dissociates from the receptor **followed by dissociation of the α from the ßγ subunits.** The subunits activate intracellular targets, which can be either an ion channel or an enzyme. Hormones that use this type of receptor include TSH, vasopressin, or antidiuretic hormone, and catecholamines.

The 2 main enzymes that interact with G proteins are adenylate cyclase and phospholipase C, and this selectivity of interaction is dictated by the type of G protein with which the receptor is associated. On the basis of the $G\alpha$ subunit, G proteins can be classified into 4 families associated with different effector proteins. The signaling pathways of 3 of these have been extensively studied. The $G\alpha_s$ activates adenylate cyclase, $G\alpha_i$ inhibits adenylate cyclase, and $G\alpha_q$ activates phospholipase C; the second-messenger pathways used by $G\alpha_{12}$ have not been completely elucidated.

The interaction of $G\alpha_s$ with adenylate cyclase and its activation result in increased conversion of adenosine triphosphate to cyclic 3′,5′-adenosine monophosphate (cAMP), with the opposite response elicited by binding to $G\alpha_i$-coupled receptors. The rise in intracellular cAMP activates protein kinase A, which in turn phosphorylates effector proteins, responsible for producing cellular responses. The action of cAMP is terminated by the breakdown of cAMP by the enzyme phosphodiesterase. In addition, the cascade of protein activation can also be controlled by phosphatases; which dephosphorylate proteins. Phosphorylation of proteins does not necessarily result in activation of an enzyme. In some cases, phosphorylation of a given protein results in inhibition of its activity.

$G\alpha_q$ activation of phospholipase C results in the hydrolysis of phosphatidylinositol bisphosphate and the production of diacylglycerol (DAG) and inositol trisphosphate (IP_3). DAG activates protein kinase C, which phosphorylates effector proteins. IP_3 binds to calcium channels in the endoplasmic reticulum, leading to an increase of Ca^{2+} influx into the cytosol. Ca^{2+} can also act as a second messenger by binding to cytosolic proteins. One important protein in mediating the effects of Ca^{2+} is **calmodulin**. Binding of Ca^{2+} to calmodulin results in the activation of proteins, some of which are kinases, leading to a cascade of phosphorylation of effector proteins and cellular responses. An example of a hormone that uses Ca^{2+} as a signaling molecule is oxytocin discussed in Chapter 2.

Receptor protein tyrosine kinases—Receptor protein tyrosine kinases are usually single transmembrane proteins that have intrinsic enzymatic activity (Figure 1–6). Examples of hormones that use these types of receptors are

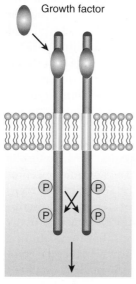

Figure 1–6. Receptor kinase and receptor-linked kinase receptors. Receptor kinases have intrinsic tyrosine or serine kinase activity, which is activated by binding of the hormone to the amino terminal of the cell membrane receptor. The activated kinase recruits and phosphorylates downstream proteins, producing a cellular response. One hormone that uses this receptor pathway is insulin. Receptor-linked tyrosine kinase receptors do not have intrinsic activity in their intracellular domain. They are closely associated with kinases that are activated with binding of the hormone. Examples of hormones using this mechanism are growth hormone and prolactin.

Growth factor

Proliferation
differentiation
survival

insulin and growth factors. Hormone binding to these receptors activates their intracellular kinase activity, resulting in phosphorylation of tyrosine residues on the catalytic domain of the receptor itself, increasing its kinase activity. Phosphorylation outside the catalytic domain creates specific binding or docking sites for additional proteins that are recruited and activated, initiating a downstream signaling cascade. Most of these receptors consist of single polypeptides, although some, like the insulin receptor, are dimers consisting of 2 pairs of polypeptide chains.

Hormone binding to cell surface receptors results in rapid activation of cytosolic proteins and cellular responses. Through protein phosphorylation, hormone binding to cell surface receptors can also alter the transcription of specific genes through the phosphorylation of transcription factors. An example of this mechanism of action is the phosphorylation of the transcription factor cyclic 3′,5′-adenosine monophosphate response element binding protein (CREB) by protein kinase A in response to receptor binding and adenylate cyclase activation. This same transcription factor (CREB) can be phosphorylated by calcium-calmodulin following hormone binding to receptor tyrosine kinase and activation of phospholipase C. Therefore, hormone binding to cell surface receptors can elicit immediate responses when the receptor is coupled to an ion channel or through the rapid phosphorylation of preformed cytosolic proteins, and it can also activate gene transcription through phosphorylation of transcription factors.

Intracellular Receptors

Receptors in this category belong to the **steroid receptor superfamily** (Figure 1–7). These receptors are transcription factors that have binding sites for the hormone (ligand) and for DNA and function as ligand (hormone)-regulated transcription factors. Hormone-receptor complex formation and binding to DNA result in either activation or repression of gene transcription. Binding to intracellular hormone receptors requires that the hormone be hydrophobic and cross the plasma membrane. Steroid hormones and the steroid derivative vitamin D_3 fulfill this requirement (see Figure 1–7). Thyroid hormones must be actively transported into the cell.

The distribution of the unbound intracellular hormone receptor can be cytosolic or nuclear. Hormone-receptor complex formation with cytosolic receptors produces a conformational change that allows the hormone-receptor complex to enter the nucleus and bind to specific DNA sequences to regulate gene transcription. Once in the nucleus, the receptors regulate transcription by binding, generally as dimers, to hormone response elements normally located in regulatory regions of target genes. In all cases, hormone binding leads to a nearly complete nuclear localization of the hormone-receptor complex. Unbound intracellular receptors may be located in the nucleus, as in the case of thyroid hormone receptors. The unoccupied thyroid receptor represses transcription of genes. Binding of thyroid hormone to the receptor activates gene transcription.

Intracellular receptors

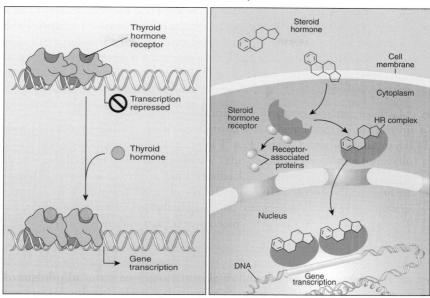

Figure 1–7. Intracellular receptors. Two general types of intracellular receptors can be identified. The unoccupied thyroid hormone receptor is bound to DNA and it represses transcription. Binding of thyroid hormone to the receptor allows for gene transcription to take place. Therefore, thyroid hormone receptor, acts as a repressor in the absence of the hormone, but hormone binding converts it to an activator that stimulates transcription of thyroid-hormone inducible genes. The steroid receptor, such as that used by estrogen, progesterone, cortisol, and aldosterone, is not able to bind to DNA in the absence of the hormone. Following steroid hormone binding to its receptor, the receptor dissociates from receptor-associated chaperone proteins. The hormone–receptor (HR) complex translocates to the nucleus, where it binds to its specific responsive element on the DNA and initiates gene transcription. (Modified with permission from Gruber et al. Mechanisms of disease: production and actions of estrogens. *N Engl J Med.* 2002;346(5):340. Copyright © Massachusetts Medical Society. All rights reserved.)

Hormone Receptor Regulation

Hormones can influence responsiveness of the target cell by modulating receptor function. Target cells are able to detect changes in hormone signal over a very wide range of stimulus intensities. This requires the ability to undergo a reversible process of adaptation or **desensitization**, whereby a prolonged exposure to a hormone decreases the cells' response to that level of hormone. This allows cells to respond to *changes* in the concentration of a hormone (rather than to the absolute concentration of the hormone) over a very wide range of hormone concentrations. Several mechanisms can be involved in desensitization to a hormone. Hormone binding to cell-surface receptors, for example, may induce their endocytosis and temporary sequestration in endosomes. Such hormone-induced receptor endocytosis can lead to the destruction of the receptors in lysosomes, a process that leads to *receptor downregulation*. In other cases, desensitization results from a rapid inactivation of the receptors for example, as a result of a receptor phosphorylation. Desensitization can also be caused by a change in a protein involved in signal transduction following hormone binding to the receptor or by the production of an inhibitor that blocks the transduction process. In addition, a hormone can downregulate or decrease the expression of receptors for another hormone and reduce that hormone's effectiveness.

Hormone receptors can also undergo upregulation. Upregulation of receptors involves an increase in the number of receptors for the particular hormone and frequently occurs when the prevailing levels of the hormone have been low for some time. The result is an increased responsiveness to the physiologic effects of the hormone at the target tissue when the levels of the hormone are restored or when an agonist to the receptor is administered. A hormone can also upregulate the receptors for another hormone, increasing the effectiveness of that hormone at its target tissue. An example of this type of interaction is the upregulation of cardiac myocyte adrenergic receptors following sustained elevations in thyroid hormone levels.

CONTROL OF HORMONE RELEASE

The secretion of hormones involves synthesis or production of the hormone and its release from the cell. In general, the discussion of regulation of hormone release in this section refers to both synthesis and secretion; specific aspects pertaining to the differential control of synthesis and release of specific hormones will be discussed in the respective chapters when they are considered of relevance.

Plasma levels of hormones oscillate throughout the day, showing peaks and troughs that are hormone specific (Figure 1–8). This variable pattern of hormone release is determined by the interaction and integration of multiple control mechanisms, which include hormonal, neural, nutritional, and environmental factors that regulate the constitutive (basal) and stimulated (peak levels) secretion of hormones. The periodic and pulsatile release of hormones is critical in maintaining normal endocrine function and in exerting physiologic effects at the target organ. The important role of the hypothalamus, and particularly of the photo-neuro-endocrine system in control of hormone pulsatility is discussed in Chapter 2. Although the mechanisms that determine the pulsatility and periodicity of hormone release are not completely understood for all the different hormones, 3 general mechanisms can be identified as common regulators of hormone release.

Neural Control

Control and integration by the central nervous system is a key component of hormonal regulation and is mediated by direct neurotransmitter control of

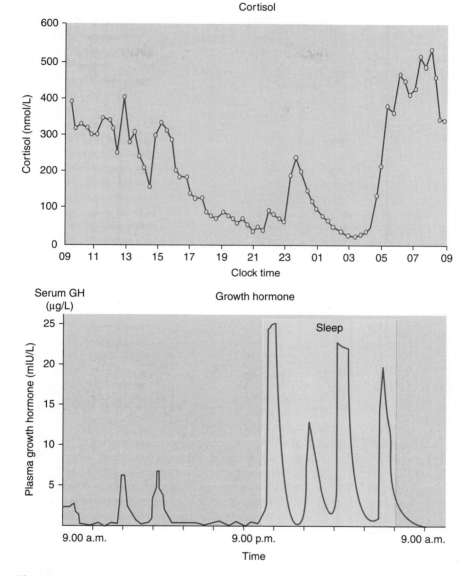

Figure 1–8. Patterns of hormone release. Plasma hormone concentrations fluctuate throughout the day. Therefore plasma hormone measurements are not always a reflection of the function of a given endocrine system. Both cortisol and growth hormone (GH) undergo considerable variations in blood levels throughout the day. These can, in addition, be affected by sleep deprivation, light, stress, and disease and are dependent on their secretion rate, rate of metabolism and excretion, metabolic clearance rate, circadian pattern, fluctuating environment stimuli, internal endogenous oscillators as well as on biologic shifts induced by illness, night work, sleep, changes in longitude, and prolonged bed rest. (Reproduced with permission from Melmed S. Acromegaly. *N Engl J Med.* 2006;355(24):2558. Copyright © Massachusetts Medical Society. All rights reserved.)

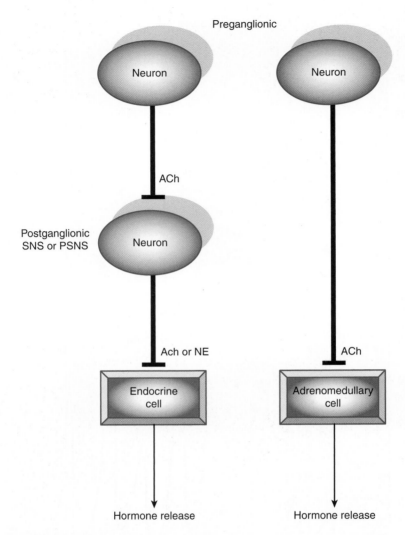

Figure 1–9. Neural control of hormone release. Endocrine function is under tight regulation by the nervous system leading to the term *neuroendocrine*. Hormone release by endocrine cells can be modulated by postganglionic neurons from the sympathetic (SNS) or parasympathetic nervous system (PSNS) using acetylcholine (Ach) or norepinephrine (NE) as neurotransmitters or directly by preganglionic neurons using acetylcholine as a neurotransmitter. Therefore, pharmacologic agents that interact with the production or release of neurotransmitters will affect endocrine function.

endocrine hormone release (Figure 1–9). The central role of the hypothalamus in neural control of hormone release is discussed in Chapter 2 and is exemplified by dopaminergic control of pituitary prolactin release. Neural control also plays an important role in the regulation of peripheral endocrine hormone release. Endocrine organs such as the pancreas receive sympathetic and parasympathetic input, which contributes to the regulation of insulin and glucagon release. The neural control of hormone release is best exemplified by the sympathetic regulation of the adrenal gland, which functions as a modified sympathetic ganglion receiving direct neural input from the sympathetic nervous system. Release of acetylcholine from preganglionic sympathetic nerve terminals at the adrenal medulla stimulates the release of epinephrine into the circulation (see Figure 1–9).

Hormonal Control

Hormone release from an endocrine organ is frequently controlled by another hormone (Figure 1–10). When the outcome is stimulation of hormone release, the hormone that exerts that effect is referred to as a tropic hormone (see Figure 1–10), as is the case for most of the hormones produced and released from the anterior pituitary. One example of this type of hormone release control is the regulation of glucocorticoid release by ACTH. Hormones can also suppress another hormone's release. An example of this is the inhibition of growth hormone release by somatostatin.

Hormonal inhibition of hormone release plays an important role in the process of **negative feedback regulation** of hormone release, described below and in Figure 1–12. In addition, hormones can stimulate the release of a second hormone in what is known as a feed-forward mechanism; as in the case of estradiol-mediated surge in luteinizing hormone at midmenstrual cycle (see Chapter 9).

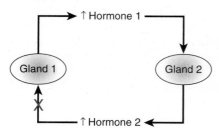

Hormonal control of hormone release

• Hormone made by gland 1 stimulates
  production of hormone from gland 2
• Hormone 2 suppresses production
  of hormone 1

↑ Hormone 1

Gland 1   Gland 2

↑ Hormone 2

Figure 1–10. Hormonal control of hormone release. In some cases, the endocrine gland is itself a target organ for another hormone. Hormones of this type are termed *tropic hormones,* and they are all released from the anterior pituitary gland (adenohypophysis). Examples of endocrine glands controlled principally by tropic hormones include the thyroid gland and the adrenal cortex.

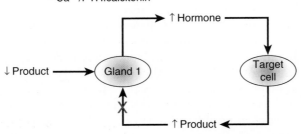

Figure 1–11. Nutrient or ion regulation of hormone release. This is the simplest form of control mechanism, where the hormone is directly influenced by the circulating blood levels of the substrate that the hormone itself controls. This sets up a simple control loop in which the substrate is controlling release of the hormone, which by its action(s) is altering the level of the substrate. Examples of this type of control are calcitonin and parathyroid hormone (substrate is calcium), aldosterone (substrate is potassium), and insulin (substrate is glucose). This control mechanism is possible because of the ability of endocrine cells to sense the changes in substrate concentrations. PTH, parathyroid hormone.

Nutrient or Ion Regulation

Plasma levels of nutrients or ions can also regulate hormone release (Figure 1–11). In all cases, the particular hormone regulates the concentration of the nutrient or ion in plasma either directly or indirectly. Examples of nutrient and ion regulation of hormone release include the control of insulin release by plasma glucose levels and the control of parathyroid hormone release by plasma calcium and phosphate levels.

In several instances, release of 1 hormone can be influenced by more than 1 of these mechanisms. For example, insulin release is regulated by nutrients (plasma levels of glucose and amino acids), neural (sympathetic and parasympathetic stimulation), and hormonal (somatostatin) mechanisms. The ultimate function of these control mechanisms is to allow the neuroendocrine system to adapt to a changing environment, integrate signals, and maintain homeostasis. The responsiveness of target cells to hormonal action leading to regulation of hormone release constitutes a **feedback** control mechanism. A dampening or inhibition of the initial stimulus is called **negative feedback** (Figure 1–12). Stimulation or enhancement of the original stimulus is called **positive feedback**. Negative feedback is the most common control mechanism regulating hormone release. The integrity of the system ensures that adaptive changes in hormone levels do not lead to pathologic conditions. Furthermore, the control mechanism plays an important role in short- and long-term adaptations to changes in the environment. Three levels of

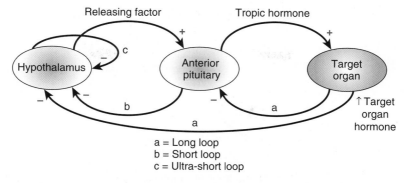

Figure 1–12. Feedback mechanisms. Three levels of feedback mechanisms controlling hormone synthesis can be identified: long loop, short loop, and ultrashort loop. Hormones under negative feedback regulation stimulate the production of another hormone by their target organ. The increasing circulating levels of that hormone then inhibit further production of the initial hormone. Hypothalamic-releasing factors stimulate the release of tropic hormones from the anterior pituitary. The tropic hormone stimulates the production and release of hormone from the target organ. The hormone produced by the target organ can inhibit the release of the tropic hormone and of the hypophysiotrophic factor by a long-loop negative feedback. The tropic hormone can inhibit the release of the hypothalamic factor in a short-loop negative feedback. The hypophysiotrophic factor can inhibit its own release in an ultrashort negative feedback mechanism. The accuracy of this control mechanism allows the use of circulating levels of hormones, tropic hormones, and nutrients for assessment of the functional status of the specific endocrine organ in question.

feedback can be identified: long loop, short loop, and ultra-short loop. These are depicted in Figure 1–12.

ASSESSMENT OF ENDOCRINE FUNCTION

In general, disorders of the endocrine system result from alterations in hormone secretion or target cell responsiveness to hormone action. Alterations in target cell response can be caused by increased or decreased biologic responsiveness to a particular hormone (Figure 1–13). The initial approach to assessment of endocrine function is measurement of plasma hormone levels.

Hormone Measurements

Hormone concentrations in biologic fluids are measured using immunoassays. These assays rely on the ability of specific antibodies to recognize specific hormones. Specificity for hormone measurement depends on the ability of the antibodies to recognize antigenic sites of the hormone. Hormone levels can be measured in plasma, serum, urine, or other biologic samples. Hormone determinations in

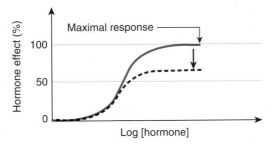

A. Decreased hormone responsiveness

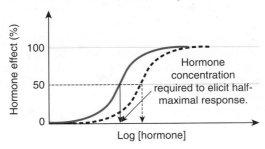

B. Decreased hormone sensitivity

Figure 1–13. Alterations in hormone biologic response. **A**. The maximal response produced by saturating doses of the hormone may be decreased because of a decreased number of hormone receptors, decreased concentration of enzyme activated by the hormone, increased concentration of noncompetitive inhibitor, or decrease in the number of target cells. When there is a decrease in responsiveness, no matter how high the hormone concentration, maximal response is not achieved. **B**. The sensitivity of tissues or cells to hormone action is reflected by the hormone concentration required to elicit half-maximal response. Decreased hormone sensitivity requires higher hormone concentrations to produce 50% of maximal response as shown in the dotted lines. This can be caused by decreased hormone-receptor affinity, decreased hormone receptor number, increased rate of hormone degradation, and increased antagonistic or competitive hormones.

urine collected over 24 hours provide an integrated assessment of the production of a hormone or metabolite, which may vary considerably throughout the day as is the case for cortisol.

Interpretation of Hormone Measurements

Because of the variability in circulating hormone levels resulting from pulsatile release, circadian rhythms, sleep/wake cycle, and nutritional status, interpretation of isolated plasma hormone measurements should always be done with caution and with understanding of the integral components of the hormone axis in question. These will be identified for each of the hormone systems discussed. Plasma hormone measurements reflect endocrine function only when interpreted in the right context. An abnormality in endocrine function is identified through measurements of hormone levels, hormone-nutrient or hormone-tropic hormone pairs, or by functional tests of hormone status together with the clinical assessment of the individual. It is important to keep in mind that the circulating levels of a particular hormone reflect the immediate state of the individual. Regulation of hormone release is a dynamic process that is constantly changing to adapt to the needs of the individual to maintain homeostasis. For example, plasma insulin levels reflect the fed or fasted state; estrogen and progesterone levels reflect the stage of the menstrual cycle. In addition, hormone levels can reflect the time of day during which they were obtained. For example, because of the circadian rhythm of cortisol release, cortisol levels will be higher early in the morning than in late afternoon. Age, health status, gender, and sleep patterns are among the many factors that influence hormone levels. Diseases and 24-hour light periods like those in an intensive care unit alter the pulsatility and rhythm of hormone release.

Some general aspects that should be considered when interpreting hormone measurements are as follows:

• Hormone levels should be evaluated with their appropriate regulatory factors (eg, insulin with glucose, calcium with parathyroid hormone, thyroid hormone with TSH).

• Simultaneous elevation of pairs (elevation of both the hormone and the substrate that it regulates such as elevated plasma glucose and insulin levels) suggests a hormone-resistance state.

• Urinary excretion of hormone or hormone metabolites over 24 hours, in individuals with normal renal function, may be a better estimate of hormone secretion than one-time plasma-level measurement.

• Target hormone excess should be evaluated with the appropriate tropic hormone to rule out ectopic hormone production, which is usually caused by a hormone-secreting tumor.

The possible interpretations of altered hormone and regulatory factor pairs are summarized in Table 1–1. Increased tropic hormone levels with low target hormone levels indicate primary failure of the target endocrine organ. Increased tropic hormone levels with increased target gland hormone levels indicate autonomous secretion of tropic hormone or inability of target gland hormone to suppress tropic hormone release (impaired negative feedback mechanisms). Low tropic hormone levels with low target gland hormone levels indicate a tropic hormone deficiency, as seen with pituitary failure. Low tropic hormone levels with high target gland hormone levels indicate autonomous hormone secretion by the target endocrine organ.

Table 1–1. Interpretation of hormone levels

Pituitary hormone level	Target hormone level		
	Low	**Normal**	**High**
High	Primary failure of target endocrine organ		Autonomous secretion of pituitary hormone or resistance to target hormone action
Normal		Normal range	
Low	Pituitary failure		Autonomous secretion by target endocrine organ

Dynamic Measurements of Hormone Secretion

In some cases, detection of abnormally high or low hormone concentrations may not be sufficient to conclusively establish the site of endocrine dysfunction. Dynamic measures of endocrine function provide more information than that obtained from hormone-pair measurements and rely on the integrity of the feedback control mechanisms that regulate hormone release. These tests of endocrine function are based on either stimulation or suppression of the endogenous hormone production.

STIMULATION TESTS

Stimulation tests are designed to determine the capacity of the target gland to respond to its control mechanism, either a tropic hormone or a substrate that stimulates its release. Examples of these tests are the use of ACTH to stimulate cortisol release (see Chapter 6) and the use of an oral glucose load to stimulate insulin release (see Chapter 7).

SUPPRESSION TESTS

Suppression tests are used to determine whether the negative feedback mechanisms that control that hormone's release are intact. Examples are the use of dexamethasone, a synthetic glucocorticoid, to suppress pituitary ACTH and adrenal cortisol release.

Hormone-Receptor Measurements

The measurement of hormone-receptor presence, number, and affinity has become a useful diagnostic tool, particularly in instituting hormone therapy for the treatment of some tumors. Receptor measurements made in tissue samples obtained surgically allow determinations of tissue responsiveness to hormone and prediction of tumor responsiveness to hormone therapy. An example is the assessment of estrogen receptors in breast tumors to determine the applicability of hormone therapy.

KEY CONCEPTS

Hormones are classified into protein, amino acid–derived, and steroid based on their chemistry.

Binding proteins regulate hormone availability and prolong hormone half-life.

Physiologic effects of hormones require binding to specific receptors in target organs.

Hormone release is under neural, hormonal, and product regulation.

Hormones can control their own release through feedback regulation.

Interpretation of hormone levels requires consideration of hormone pairs or of the nutrient or factor controlled by the hormone.

STUDY QUESTIONS

1–1.   *Which of the following statements concerning a particular hormone (hormone X) is correct?*

   a. It will bind to cell membrane receptors in all cell types.

   b. It is lipid soluble and has an intracellular receptor.

   c. It circulates bound to a protein, and this shortens its half-life.

   d. It is a small peptide; therefore, its receptor localization will be in the nucleus.

1-2.   Which of the following would be expected to alter hormone levels?
    a. Changes in mineral and nutrient plasma levels
    b. Pituitary tumor
    c. Transatlantic flight
    d. Training for the Olympics
    e. All of the above

1-3.   Which of the following statements concerning hormonal regulation is correct?
    a. A hormone does not inhibit its own release.
    b. The substrate a hormone regulates does not affect that hormone's release.
    c. Negative feedback regulation occurs only at the level of the anterior pituitary.
    d. Feedback inhibition may be exerted by nutrients and hormones.

1-4.   The structure of a newly discovered hormone shows that it is a large peptide with a glycosylated subunit. The hormone is likely to:
    a. Bind to DNA and affect gene transcription
    b. Bind to adenylate cyclase and stimulate protein kinase C
    c. Bind to a cell membrane receptor
    d. Be secreted intact in the urine

SUGGESTED READINGS

Aranda A, Pascual A. Nuclear hormone receptors and gene expression. *Physiol Rev.* 2001;81:1269.
Morris AJ, Malbon CC. Physiological regulation of G protein-linked signaling. *Physiol Rev.* 1999;79:1373.

The Hypothalamus and Posterior Pituitary Gland

2

OBJECTIVES

▶ Describe the physiologic and anatomic relationships between the hypothalamus and the anterior and the posterior pituitary.

▶ Understand the integration of hypothalamic and pituitary function and identify the 2 different pathways used for hypothalamic-pituitary interactions.

▶ Identify the appropriate hypothalamic releasing and inhibitory factors controlling the secretion of each of the anterior pituitary hormones.

▶ Differentiate between the routes of transport of hypothalamic neuropeptides to the posterior and anterior pituitary.

▶ Identify the mechanisms that control the release of oxytocin and arginine vasopressin (AVP).

▶ Understand the physiologic target organ responses and the cellular mechanisms of oxytocin and AVP action.

The hypothalamus is the region of the brain involved in coordinating the physiologic responses of different organs that together maintain homeostasis. It does this by integrating signals from the environment, from other brain regions, and from visceral afferents and then stimulating the appropriate neuroendocrine responses. In doing so, the hypothalamus influences many aspects of daily function, including food intake, energy expenditure, body weight, fluid intake and balance, blood pressure, thirst, body temperature, and the sleep cycle. Most of these hypothalamic responses are mediated through hypothalamic control of pituitary function (Figure 2–1). This control is achieved by 2 mechanisms: (1) release of hypothalamic neuropeptides synthesized in hypothalamic neurons and transported through the hypothalamo-hypophysial tract to the posterior pituitary, and (2) neuroendocrine control of the anterior pituitary through the release of peptides that mediate anterior pituitary hormone release (hypophysiotropic hormones) (Figure 2–2). Because of this close interaction between the hypothalamus and the pituitary in the control of basic endocrine physiologic function, they are presented as an integrated topic.

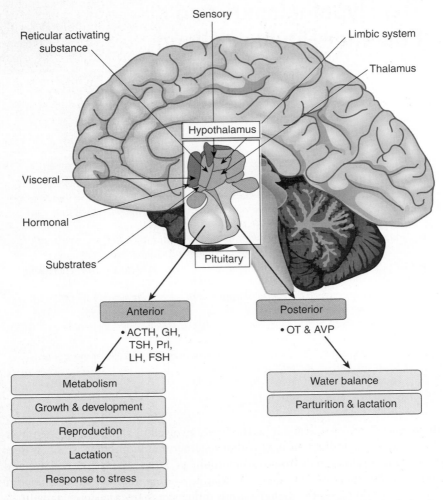

Figure 2–1. Neuroendocrine regulation of homeostasis. The release of hypothalamic neuropeptides is regulated by afferent signals from other brain regions, from visceral afferents, and by circulating levels of substrates and hormones. The sleep/awake state of the individual, variations in light, noise, fear, anxiety, and visual images all are examples of signals that are integrated by the hypothalamus and that are involved in the regulation of hypothalamic neuropeptide release and control of pituitary function. The hormones released from the anterior and posterior pituitary regulate vital body functions to maintain homeostasis. ACTH, adrenocorticotropic hormone; AVP, arginine vasopressin; FSH, follicle-stimulating hormone; GH, growth hormone; LH, luteinizing hormone; OT, oxytocin; Prl, prolactin; TSH, thyroid-stimulating hormone.

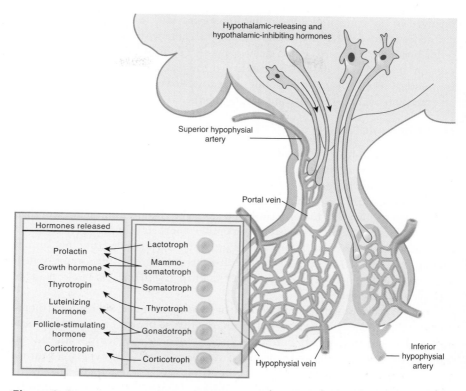

Figure 2–2. Anatomical and functional relationship between the hypothalamus and the pituitary. The hypothalamus is anatomically and functionally linked with the anterior and posterior pituitary. They are closely related because of the portal system of blood supply. The superior, medial, and inferior hypophyseal arteries provide arterial blood supply to the median eminence and the pituitary. Magnocellular neurons of the supraoptic (SON) and paraventricular (PVN) nuclei have long axons that terminate in the posterior pituitary. The axons of parvicellular neurons terminate in the median eminence where they release their neuropeptides. The long portal veins drain the median eminence, transporting the peptides from the primary capillary plexus to the secondary plexus that provides blood supply to the anterior pituitary. (Adapted with permission from Melmed S. Medical progress: acromegaly. *N Engl J Med*. 2006;355(24): 2558–2573. Copyright © Massachusetts Medical Society. All rights reserved.)

FUNCTIONAL ANATOMY

The hypothalamus is the part of the diencephalon located below the thalamus and between the lamina terminalis and the mamillary bodies forming the walls and the floor of the third ventricle. At the floor of the third ventricle, the 2 halves of the hypothalamus are rejoined to form a bridge-like region known as the *median eminence* (see Figure 2–2). The median eminence is important because this is where axon terminals of hypothalamic neurons release neuropeptides involved in the control of anterior pituitary function. In addition, the median eminence is traversed by the axons of hypothalamic neurons ending in the posterior pituitary. The median eminence funnels down to form the infundibular portion of the neurohypophysis (also called the *pituitary* or *infundibular stalk*). In practical terms, the neurohypophysis or posterior pituitary can be considered an extension of the hypothalamus.

Hypothalamic Nuclei

In the hypothalamus, the neuronal bodies are organized in nuclei. These are clusters or groups of neurons that have projections reaching other brain regions as well as ending in other hypothalamic nuclei. This intricate system of neuronal connections allows continuous communication between the hypothalamic neurons and other brain regions. The hypothalamic nuclei can be classified on the basis of their anatomic location or the principal neuropeptide that their cells produce. However, these are not discrete definitions of cell groups; some hypothalamic nuclei may contain more than 1 neuronal cell type. It is best to consider the groups of neurons as clusters of neurons and not as well-defined and delineated nuclei made of a single neuronal type.

Some of the neurons that make up the hypothalamic nuclei are neurohormonal in nature. *Neurohormonal* refers to the ability of these neurons to synthesize neuropeptides that function as hormones and to release these neuropeptides from axon terminals in response to neuronal depolarization. Two types of neurons are important in mediating the endocrine functions of the hypothalamus: the **magnocellular** and the **parvicellular** neurons (Figure 2–3). The magnocellular neurons are predominantly located in the paraventricular and supraoptic nuclei of the hypothalamus and produce large quantities of the neurohormones **oxytocin** and **arginine vasopressin** (AVP). The unmyelinated axons of these neurons form the **hypothalamo-hypophysial tract**, the bridge-like structure that traverses the median eminence and ends in the posterior pituitary. Oxytocin and AVP are released from the posterior pituitary in response to an action potential. Parvicellular neurons have projections that terminate in the median eminence, brainstem, and spinal cord. These neurons release small amounts of releasing or inhibiting neurohormones (**hypophysiotropic hormones**) that control anterior pituitary function.

Blood Supply

The specialized capillary network that supplies blood to the median eminence, infundibular stalk, and pituitary plays an important role in the transport of hypophysiotropic neuropeptides to the anterior pituitary. Hypophysiotropic peptides released near the median eminence are transported down the infundibular stalk to the anterior pituitary, where they exert their physiologic effects. Branches from the internal carotid artery provide the blood supply to the pituitary. The superior hypophysial arteries form the primary capillary plexus that supplies blood to the median eminence. From this capillary network, the blood is drained in parallel veins called *long hypophysial portal veins* down the infundibular stalk into

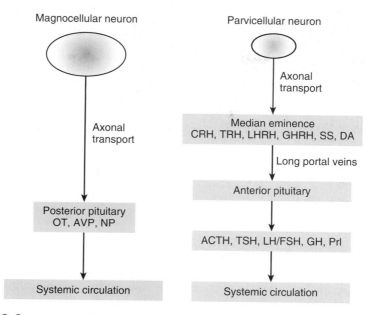

Figure 2–3. Magnocellular neurons are larger in size and produce large quantities of neurohormones. Located predominantly in the paraventricular and supraoptic nuclei of the hypothalamus, their unmyelinated axons form the hypothalamohypophyseal tract that traverses the median eminence ending in the posterior pituitary. They synthesize the neurohormones oxytocin and vasopressin, which are transported in neurosecretory vesicles down the hypothalamohypophyseal tract and stored in varicosities at the nerve terminals in the posterior pituitary. Parvicellular neurons are small in size and have projections that terminate in the median eminence, brain stem, and spinal cord. They release small amounts of releasing or inhibiting neurohormones (hypophysiotrophic hormones) that control anterior pituitary function will be discussed in the next chapter. These are transported in the long portal veins to the anterior pituitary where they stimulate the release of pituitary hormones into the systemic circulation. ACTH, adrenocorticotropic hormone; AVP, arginine vasopressin; CRH, corticotropin-releasing hormone; DA, dopamine; FSH, follicle-stimulating hormone; GH, growth hormone; GHRH, growth hormone-releasing hormone; LH, luteinizing hormone; LHRH, luteinizing hormone-releasing hormone; NP, neurophysins; OT, oxytocin; Prl, prolactin; SS, somatostatin; TRH, thyrotropin-releasing hormone; TSH, thyroid-stimulating hormone.

the secondary plexus (see Figure 2–2). The hypophysiotropic peptides released at the median eminence enter the primary plexus capillaries. From there, they are transported to the anterior pituitary via the long hypophysial portal veins to the secondary plexus. The secondary plexus is a network of fenestrated sinusoid capillaries that provides the blood supply to the **anterior pituitary** or adenohypophysis. Because of the fenestrated architecture of these capillary vessels, the neuropeptides easily diffuse out of the circulation to reach the cells of the anterior pituitary. The cells of the anterior pituitary express specific cell surface G protein–coupled receptors (see Chapter 1, Figure 1–5) that bind the neuropeptides, activating intracellular second-messenger cascades that produce the release of anterior pituitary hormones.

The blood supply to the posterior pituitary and to the pituitary stalk is provided mostly by the middle and inferior hypophysial arteries and, to a lesser extent, by the superior hypophysial arteries. Short portal vessels provide venous connections that originate in the neural lobe and pass across the intermediate lobe of the pituitary to the anterior lobe. This structure allows neuropeptides released from the posterior pituitary to have access to cells in the anterior pituitary, so that the functions of the 2 main regions of the pituitary cannot be dissociated from each other. Blood from the anterior and posterior pituitary drains into the intercavernous sinus and then into the internal jugular vein, entering the systemic venous circulation.

Hypothalamic Neuropeptides

As described earlier, 2 general types of neurons constitute the endocrine hypothalamus: the magnocellular neurons, with axons terminating in the posterior pituitary; and the parvicellular neurons, with axons terminating in the median eminence. The neuropeptides released from the parvicellular neuron terminals in the median eminence (corticotropin-releasing hormone, growth hormone–releasing hormone, thyrotropin-releasing hormone, dopamine, luteinizing hormone–releasing hormone, and somatostatin) control anterior pituitary function (Table 2–1). The hypothalamic hypophysiotropic peptides stimulate the release of anterior pituitary hormones. The products released from both the anterior pituitary (**adrenocorticotropic hormone [ACTH], prolactin, growth hormone [GH], luteinizing hormone [LH], follicle-stimulating hormone [FSH], and thyroid-stimulating hormone [TSH]**) and the posterior pituitary (oxytocin and AVP) are transported in the venous blood draining the pituitary that enters the intercavernous sinus and the internal jugular veins to reach the systemic circulation (see Figure 2–2). Their control and regulation will be discussed repeatedly throughout this book whenever the specific hormone systems to which they belong are described. Several neuropeptides have been isolated from the hypothalamus, and many continue to be discovered. However, only those that have been demonstrated to control anterior pituitary function (hypophysiotropic hormones) and, therefore, play an important role in endocrine physiology will be discussed.

Regulation of Hormone Release

Because the hypothalamus receives and integrates afferent signals from multiple brain regions, it does not function in isolation from the rest of the central nervous system (see Figure 2–1). Some of these afferent signals convey sensory information about the individual's environment such as light, heat, cold, and noise. Among the environmental factors, light plays an important role in generating the circadian rhythm of hormone secretion. This endogenous rhythm

Table 2–1. Key aspects of hypophysiotropic hormones

Hypophysiotropic hormone	Predominant hypothalamic nuclei	Anterior pituitary hormone controlled	Target cell
Thyrotropin-releasing hormone	Paraventricular nuclei	Thyroid-stimulating hormone and prolactin	Thyrotroph
Luteinizing hormone-releasing hormone	Anterior and medial hypothalamus; preoptic septal areas	Luteinizing hormone and follicle-stimulating hormone	Gonadotroph
Corticotropin-releasing hormone	Medial parvicellular portion of paraventricular nucleus	Adrenocorticotropic hormone	Corticotroph
Growth hormone-releasing hormone	Arcuate nucleus, close to median eminence	Growth hormone	Somatotroph
Somatostatin or growth hormone-inhibiting hormone	Anterior paraventricular area	Growth hormone	Somatotroph
Dopamine	Arcuate nucleus	Prolactin	Lactotroph

The 6 recognized hypophysiotropic factors and the predominant locations of their cells of origin are listed in the left columns. The right columns list the anterior pituitary hormone that each hypophysiotropic factor regulates and the cell that releases the specific hormones.

is generated through the interaction between the retina, the hypothalamic supra-chiasmatic nucleus, and the pineal gland through the release of melatonin. Melatonin is a hormone synthesized and secreted by the pineal gland at night. Its rhythm of secretion is entrained to the light/dark cycle. Melatonin conveys information concerning the daily cycle of light and darkness to body and participates in the organization of circadian rhythms. Other signals perceived by the hypothalamus are visceral afferents that provide information to the central nervous system from peripheral organs such as the intestines, the heart, the liver, and the stomach. One can think of the hypothalamus as a center for integration of the information that the body is continuously processing. The neuronal signals are transmitted by various neurotransmitters released from the afferent fibers, including glutamate, norepinephrine, epinephrine, serotonin, acetylcholine, histamine, γ-aminobutyric acid, and dopamine. In addition, circulating hormones produced by endocrine organs and substrates such as glucose can regulate hypothalamic neuronal function. All of these neurotransmitters, substrates, and hormones can influence hypothalamic hormone release. Therefore, hypothalamic hormone release is under environmental, neural, and hormonal regulation. The ability of the hypothalamus to integrate these signals makes it a center of command for regulating endocrine function and maintaining homeostasis.

Hormones can signal the hypothalamus to either inhibit or stimulate hypophysiotropic hormone release. This control mechanism of negative (or positive) feedback regulation, discussed in detail in Chapter 1, consists of the ability of a hormone to regulate its own cascade of release (see Figure 1–11). For example, as discussed in greater detail in Chapter 6, cortisol produced from the adrenal gland can inhibit the release of CRH, thus inhibiting the production of proopiomelanocortin and ACTH and consequently decreasing adrenal gland synthesis of cortisol. This loop of hormonal control and regulation of its own synthesis is critical in maintaining homeostasis and preventing disease. A shorter loop of negative feedback inhibition also exists, which depends on the inhibition of hypophysiotropic neuropeptide release by the pituitary hormone that it stimulates. In this case, an example would be the ability of ACTH to inhibit CRH release by the hypothalamus. Some neuropeptides also possess an ultrashort feedback loop, in which the hypophysiotropic neuropeptide itself is able to modulate its own release. As an example, oxytocin stimulates its own release, creating a positive feedback regulation of neuropeptide release. These feedback loops are illustrated in Figure 1–12, Chapter 1.

This continuous regulation of hormonal release is dynamic; it is continuously adapting to changes in the environment and in the internal milieu of the individual. Throughout a given day, the hypothalamus integrates a multitude of signals to ensure that the rhythms of hormone release are kept in pace with the needs of the organism. Disruption of these factors can alter the patterns of hormone release. For example, a patient in the intensive care unit, where the lights are on throughout the 24 hours of the day, will have a disrupted cycle of hormone release. Other situations that disrupt the normal cycles of hormone release are travel across time zones, night-shift employment, and aging.

HORMONES OF THE POSTERIOR PITUITARY

The posterior pituitary is an extension of the hypothalamus and contains the axon terminals of magnocellular neurons located in the supraoptic and paraventricular nuclei (see Figures 2–2 and 2–3). These neurons generate and propagate action potentials, producing membrane depolarization and exocytosis of the contents of their secretory granules. The neuropeptides produced by the magnocellular neurons, and consequently released from the posterior pituitary, are oxytocin and AVP. As the axons leave the supraoptic and paraventricular nuclei, they give rise to collaterals, some of which terminate in the median eminence.

Oxytocin and AVP are closely related peptides consisting of 9 amino acids (nonapeptides) with ring structures (Figure 2–4). They are synthesized as part of a larger precursor protein, consisting of a signal peptide, the hormone, a peptide called *neurophysin 2*, and a glycopeptide called *copeptin*. Following cleavage of the signal peptide in the endoplasmic reticulum, the remaining precursor folds, dimerizes, exits from the Golgi apparatus, and moves down the neurohypophyseal axons packaged within neurosecretory vesicles (see Figure 2–4).

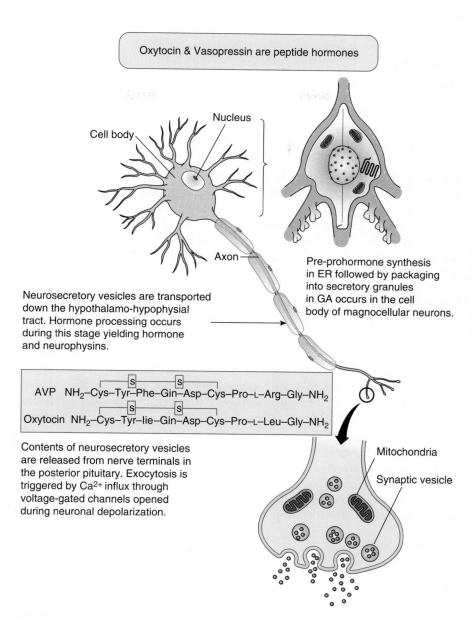

Oxytocin & Vasopressin are peptide hormones

Nucleus

Cell body

Axon

Pre-prohormone synthesis in ER followed by packaging into secretory granules in GA occurs in the cell body of magnocellular neurons.

Neurosecretory vesicles are transported down the hypothalamo-hypophysial tract. Hormone processing occurs during this stage yielding hormone and neurophysins.

AVP NH_2–Cys–Tyr–Phe–Gin–Asp–Cys–Pro–L–Arg–Gly–NH_2

Oxytocin NH_2–Cys–Tyr–Ile–Gin–Asp–Cys–Pro–L–Leu–Gly–NH_2

Contents of neurosecretory vesicles are released from nerve terminals in the posterior pituitary. Exocytosis is triggered by Ca^{2+} influx through voltage-gated channels opened during neuronal depolarization.

Mitochondria

Synaptic vesicle

Figure 2–4. Synthesis and processing of oxytocin (OT) and arginine vasopressin (AVP). OT and AVP are synthesized in the endoplasmic reticulum (ER) of hypothalamic magnocellular neurons as pre-prohormones. In the Golgi apparatus (GA), they are packaged in secretory granules and are transported down the hypothalamo-hypophysial tract. During transport, the precursor hormones are processed, yielding the final hormone and the respective neurophysins. The contents of the neurosecretory vesicles are released by exocytosis from the axon terminals in the posterior pituitary. Exocytosis is triggered by the influx of Ca^{2+} through voltage-gated channels that are opened during neuronal depolarization. The increase in Ca^{2+} allows docking of the secretory vesicles on the axonal plasma membrane and release of the neuropeptides into the interstitial space.

Within the neurosecretory vesicles, as they migrate down the axons, the precursor protein undergoes post-translational processing, producing the peptides AVP, oxytocin, neurophysins (defined below), and copeptin all of which are stored in the vesicles. The release of the contents of the vesicles is triggered by the neuronal influx of calcium ions through voltage-gated calcium channels, which open as the wave of depolarization reaches the axon terminals. The increase in intracellular calcium triggers the movement and docking of the secretory vesicles on the plasma membrane, resulting in exocytosis of the vesicle contents into the extracellular space. These neuropeptides enter the systemic circulation through venous drainage of the posterior pituitary into the intercavernous sinus and internal jugular vein. In the systemic circulation, oxytocin and AVP circulate unbound. They are rapidly cleared from the circulation by the kidney and, to a lesser extent, by the liver and brain. Their half-life is short and is estimated to range between 1 and 5 minutes.

Neurophysins

Neurophysins are by-products of post-translational prohormone processing in the secretory vesicles. The release of AVP and oxytocin is accompanied by the release of neurophysins from the secretory granules. Although the exact function of these by-products is not clear, it appears that neurophysins play an important role in AVP release. This role has become more evident since the identification of the inherited disease of familial neurogenic diabetes insipidus (DI). This disease is characterized by AVP deficiency caused by mutations in neurophysins and improper targeting of the hormone to neurosecretory granules. Neurophysins thus have an important role in the transport of AVP from the cell bodies of magnocellular neurons to their final release from the posterior pituitary. Impairment in hormone targeting leads to retention of the mutated neuropeptide precursor in the endoplasmic reticulum of the magnocellular neurons, and these cells progress to programmed cell death (apoptosis).

Oxytocin

The neuropeptide oxytocin is synthesized by magnocellular neurons in the supraoptic and paraventricular nuclei of the hypothalamus and is released from the posterior pituitary into the peripheral circulation. The release of oxytocin is stimulated by sucking during breast-feeding (lactation) and stretch of the cervix during childbirth (parturition) (Figure 2–5).

PHYSIOLOGIC EFFECTS OF OXYTOCIN

The 2 main target organs for oxytocin's physiologic effects are the lactating breast and the uterus during pregnancy (see Figure 2–5). In the lactating breast, oxytocin stimulates milk ejection by producing contraction of the myoepithelial cells that line the alveoli and ducts in the mammary gland. In the pregnant uterus, oxytocin produces rhythmic smooth muscle contractions to help induce labor and to promote regression of the uterus following delivery (see Chapter 9). Oxytocin analogs may be used clinically during labor and delivery to promote uterine contractions

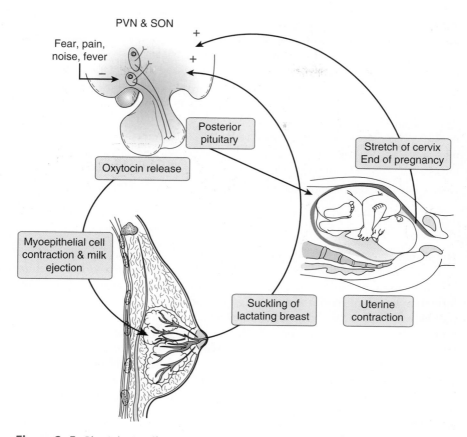

PVN & SON

Fear, pain, noise, fever

Posterior pituitary

Oxytocin release

Stretch of cervix
End of pregnancy

Myoepithelial cell contraction & milk ejection

Suckling of lactating breast

Uterine contraction

Figure 2–5. Physiologic effects and regulation oxytocin release. The release of oxytocin is stimulated by the distention of the cervix toward the term of pregnancy as well as by the contraction of the uterus during parturition. The signals are transmitted to the paraventricular (PVN) and supraoptic (SON) nuclei of the hypothalamus where they provide a positive feedback regulation of oxytocin release. The increased number in oxytocin receptors, the increase number in gap junctions between smooth muscle cells, and the increased synthesis of prostaglandins enhance the responsiveness of the uterine muscle. The suckling of the nipple of the lactating breast also stimulates oxytocin release. The afferent sensory signals elicit an increase in oxytocin release into the circulation.

and during the postpartum period to help decrease bleeding and return the uterus to its normal size (uterine involution) (Table 2–2).

The physiologic effects of oxytocin in the pregnant uterus are augmented by a dramatic increase in sensitivity to the hormone during the onset of labor. This increased sensitivity to oxytocin is caused by an increased density (upregulation) of oxytocin receptors in the uterine muscle. Receptor levels can be 200 times greater at the onset of labor than in the nonpregnant uterus. Because of this increase, levels of oxytocin that would normally not be effective can produce forceful

Table 2–2. Key aspects of posterior pituitary hormones

	Oxytocin	Arginine vasopressin
Receptor	$G_{q/11}$ protein-coupled	G protein-coupled (V_1R, $G_{q/11}$, V_2R, G_s)
Second messenger	Phospholipase C $\uparrow [Ca^{2+}]_i$	(V_1R) Phospholipase C $\uparrow [Ca^{2+}]_i$ (V_2R) Adenylate cyclase cAMP
Target organ or cells	Uterus Mammary myoepithelial cells	V_2R; kidney collecting ducts V_1R; smooth muscle cells
Physiologic effects	Uterine contraction Milk ejection	Increased H_2O permeability Vasoconstriction

cAMP, cyclic adenosine monophosphate.

uterine contractions toward the end of pregnancy. The increased density of oxytocin receptors is mediated by steroid hormone regulation of oxytocin-receptor synthesis. Responsiveness of the uterus is also enhanced by increased gap-junction formation between smooth muscle cells, facilitating conduction of action potentials between one cell and the next; and by increased synthesis of prostaglandin, a known stimulator of uterine contraction toward the end of gestation. All of these factors enhance myometrial contractile activity in response to oxytocin at term (see Chapter 9). Additional secondary effects that have been attributed to oxytocin are potentiation of the release of ACTH by CRH, interaction with the AVP receptor to produce vasoconstriction, stimulation of prolactin release, and an influence on maternal behavior and amnesia.

CONTROL OF OXYTOCIN RELEASE

The principal stimulus for oxytocin release is mechanical stimulation of the uterine cervix by the fetus near the end of gestation. Oxytocin release is also stimulated by the forceful contractions of the uterus during the fetal expulsion reflex. Hence, the contractile activity of the uterus acts through positive feedback mechanisms during parturition to stimulate oxytocin neurons, and this further increases the secretion of oxytocin. Before the oxytocin neurons can secrete oxytocin, they must be released from inhibition by other neurons containing endogenous opioids, nitric oxide, and γ-aminobutyric acid. This modulation of oxytocin release is partly caused by the declining blood levels of progesterone and increasing levels of estrogen during late pregnancy. The neurotransmitters involved in stimulating oxytocin release are thought to be acetylcholine and dopamine.

Oxytocin release is also triggered by stimulation of tactile receptors in the nipples of the lactating breast by suckling (see Figure 2–5). Breast-feeding generates sensory impulses that are transmitted to the spinal cord and then to the oxytocin-producing neurons in the hypothalamus. The information transmitted by these sensory afferents produces intermittent synchronized burst-firing of oxytocin neurons, resulting in pulsatile release of oxytocin and increases in blood oxytocin concentrations.

In addition to its secretion from neurohypophysial terminals in the posterior pituitary, oxytocin is released within the hypothalamic supraoptic and paraventricular nuclei. The function of this intrahypothalamic release of oxytocin is to control the activity of oxytocin neurons in an autocrine fashion by a positive feedback mechanism, increasing the neurohypophysial release of oxytocin. The release of oxytocin is inhibited by severe pain, increased body temperature, and loud noise. Note how the environmental, hormonal, and neural mechanisms of hypothalamic hormone regulation are in play to regulate oxytocin release at the appropriate time of gestation and in response to the relevant stimuli. The role of oxytocin in males is not clear, although recent studies have suggested that it may participate in ejaculation.

OXYTOCIN RECEPTORS

The physiologic effects of oxytocin are achieved by binding to cell membrane $G_{q/11}$ protein–coupled oxytocin receptors expressed in the uterus, mammary glands, and brain (Figure 2–6). Binding of oxytocin to the receptor

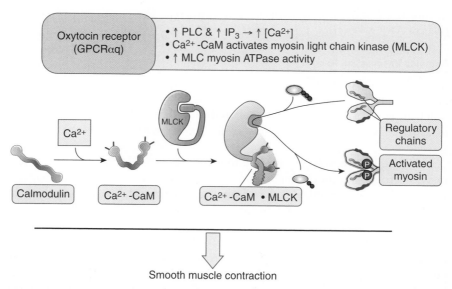

Figure 2–6. Receptor-mediated oxytocin effects. Oxytocin binds to cell membrane $G_{aq/11}$ protein–coupled receptors expressed in the uterus, mammary glands, and brain. Binding of oxytocin to the receptor activates phospholipase C (PLC), producing an increase in inositol trisphosphate (IP_3) and 1,2-diacylglycerol, which in turn results in an increase in cytosolic calcium concentrations. Calcium binds to calmodulin (CaM) and the Ca^{2+}-CaM complex activates myosin light chain kinase (MLCK), which in turn phosphorylates (activating) myosin regulatory chains. The phosphorylated myosin filament combines with the actin filament leading to smooth muscle contraction. ATPase, adenosine triphosphatase; MLC, myosin light chain.

activates phospholipase C, producing an increase in inositol trisphosphate and 1,2-diacylglycerol, which in turn results in an increase in cytosolic calcium concentrations leading to smooth muscle contraction.

DISORDERS OF OXYTOCIN PRODUCTION

Diseases resulting from oxytocin excess have not been described. Although oxytocin deficiency causes difficulty with nursing because of impaired milk ejection, it is not associated with altered fertility or delivery. Normal oxytocin levels have been detected in women with DI (AVP deficiency).

Arginine Vasopressin

AVP, also known as *antidiuretic hormone* (ADH), is the other neuropeptide produced by magnocellular neurons of the hypothalamus and released from the posterior pituitary. The principal effect of AVP is to increase water reabsorption by enhancing permeability to water in the distal convoluted tubules and the medullary collecting ducts in the kidney. In addition, AVP increases vascular resistance. This function of AVP may be important during periods of severe lack of responsiveness to other vasoconstrictors, as may occur during severe blood loss (hemorrhagic shock) or systemic infection (sepsis). The circulating concentrations of AVP range from 1.5 to 6 ng/L.

ARGININE VASOPRESSIN RECEPTORS

The cellular effects of AVP are mediated by binding to G protein–coupled membrane receptors. Three AVP receptors have been characterized thus far, which differ in terms of where they are expressed as well as in the specific G proteins to which they are coupled and, thus, in the second-messenger systems that they activate.

V_1R (also known as V_{1a}) is coupled to $G_{q/11}$ and is specific for AVP. It is found in the liver, smooth muscle, brain, and adrenal glands. It activates phospholipases C, D, and A_2 and stimulates the hydrolysis of phosphatidylinositol, resulting in an increase in intracellular calcium concentrations. The vasopressor effects of AVP are mediated through the V_1R.

V_2R is coupled to G_s and is expressed in the kidney. Binding of AVP to the V_2R receptor activates adenylate cyclase and increases cyclic 3′,5′-adenosine monophosphate (cAMP) formation and aquaporin 2 (AQP2) phosphorylation and insertion into the luminal membrane. The water reabsorptive effects of AVP are mediated through the V_2R.

V_3R (also known as V_{1b}) is coupled to $G_{q/11}$ and is expressed in the majority of anterior pituitary corticotroph cells and in several tissues, including the kidney, thymus, heart, lung, spleen, uterus, and breast. Binding of AVP to the V_3R receptor stimulates the activity of phospholipase C, resulting in an increase in intracellular calcium.

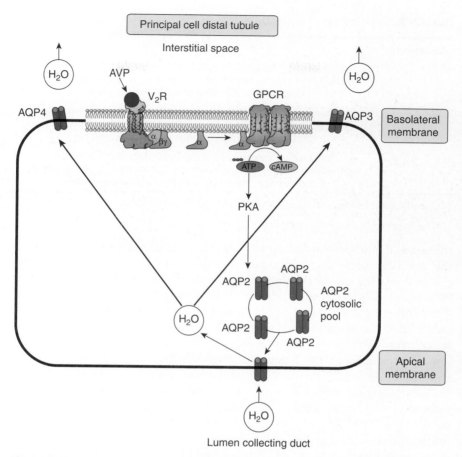

Figure 2–7. Cellular mechanism of arginine vasopressin (AVP) water conservation. The principal function of AVP is to increase water reabsorption and to conserve water. AVP binds to the V_2 G protein–coupled receptor (V_2R) in the principal cells of the distal tubule. This triggers the activation of adenylate cyclase and the formation of cyclic 3′,5′-adenosine monophosphate (cAMP), leading to activation of protein kinase A (PKA). PKA phosphorylates the water channel aquaporin 2 (AQP2), leading to the insertion of AQP2 into the luminal cell membrane. The insertion of water channels into the membrane increases the permeability to water. Water reabsorbed through these water channels leaves the cell through aquaporin 3 (AQP3) and aquaporin 4 (AQP4), which are constitutively expressed in the basolateral membrane of the principal cells. GPCR, G protein–coupled receptor.

Physiologic Effects of Arginine Vasopressin

The main target site of ADH is the collecting duct in the kidney (Figure 2–7). Water permeability in the collecting duct is relatively low compared with that in the proximal tubule and the thin descending limb of Henle's loop. In the proximal tubule and the descending limb of Henle's loop,

Table 2–3. Key features of aquaporins

Aquaporin	Features
AQP1	Constitutively expressed in apical and basolateral membranes of epithelial cells of proximal tubules and descending limb of Henle's loop. Involved in 90% of water reabsorption.
AQP2	Exclusively expressed in the collecting ducts. The only aquaporin directly regulated by ADH. Binding to the V_2 AVP receptor stimulates insertion into the luminal membrane.
AQP3, AQP4	Constitutively expressed in the basolateral membranes of epithelial cells in the collecting ducts. Enhance water reabsorption following AQP2 insertion into the luminal membrane.

ADH, antidiuretic hormone; AQP, aquaporin; AVP, arginine vasopressin.

the water channel protein aquaporin 1 (AQP1) is constitutively expressed both in the apical (luminal) and basolateral (interstitial) membranes of epithelial cells (Table 2–3). The proximal tubule is responsible for reabsorbing approximately 90% of filtered water. Reabsorption of the remaining 10% of filtered water in the distal collecting ducts is under tight control by AVP. Although it may seem that only a small fraction of the total filtered water reabsorption is under AVP control, water permeability of the collecting duct can be dramatically increased (within a few minutes) through the production of cAMP following AVP binding to V_2 receptors in the basolateral membrane of the principal cells (see Figure 2–7).

The importance of AVP is better understood in terms of the total amount of urine that would be excreted in its absence. For example, in a healthy individual an average of 180 L of glomerular filtrate is formed per day. Thus, without AVP-mediated reabsorption of 10% of filtered water in the distal collecting ducts, urine output would be close to 18 L/d. This is 10-fold higher than the volume of urine output (1.5–2 L/d) under normal conditions.

The increase in cAMP that is stimulated by AVP binding to the receptor located in the basolateral membrane activates protein kinase A and subsequently the phosphorylation of AQP2, another protein. Phosphorylation of AQP2 is essential for its movement from cytoplasmic pools and its insertion in the luminal (apical) epithelial cell membrane of the collecting duct cells. The result is an increase in the number of functional water channels in the luminal membrane, making it more permeable to water. Thus, AVP-mediated insertion of AQP2 into the luminal membrane results in water conservation and urine concentration. This event is a short-term regulation of water permeability in response to an increase in circulating levels of AVP. In addition, AVP is thought to regulate water permeability over hours to days as a result of an increase in the total cellular amount of AQP2 caused by increased protein synthesis.

AQP2, one of several members of the aquaporin family, is exclusively expressed in the collecting ducts of the kidney. It is the only aquaporin that is directly regulated by ADH via the V_2 AVP receptor. Water that diffuses into the cells through AQP2 exits through the basolateral side through aquaporin 3 (AQP3) and 4 (AQP4) eventually entering the vasculature. AQP3 and AQP4 are constitutively expressed in the basolateral membranes of the collecting ducts.

Water reabsorption through this mechanism is driven by the hydroosmotic gradient generated by a countercurrent mechanism in the renal medulla. The result is an increase in the concentration and reduction of urine volume, which minimizes urinary water loss. This antidiuretic mechanism may increase urine osmolarity to approximately 1200 mmol/L and reduce urine flow to approximately 0.5 mL/min. Without AVP-mediated effects, the principal cells of the collecting duct are impermeable to water, resulting in large volumes of diluted urine entering the collecting tubules from the ascending limb of the loop of Henle. As mentioned above, this could translate into excessive urine output and reduced urine osmolarity.

AVP also binds the V_1 receptor, expressed in vascular smooth muscle, producing contraction and increasing peripheral vascular resistance (Figure 2–8). The hormone is known as *vasopressin* because of these vasoconstrictor effects. In particular, renal medullary blood flow has been demonstrated to be under AVP regulation. AVP circulates unbound and is distributed in a volume approximately equal to that of the extracellular space. Because of its relatively low molecular weight, AVP permeates peripheral and glomerular capillaries readily, so the urinary excretion rate of AVP is extraordinarily high.

AVP vasculature effects

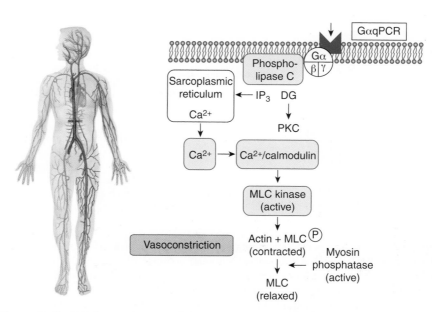

Figure 2–8. Cellular mechanism of AVP vasoconstrictor effects. AVP also known as vasopressin binds the V_1 receptor, expressed in vascular smooth muscle, producing contraction and increasing peripheral vascular resistance. DG, diacylglycerol; IP_3, inositol trisphosphate; MLC, myosin light chain; PCR, protein-coupled receptor; PKC, protein kinase C.

CONTROL OF ARGININE VASOPRESSIN RELEASE

AVP is released into the circulation following either an increase in plasma osmolarity or a decrease in blood volume (Figure 2–9). Under physiologic conditions, the most important stimulus for AVP release is the "effective" plasma osmolarity. The changes in osmotic pressure are detected by special osmoreceptor neurons located in the hypothalamus and in 3 structures associated with the lamina terminalis: the subfornical organ, the median preoptic nucleus, and the organum vasculosum lamina terminalis. Dehydration produces loss of intracellular water from the osmoreceptors, resulting in cell shrinkage, which signals the AVP magnocellular neurons to stimulate AVP release. Release of AVP occurs

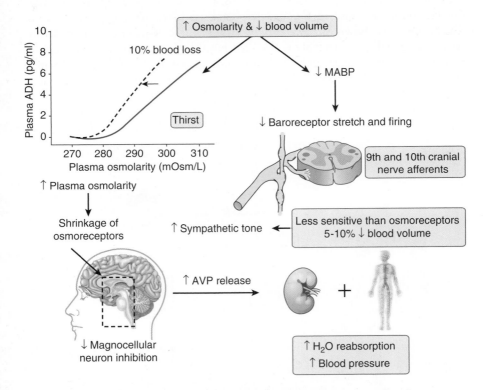

Figure 2–9. Integration of signals that trigger arginine vasopressin (AVP) release. Release of AVP is stimulated by an increase in plasma osmolarity and by a decrease in blood volume. Small changes in plasma osmolarity above a threshold of 280–284 mOsm/L produce an increase in antidiuretic hormone (ADH) release before the stimulation of thirst. A decrease in blood volume sensitizes the system and increases the responsiveness to small changes in plasma osmolarity. Blood loss and a decrease in mean arterial blood pressure (MABP) greater than 10% signal the hypothalamus to increase the release of AVP. The afferent signals are transmitted by the 9th and 10th cranial nerves. These signals increase sympathetic tone, therefore decreasing magnocellular neuron inhibition and stimulating AVP release.

even before the sensation of thirst. Therefore, on a hot day, an increase in AVP has already been initiated, and AVP is at work conserving fluid even before one feels the desire to drink water. In contrast, hypotonic stimuli, such as excess fluid intake or intravenous fluid administration in a hospital setting, result in cell swelling and stretching and hyperpolarization of the magnocellular neurons, which result in decreased depolarization and firing and consequently decreased release of AVP. The sensitivity of this system is quite high. That is, very small changes in plasma osmolarity (as little as 1% change) above the osmotic threshold of 280–284 mOsm/L produce significant increases in AVP release.

AVP secretion is also stimulated by a decrease in blood pressure of greater than 10% (see Figure 2–9). Decreases in blood volume or blood pressure are detected by pressure-sensitive receptors in the cardiac atria, aorta, and carotid sinus. Factors that reduce cardiac output, such as a decrease in blood volume, orthostatic hypotension, and positive-pressure breathing, are all potent stimuli for AVP release. A decrease in blood pressure decreases the stretch of the baroreceptors and decreases their firing rate. These signals are transmitted to the central nervous system by neurons of the vagus and glossopharyngeal nerves. The reduced stimulation produces a decrease in tonic inhibition of AVP release, leading to an increase in AVP release from the magnocellular neurosecretory neurons. In addition to signaling the brain to stimulate the release of AVP, the decrease in blood pressure is also perceived by the macula densa in the kidney. This results in stimulation of renin release from the juxtaglomerular apparatus in the kidney. Renin catalyzes the conversion of angiotensinogen produced in the liver to angiotensin I, which is then converted to angiotensin II, by angiotensin-converting enzyme. The resulting rise in circulating levels of angiotensin II sensitizes the osmoreceptors, leading to enhanced AVP release. This is another example of hormonal regulation of hypothalamic neuropeptide release.

The volume-induced sensitization of AVP release results in a more accentuated AVP response to changes in plasma osmolarity. However, AVP secretion is far more sensitive to small changes in plasma osmolarity than to changes in blood volume. AVP is barely detectable below a certain plasma osmolarity (287 mOsm/L) threshold. Above this threshold, the plasma AVP concentration increases steeply in direct proportion to plasma osmolarity. An increase in osmolarity of only 1% will change AVP by an average of 1 pg/mL, an amount sufficient to significantly alter urine concentration and output. Circulating levels of AVP may reach 15–20 pg/mL under a strong osmotic stress. Because of this extraordinary sensitivity, the osmoreceptor plays the primary role in mediating the antidiuretic response to changes in water balance. In contrast, the response to pressure-volume changes is exponential. Reductions in plasma volume by 5%–10% usually have little effect on AVP levels, whereas decreases of 20%–30% result in intense hormone secretion, bringing AVP concentrations to a level many times higher than that required to produce maximum antidiuresis (up to 50–100 pg/mL). In other words, small changes in plasma osmolarity are more effective than small changes in blood pressure and volume in stimulating AVP release. Release of AVP can be modulated by estrogen and progesterone, opiates, nicotine, alcoholic beverages, and atrial natriuretic factor.

DISORDERS OF ARGININE VASOPRESSIN PRODUCTION

Either deficiency or excess of AVP can result in clinical disease. Deficiency of ADH release results in DI, a clinical syndrome resulting from the inability to form concentrated urine. Excess AVP release is known as *syndrome of inappropriate antidiuretic hormone secretion* (SIADH). The concentrations of AVP may be altered in various chronic pathophysiologic conditions, including congestive heart failure, liver cirrhosis, and nephritic syndrome.

Diabetes insipidus—DI is characterized by the excretion of abnormally large volumes (30 mL/kg of body weight per day for adult subjects) of dilute (<250 mmol/kg) urine and excessive thirst. Three basic defects have been identified in the etiology. Only the first 2 pertain to alterations related to components of the AVP system itself. The third, excess water intake does not involve alterations in ADH release.

Decreased arginine vasopressin release—Neurogenic (central or hypothalamic) DI is the most common defect and is caused by a decrease in AVP release resulting from diseases affecting the hypothalamic-neurohypophysial axis. Three causes can be identified: traumatic, inflammatory or infectious, and cancer related.

Decreased renal responsiveness to arginine vasopressin—Renal (nephrogenic) DI results from renal insensitivity to the antidiuretic effect of AVP. AVP production and release are not affected, but responsiveness at the distal tubule is impaired. Nephrogenic DI can be inherited or acquired and is characterized by an inability to concentrate urine despite normal or elevated plasma concentrations of AVP. Approximately 90% of cases are males with the X-linked recessive form of the disease who have mutations in the AVP type-2 receptor gene. A small number of cases of inherited nephrogenic DI are caused by mutations in the AQP2 water channel gene. Acquired nephrogenic DI can result from lithium treatment, hypokalemia, and postobstructive polyuria.

Differential diagnosis—The differential diagnosis of DI relies on an understanding of the physiologic regulation of AVP release and its effects on the kidney. Plasma levels of AVP are interpreted together with the indirect assessment of antidiuretic activity triggered by a dehydration test. This test determines the ability of the body to increase the production and release of AVP during water deprivation. Fluids are withheld from the individual, and the rise in urine osmolarity, which indicates the response of the body to conserve fluid, is measured. Normal function consists of an increase in urine osmolarity and a decrease in urine output during water deprivation alone.

Another way of testing the system is by a challenge test with synthetic AVP. Individuals with normal pituitary function do not exhibit a further increase in urine osmolarity following the administration of a synthetic AVP analog (desmopressin). Individuals with central DI have a greater than 9% increase in urine osmolarity following desmopressin administration, indicating that the body is not capable of producing maximal release of AVP and consequently does a better job when a synthetic analog of AVP is administered. Another approach to diagnosing central DI is also based on the physiologic regulation of AVP release and uses the response to osmotic stimulation produced by the intravenous infusion of hypertonic (5%) saline solution. These examples illustrate that understanding the etiology of the disease requires an understanding of the normal physiologic regulation of the endocrine system in question.

 Syndrome of inappropriate antidiuretic hormone secretion—An increase or excess in the release of ADH, in the absence of a physiologic stimuli for its release (thus the name inappropriate) is known as SIADH. This may be the result of brain injury or tumor production of AVP. The tumor can be located in the brain, but malignancies of other organs, such as the lung, have also been shown to produce high levels of AVP. The excess production of AVP results in the production of very small volumes of concentrated urine and dilutional hyponatremia. Management of this condition entails fluid restriction and, in some cases, the use of saline solutions to restore adequate plasma sodium levels.

KEY CONCEPTS

 Hypothalamic peptides released at the median eminence are transported to the anterior pituitary, where they regulate the release of anterior pituitary hormones.

 The hypothalamus integrates information from various brain regions, the environment, and peripheral organs and mediates systemic responses that help maintain homeostasis.

 Oxytocin and AVP are neuropeptides made in hypothalamic neurons and released from the posterior pituitary into the systemic circulation.

 Prohormone posttranslational modification and processing of oxytocin and AVP occur inside the secretory granules during axonal transport and generate neurophysins.

 AVP binds to the V_2 receptor in tubular collecting-duct epithelial cells, stimulating the insertion of AQP2 into the apical (luminal) membrane leading to increased water reabsorption.

 The release of AVP is more sensitive to small changes in plasma osmolarity than to small changes in blood volume.

 Deficiency of AVP results in the production of large volumes of dilute urine.

 Excess AVP release results in small volumes of concentrated urine and hemodilution leading to hyponatremia.

STUDY QUESTIONS

2–1. A 55-year-old male trauma victim has been a patient in the surgical intensive care unit for the past 6 days. During rounds, he appears semi-conscious, his heart rate is 85 beats per minute, blood pressure is 120/90 mm Hg, and respiratory rate is 18 breaths per minute. Records indicate his urine output to average 15 L/24 h. You suspect he has a neuroendocrine abnormality of traumatic origin. Which set of laboratory values would be compatible with your differential diagnosis?

	Serum Na (135–145 mEq/L)	Serum osmolarity (280–310 mOsm/L)
A	125	245
B	156	356
C	136	356
D	160	250
E	125	380

2–2. You request additional tests on the urine of this patient. Which of the following would you expect to be the set of results compatible with his condition?

	Urine Na (20–40 mEq/L)	Urine osmolarity (<150 mOsm/L)
A	45	140
B	10	100
C	15	300
D	25	150
E	40	200

2–3. This patient's problem is most likely associated with:
   a. Increased production and release of arginine vasopressin
   b. Increased urinary release of cAMP
   c. Decreased free water reabsorption
   d. Increased sodium reabsorption

2–4. Rupture of membranes, without active labor in a 32-year-old patient during her 40th week of gestation leads you to start induction of labor and delivery with an intravenous drip of oxytocin analog (Pitocin). Which of the following best summarizes the uterine changes (increases ↑ or decreases ↓) that have occurred during pregnancy that will contribute to enhanced responsiveness to Pitocin?

	Prostaglandin synthesis	β-adrenergic receptor expression	Gap junction formation	Oxytocin receptor expression
A	↑	↑	↓	↑
B	↓	↑	↑	↓
C	↑	↓	↑	↑
D	↓	↑	↓	↑
E	↑	↓	↓	↓

2–5.   A 74-year-old male patient recovering from a surgical procedure complains of
       headache, difficulty concentrating, impaired memory, muscle cramps, and weak-
       ness of 48 hours duration. On examination, vital signs are all within normal range,
       and there are no signs of dehydration or of edema. Laboratory values report serum
       sodium of 130 mmol/L. Which of the following would be compatible with a differ-
       ential diagnosis of syndrome of inappropriate ADH secretion?

   a. Low plasma AVP levels

   b. Serum osmolarity of 275 mOsm/L

   c. Plasma glucose 300 mg/dL

   d. Urinary osmolarity >400 mOsm/L

SUGGESTED READINGS

Bourque CW, Oliet SHR. Osmoreceptors in the central nervous system. *Annu Rev Physiol.* 1997;59:601.

de Bree FM. Trafficking of the vasopressin and oxytocin prohormone through the regulated secretory
   pathway. *J Neuroendocrinol.* 2000;12:589.

Gimpl G, Fahrenholz F. The oxytocin receptor system: structure, function, and regulation. *Physiol Rev.*
   2001;81:629.

Melmed S. Medical progress: acromegaly. *N Engl J Med.* 2006;355(24):2558–2573.

Anterior Pituitary Gland

3

OBJECTIVES

▶ Identify the 3 families of anterior pituitary hormones and their main structural differences.

▶ Understand the mechanisms that regulate anterior pituitary hormone production and describe the actions of tropic hormones on target organs.

▶ Diagram the short-loop and long-loop negative feedback control of anterior pituitary hormone secretion.

▶ Predict the changes in secretory rates of hypothalamic anterior pituitary and target gland hormones caused by oversecretion or undersecretion of any of these hormones or receptor deficit for any of these hormones.

▶ Explain the importance of pulsatile and diurnal hormone secretion.

The anterior pituitary, or adenohypophysis, plays a central role in the regulation of endocrine function through the production and release of **tropic hormones** (Figure 3–1). The function of the anterior pituitary, and thereby the production of tropic hormones, is under hypothalamic regulation by the hypophysiotropic neuropeptides released in the median eminence, as discussed in Chapter 2 and summarized in Table 3–1. The tropic hormones produced by the anterior pituitary are released into the systemic circulation, from where they reach their target organs to produce a physiologic response, most frequently involving the release of a target organ hormone (see Figure 3–1). The hormones produced by the target organs affect anterior pituitary function as well as the release of hypophysiotropic neuropeptides, maintaining an integrated feedback control system of endocrine function (see Chapter 1, Figure 1–12).

FUNCTIONAL ANATOMY

The pituitary, or hypophysis, consists of an anterior and a posterior lobe that differ from one another in their embryologic origin, mode of development, and structure. The anterior lobe, also known as the **adenohypophysis**, is the larger and consists of a pars anterior and a pars intermedia, or intermediate lobe, separated from each other by a narrow cleft, the remnant of Rathke's pouch. The pars intermedia is of minor importance in human physiology. The anterior pituitary is a

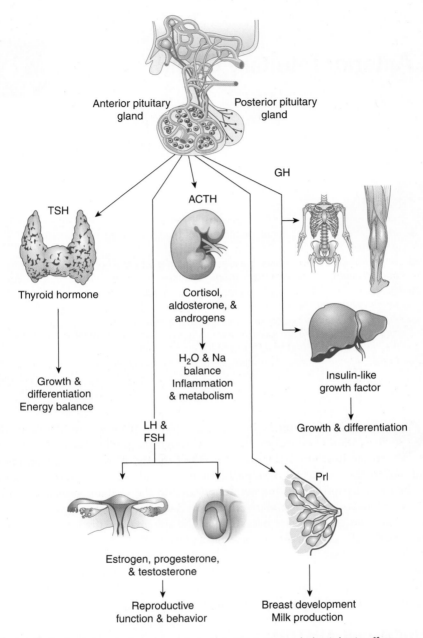

Figure 3–1. Anterior pituitary hormones, target organs, and physiologic effects. Thyroid-stimulating hormone (TSH) stimulates the thyroid gland to produce and release thyroid hormones that regulate growth, differentiation, and energy balance. Luteinizing hormone (LH) and follicle-stimulating hormone (FSH) stimulate gonadal production of sex steroids, which mediate reproductive function and behavior. Adrenocorticotropic hormone (ACTH) stimulates the adrenal glands to produce steroid hormones, which regulate water and sodium balance, inflammation, and metabolism. Prolactin (Prl) stimulates breast development and milk production. Growth hormone (GH) exerts direct effects on tissue growth and differentiation and indirect effects through the stimulation of insulin-like growth factor 1 production, which mediates some of the growth and differentiation effects of GH.

Table 3–1. Anterior pituitary cell type, regulatory hypothalamic factor, and hormone product

Anterior pituitary cells	Hypothalamic factor	Pituitary hormone produced
Lactotrophs	Dopamine	Prolactin
Corticotrophs	CRH	POMC: ACTH, β-LPH, α-MSH, β-endorphin
Thyrotrophs	TRH	Thyroid-stimulating hormone
Gonadotrophs	GnRH	LH and FSH
Somatotrophs	GHRH	Growth hormone

ACTH, adrenocorticotropic hormone; CRH, corticotropin-releasing hormone; FSH, follicle-stimulating hormone; GHRH, growth hormone-releasing hormone; GnRH, gonadotropin-releasing hormone; LH, luteinizing hormone; LPH, lipotropin; MSH, melanocyte-stimulating hormone; POMC, proopiomelanocortin; TRH , thyrotropin-releasing hormone.

highly vascularized structure consisting of epithelial cells derived from the ecto-dermal lining of the roof of the mouth. The pituitary cells that line the capillaries produce the tropic hormones: adrenocorticotropic hormone (**ACTH**), thyroid-stimulating hormone (**TSH**), growth hormone (**GH**), **prolactin,** and the gonado-tropins luteinizing hormone (**LH**) and follicle-stimulating hormone (**FSH**) (see Figure 3–1). All of these hormones are released into the systemic circulation.

The cells of the anterior pituitary are named according to the hormone that they produce. According to their specific distribution, they may be more or less susceptible to traumatic injury. For example, the gonadotrophs and somato-trophs (GH-producing cells) are more numerous in the posterolateral region of the anterior pituitary, making them vulnerable to mechanical damage of the pituitary. The corticotrophs (ACTH-producing cells) and the thyrotrophs (TSH-producing cells) are located predominantly in the anteromedial region, making them more resilient to traumatic injury. The lactotrophs (prolactin-producing cells) are dispersed throughout the pituitary, and this too is a resil-ient cell population. The posterior pituitary is of nervous origin. It consists of unmyelinated nerve fibers and axon terminals of magnocellular hypothalamic neurons, with bodies located primarily in the supraoptic and paraventricular hypothalamic nuclei. The neurohormones released from the posterior pituitary have been discussed in Chapter 2. This chapter will focus on the endocrine function of the anterior pituitary.

HYPOTHALAMIC CONTROL OF ANTERIOR PITUITARY HORMONE RELEASE

The production of pituitary tropic hormones is under direct regulation by the hypothalamic neurohormones released from neuronal terminals in the median eminence. The neurohormones are delivered to the anterior pituitary through a specialized capillary network, described in Chapter 2 and illustrated in Figure 2–2. The hypothalamic neuropeptides travel down the long hypophysial portal veins to the anterior pituitary, where they bind to specific cell surface G protein–coupled receptors and activate intracellular second-messenger cascades, resulting in the release of pituitary hormone from the respective target cells.

The responsiveness of the anterior pituitary to the inhibitory or stimulatory effects of hypophysiotropic neurohormones can be modified by several factors, including hormone levels, negative feedback inhibition, and circadian rhythms as discussed in Chapter 1. The release of anterior pituitary hormones is cyclic in nature, and this cyclic pattern of hormone release is governed by the nervous system. Most rhythms are driven by an internal biologic clock located in the hypothalamic **suprachiasmatic nucleus**; this clock is synchronized or entrained by external signals such as light and dark periods. Both sleep and circadian effects interact to produce the overall rhythmic pattern of pituitary hormone release and the associated responses. Some of the 24-hour hormonal rhythms depend on the circadian clock (ie, ACTH, cortisol, and melatonin) and some are sleep related (ie, prolactin, GH, and TSH). For example, GH secretion is influenced by the first slow-wave sleep episode at the beginning of the night. Pulses of prolactin and GH are positively linked to increases in delta-wave activity, present during the deepest phases of sleep and occurring primarily during the first third of the night. Pulses of TSH and cortisol are related to superficial phases of sleep.

Although the regulation of the patterns of hormone release is not well understood, it is clear that the respective patterns of anterior pituitary hormone release play a crucial role in achieving their physiologic effects and, thus, in maintaining homeostasis. The importance of this regulation has become evident because constant or continuous exogenous hormone administration produces effects that differ from the hormone's natural physiologic effects. These observations have highlighted the importance of trying to simulate, as much as possible, the endogenous cyclic patterns of hormone release when giving hormone replacement therapy to a patient. In addition, disruption of the cyclic patterns of hormone release has been identified in disease states and is thought to play an important role in the impaired endocrine function that occurs with aging. Disruption of circadian rhythms leads to symptoms of fatigue, disorientation, altered hormone profiles, and higher morbidity. Therefore, the natural cyclic pattern of hypothalamic, pituitary, and target organ hormone release is of central importance to normal endocrine function.

HORMONES OF THE ANTERIOR PITUITARY

The hormones of the anterior pituitary can be classified into 3 families: the **glycoproteins,** those derived from proopiomelanocortin (**POMC**), and those belonging to the **GH and prolactin** family (Figure 3–2).

Anterior pituitary hormones

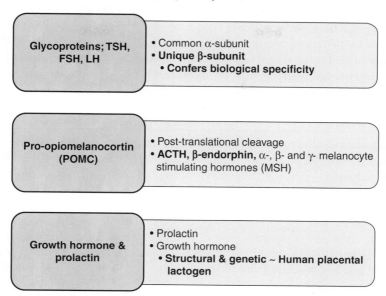

Figure 3–2. Classification of anterior pituitary hormones. Thyroid-stimulating hormone (TSH), luteinizing hormone (LH), and follicle-stimulating hormone (FSH) are glycoproteins with very similar structures. Proopiomelanocortin (POMC) is a polypeptide hormone that is posttranslationally cleaved to adrenocorticotropin (ACTH), β-endorphin, and melanocyte-stimulating hormones. Growth hormone and prolactin are structurally similar to human placental lactogen.

Glycoproteins

Glycoprotein hormones are among the largest hormones known to date. They include TSH, FSH, LH, and human chorionic gonadotropin (HCG) produced by the placenta. These hormones are heterodimeric glycoproteins consisting of a common α-subunit and a unique β-subunit, which confers the biologic specificity of each hormone.

THYROID-STIMULATING HORMONE

TSH is a glycoprotein synthesized and secreted from thyrotrophs of the anterior pituitary gland. Thyrotrophs synthesize and release TSH in response to thyrotropin-releasing hormone (TRH) stimulation. TRH is synthesized in the paraventricular nuclei of the hypothalamus, predominantly by parvicellular neurons, and is released from nerve terminals in the median eminence. TRH binds to a $G_{q/11}$ protein–coupled receptor, which activates phospholipase C, leading to increased phosphoinositide turnover, calcium mobilization, and release of TSH into the circulation. TSH binds to a G_s protein–coupled receptor in the thyroid gland, activating adenylate cyclase and leading to increased intracellular cyclic 3′,5′-adenosine monophosphate (cAMP) formation and stimulation of the protein kinase A signaling pathway. TSH stimulates all the events involved in thyroid hormone synthesis and release (see Chapter 4). In addition, it acts as a growth and survival factor for the thyroid gland. The release of TSH from the anterior pituitary gland is under negative feedback inhibition by thyroid hormone, particularly triiodothyronine, as discussed in detail in Chapter 4.

GONADOTROPINS (FOLLICLE-STIMULATING HORMONE AND LUTEININZING HORMONE)

The gonadotropic hormones LH and FSH are synthesized and secreted by gonadotrophs of the anterior pituitary in response to stimulation by gonadotropin-releasing hormone (GnRH). Most of the gonadotrophs produce both LH and FSH; with a fraction of the gonadotroph population producing LH or FSH exclusively. GnRH is synthesized and secreted by the hypothalamus in a pulsatile manner. GnRH binds to the GnRH $G_{q/11}$ protein–coupled receptor on pituitary gonadotrophs and produces activation of phospholipase C, leading to phosphoinositide turnover and Ca^{2+} mobilization and influx. This signaling cascade increases the transcription of the FSH and LH α-subunit and β-subunit genes and increases the release of FSH and LH into the circulation.

FSH and LH exert their physiologic effects on the testes and ovaries by binding to G_s protein–coupled receptors and activating adenylate cyclase. Among the target cells for gonadotropins are ovarian granulosa cells, theca interna cells, testicular Sertoli cells, and Leydig cells. The physiologic responses produced by the gonadotropins include stimulation of sex hormone synthesis (steroidogenesis), spermatogenesis, folliculogenesis, and ovulation. Therefore, their central role is the control of reproductive function in both males and females. GnRH controls the synthesis and secretion of both FSH and LH by the pituitary gonadotroph cell. Gonadotropin synthesis and release, as well as differential expression, is under both positive and negative feedback control by gonadal steroids and gonadal peptides (Figure 3–3). Gonadal hormones can decrease gonadotropin release both by decreasing GnRH release from the hypothalamus and by affecting the ability of GnRH to stimulate gonadotropin secretion from the pituitary itself. Estradiol enhances LH and inhibits FSH release, whereas inhibins A and B, gonadal glycoprotein hormones, reduce FSH secretion (see Chapter 9).

The complexity of the regulation of synthesis and release of anterior pituitary hormones is best illustrated by the cyclic nature of FSH and LH release. The pattern of GnRH pulses changes during the menstrual cycle in women, as summarized in Table 3–2 and discussed in detail in Chapter 9. During the luteal to follicular phase transition, pulses of GnRH release occur every 90–120 minutes, and FSH secretion predominates. In the mid-to-late follicular phase, GnRH frequency increases to 1 pulse every 60 minutes, favoring LH secretion over FSH. After ovulation, ovarian progesterone production predominates. Progesterone increases hypothalamic opioid activity and slows GnRH pulse secretion. This slower GnRH pulse pattern (1 pulse per 3–5 hours) favors FSH production. However, at the same time, estradiol and inhibin A produced by the corpus

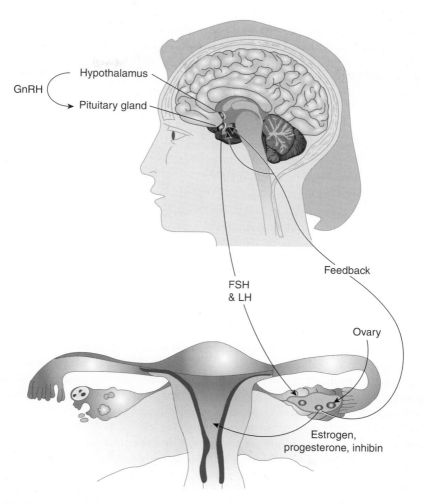

GnRH

Hypothalamus

Pituitary gland

Feedback

FSH
& LH

Ovary

Estrogen,
progesterone, inhibin

Figure 3–3. Feedback regulation of pituitary hormone release. Hypothalamic neurohormones (eg, gonadotropin-releasing hormone) stimulate the anterior pituitary to produce and release tropic hormones (eg, follicle-stimulating hormone and luteinizing hormone). Tropic hormones bind to receptors in target organs and elicit a physiologic response. In most cases, the response involves the production of a target organ hormone, which, in turn, mediates physiologic effects at the target organ (eg, uterus). In addition, the target organ hormone is involved in feedback mechanisms (negative or positive) that regulate the production and release of the tropic hormone and the hypothalamic factor that regulates pituitary hormone release.

luteum inhibit FSH release, leading to increased FSH stores. With involution of the corpus luteum and the sharp decline in estradiol, inhibin A, and progesterone, the frequency of GnRH pulse secretion is increased. In the absence of estradiol and inhibin A (inhibitors of FSH release), a selective FSH release predominates and initiates the next wave of follicular development.

Table 3–2. Regulation of gonadotropin release in ovulating females

Phase of menstrual cycle	Gonadal hormones	GnRH pulses	Gonadotropin release
Luteal to follicular transition	Low estradiol, low inhibin	90–120 min	FSH > LH
Mid to late follicular phase	Increasing estradiol and inhibin B	Increased pulsatility; 60 min	LH > FSH
Post ovulation	Increased estradiol, inhibin A, and progesterone	Decreased GnRH pulsatility	Increased FSH synthesis; inhibited release
Corpus luteum involution	Decreased estradiol, inhibin A, and progesterone	Increased GnRH pulsatility	FSH

FSH, follicle-stimulating hormone; GnRH, gonadotropin-releasing hormone; LH, luteinizing hormone.

Proopiomelanocortin-Derived Hormones

POMC is a precursor pro-hormone produced by the corticotrophs of the anterior pituitary. The production and secretion of POMC-derived hormones from the anterior pituitary are regulated predominantly by corticotropin-releasing hormone (CRH) produced in the hypothalamus and released in the median eminence. CRH binds to a G_s protein–coupled receptor whose actions are mediated through activation of adenylate cyclase and elevation of cAMP production (see Figure 3–3). Two types of remarkably homologous (approximately 70% amino acid identity) CRH receptors have been identified. Both CRH-1 and CRH-2 receptors belong to the family of transmembrane receptors that signal by coupling to G proteins and use cAMP as a second messenger. Stimulation of POMC synthesis and peptide release is mediated by the CRH-1 receptor, which is expressed in many areas of the brain as well as in the pituitary, gonads, and skin. CRH-2 receptors are expressed on brain neurons located in neocortical, limbic, and brainstem regions of the central nervous system and on pituitary corticotrophs and in peripheral tissues (eg, cardiac myocytes, gastrointestinal tract, lung, ovary, and skeletal muscle). The role of CRH-2 receptors is not completely understood.

POMC is posttranslationally cleaved to ACTH; β-endorphin, an endogenous opioid peptide; and α-, β-, and γ-melanocyte-stimulating hormones (MSHs) (see Figure 3–5). The biologic effects of POMC-derived peptides are largely mediated through melanocortin receptors (MCRs), of which 5 have been described. MC1R, MC2R, and MC5R have defined roles in the skin, adrenal steroid hormone production, and thermoregulation, respectively. MC4R is expressed in the brain and has been implicated in feeding behavior and appetite regulation. The role of MC3R is not well defined.

ADRENOCORTICOTROPIC HORMONE

The main hormone of interest produced by the cleavage of POMC is ACTH. The release of ACTH is stimulated by psychologic and physical stress such as infection, hypoglycemia, surgery, and trauma and is considered critical in mediating the stress or the adaptive response of the individual to stress (see Chapter 10). ACTH is released in small amounts, and circulating levels average 2–19 pmol/L in healthy individuals. The hormone is released in pulses, with the highest concentrations occurring at approximately 4:00 AM and the lowest concentrations in the afternoon. ACTH released into the systemic circulation binds to a G_s protein–coupled receptor, part of the MCR superfamily (MC2R), and activates adenylate cyclase, increases cAMP formation, and activates protein kinase A (Figure 3–4). The physiologic effects of ACTH at the adrenal cortex are to stimulate the production and release of glucocorticoids (cortisol) and, to a lesser extent, mineralocorticoids (aldosterone) (see Chapter 6). Although all 5 MCRs can bind ACTH to some extent, MC2R binds ACTH with the highest affinity and is expressed almost exclusively in the adrenal cortex; thus, it is considered the physiologic ACTH receptor. The release of cortisol follows the same diurnal rhythm as that of ACTH (see Chapter 1, Figure 1–8). The feedback inhibition of ACTH and of CRH release by cortisol is mediated by glucocorticoid receptor binding in the hypothalamus and in the anterior pituitary.

MELANOCYTE-STIMULATING HORMONE

α-MSH is produced by the proteolytic cleavage of POMC, mainly in the pars intermedia of the pituitary gland (Figure 3–5). Only small amounts of α-MSH are produced in the pituitary under normal conditions. Melanocortin peptides exert their effects through MC1R found in melanocytes, which are key components of the skin's pigmentary system, endothelial cells, monocytes, and keratinocytes. Binding of α-MSH to MC1R activates adenylate cyclase, which in turn causes an increase in intracellular cAMP. This is the classic pathway by which α-MSH is believed to increase melanin synthesis in melanocytes. The peripheral production of α-MSH by nonendocrine cells, particularly by melanocytes, has been described. The involvement of this paracrine system in the development of skin cancer has received considerable attention because of the localized production and paracrine actions of this peptide and the greater expression of MC1R in melanoma than in normal skin.

β-ENDORPHIN

β-Endorphin, the most abundant endogenous opioid peptide, is another product of POMC processing in the pituitary (see Figure 3–4). The physiologic effects of this opioid peptide are mediated by binding to opiate receptors. Because these receptors are expressed in multiple cell types in the brain as well as in peripheral tissues, their effects are pleiotropic. The physiologic actions of endorphins include analgesia, behavioral effects, and neuromodulatory functions. Among the effects on endocrine function is inhibition of GnRH release. Endogenous opioids have

Hypothalamic Peptides

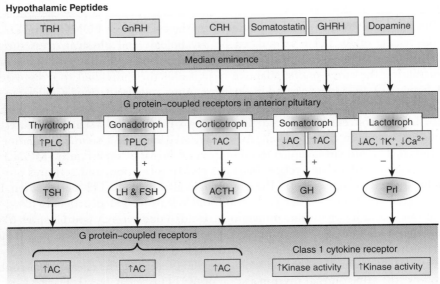

Figure 3–4. Cellular signaling pathways involved in hypothalamo-pituitary hormone-mediated effects. All hypothalamic releasing and inhibiting factors mediate their effects predominantly via G protein–coupled receptors. Anterior pituitary hormones bind to either G protein–coupled receptors (thyroid-stimulating hormone [TSH], luteinizing hormone [LH], follicle-stimulating hormone [FSH], adrenocorticotropic hormone [ACTH]) or class 1 cytokine receptors (growth hormone [GH] and prolactin [Prl]). Most of the cellular responses elicited by anterior pituitary hormones that bind to G protein–coupled receptors are mediated by modulation of adenylate cyclase activity. The cellular responses evoked by anterior pituitary binding to class 1 cytokine receptors are mediated through protein kinase activation. AC, adenylate cyclase; CRH, corticotropin-releasing hormone; GHRH, growth hormone-releasing hormone; GnRH, gonadotropin-releasing hormone; PLC, phospholipase C; TRH, thyrotropin-releasing hormone.

also been implicated in the mechanisms involved in alcohol and drug addiction and have led to therapies such as the use of naltrexone, an opiate receptor antagonist, in the management of alcohol dependency.

Growth Hormone and Prolactin Family

GROWTH HORMONE

GH is a 191 amino acid peptide hormone, with a molecular weight of approximately 22 kDa and structural similarity to prolactin and chorionic somatomammotropin, a placental-derived hormone. GH exists in various molecular isoforms, and this heterogeneity is reflected in the wide variability in GH levels

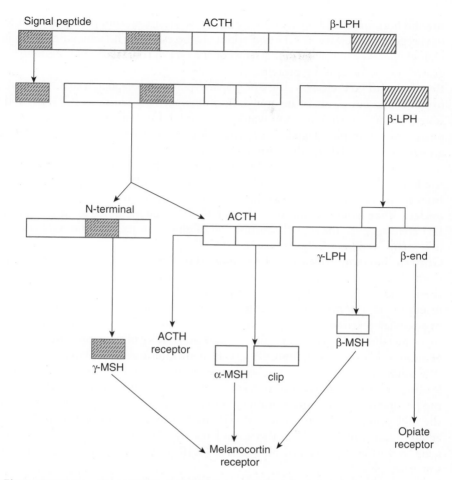

Figure 3–5. Proopiomelanocortin (POMC) processing. Corticotropin-releasing hormone stimulates the production, release, and processing of POMC, a preprohormone synthesized in the anterior pituitary. POMC is post-translationally cleaved to adrenocorticotropic hormone (ACTH); β-endorphin, an endogenous opioid peptide; and α-, β-, and γ-melanocyte-stimulating hormones (MSHs). The cellular effects of these peptides are mediated via melanocortin (ACTH and MSH) or opiate (β-endorphin) receptors. LPH, β-lipotropin.

determined by different immunoassays. However, it is the 22 kDa that is the principal form with physiologic effects found in humans. GH is released from the somatotrophs, an abundant cell type in the anterior pituitary. GH is released in pulsatile bursts, with the majority of secretion occurring nocturnally in association with slow-wave sleep (Figure 1–8). The basis of the pulsatile release of GH and the function of this pattern are not fully understood; however, nutritional, metabolic, and age-related sex steroid mechanisms, adrenal glucocorticoids, thyroid hormones, and renal and hepatic functions are all thought to contribute to the pulsatile release of GH and appear to be essential in achieving optimal biologic potency of the hormone. Most of the GH in the circulation is bound to growth hormone binding protein.

Regulation of GH release—The 2 principal hypothalamic regulators of GH release from the anterior pituitary are growth hormone-releasing hormone (GHRH) and somatostatin, which exert stimulatory and inhibitory influences, respectively, on the somatotrophs (Figure 3–6). GH release is also inhibited by insulin-like growth factor 1 (**IGF-1**), the hormone produced in peripheral tissues in response to GH stimulation. IGF-1 derived from hepatic synthesis is part of a classic negative feedback mechanism of GH release. Ghrelin a peptide released predominantly from stomach, but also expressed in the pancreas, kidney, liver, and in the arcuate nucleus of the hypothalamus (see Chapter 10) has been identified as an additional GH secretagogue. The overall contribution of ghrelin to regulation of GH release in humans is still not fully elucidated.

Growth hormone-releasing hormone—GHRH stimulates GH secretion from somatotrophs through increases in GH gene transcription and biosynthesis and somatotroph proliferation. GHRH binds to G_s protein–coupled receptors on anterior pituitary somatotrophs, activating the catalytic subunit of adenylate cyclase. The stimulation of adenylate cyclase by G_s protein leads to intracellular cAMP accumulation and activation of the catalytic subunit of protein kinase A (see Figure 3–4). Protein kinase A phosphorylates cyclic 3′,5′-adenosine monophosphate response element binding protein (CREB), leading to CREB activation and enhanced transcription of the gene encoding pituitary-specific transcription factor (Pit-1). Pit-1 activates transcription of the GH gene, leading to increased GH mRNA and protein and replenishing cellular stores of GH. Pit-1 also stimulates transcription of GHRH receptor gene, resulting in increased numbers of GHRH receptors on the responding somatotroph cell.

Somatostatin—The stimulated release of GH is inhibited by somatostatin, a peptide synthesized in most brain regions, predominantly in the periventricular nucleus, arcuate nucleus, and ventromedial nucleus of the hypothalamus. Somatostatin is also produced in peripheral organs, including the endocrine pancreas, where it also plays a role in the inhibition of hormone release. Axons from somatostatin neurons run caudally through the hypothalamus to form a discrete pathway toward the midline that enters the median eminence. Somatostatin produces its physiologic effects through binding to the G_i protein–coupled somatostatin receptors, resulting in decreased activity of adenylate cyclase, intracellular cAMP, and Ca^{2+} concentrations and stimulation of protein tyrosine phosphatase. In addition, somatostatin binding to receptors coupled to K^+ channels causes hyperpolarization of the membrane, leading to cessation of spontaneous action potential activity and a secondary reduction in intracellular Ca^{2+} concentrations. The expression of somatostatin receptors is modulated by hormones and by the nutritional state of the individual.

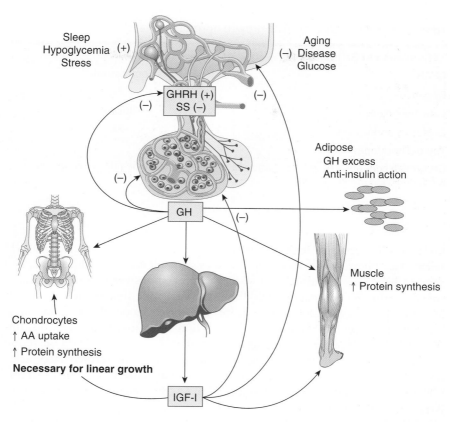

Figure 3–6. Growth hormone (GH) release and effects. GH release from the anterior pituitary is modulated by several factors. The primary controllers of GH release are growth hormone-releasing hormone (GHRH), which stimulates both the synthesis and secretion of GH, and somatostatin (SS), which inhibits GH release in response to GHRH and to other stimulatory factors such as low blood glucose concentration. GH secretion is also part of a negative feedback loop involving insulin-like growth factor 1 (IGF-1). IGF-1 suppresses secretion of GH not only by directly suppressing the somatotroph, but by stimulating release of SS from the hypothalamus. GH also feeds back to inhibit GHRH secretion and probably has a direct (autocrine) inhibitory effect on secretion from the somatotroph. Integration of all the factors that affect GH synthesis and secretion lead to a pulsatile pattern of release. GH effects in peripheral tissues are mediated directly by GH binding to its receptor and through the synthesis of IGF-1 by the liver and at the tissue level. The overall effects of GH and IGF-1 are anabolic. AA, amino acid; FFA, free fatty acid.

Other regulators—In addition to regulation by GHRH and somatostatin, GH is regulated by other hypothalamic peptides and neurotransmitters, which act by regulation of GHRH and somatostatin release, as summarized in Table 3–3. Catecholamines, dopamine, and excitatory amino acids increase

Table 3–3. Factors that regulate growth hormone release

Stimulation of GH release	Inhibition of GH release
GHRH	Somatostatin
Dopamine	IGF-1
Catecholamines	Glucose
Excitatory amino acids	FFA
Thyroid hormone	

GH, growth hormone; FFA, free fatty acids; GHRH, growth hormone-releasing hormone; IGF-1, insulinlike growth factor 1.

GHRH and decrease somatostatin release, resulting in an increase in GH release (see Figure 3–6). Hormones such as cortisol, estrogen, androgens, and thyroid hormone can also affect somatotroph responsiveness to GHRH and somatostatin and consequently GH release. Metabolic signals such as glucose and amino acids can affect GH release. Decreased blood glucose concentrations (hypoglycemia) stimulate GH secretion in humans. In fact, insulin-induced hypoglycemia is used as a clinical test to provoke GH secretion in GH-deficient children and adults. Glucose and nonesterified fatty acids decrease GH release. In contrast, amino acids, particularly arginine, increase GH release by decreasing somatostatin release. Consequently, arginine administration is also an effective challenge to elicit an increase in GH release in the clinical setting.

GH is released from the anterior pituitary into the systemic circulation. Circulating GH levels are less than 3 ng/mL, and the majority (60%) is bound to GH-binding protein. This protein is derived from proteolytic cleavage of the GH membrane receptor by metalloproteases and serves as a reservoir for GH, prolonging its half-life by decreasing its rate of degradation. The half-life of the hormone averages 6–20 minutes. GH is degraded in the lysosomes following binding to its receptor and internalization of the hormone-receptor complex.

Physiologic effects of GH—GH can have direct effects on cellular responses, by binding to the GH receptor at target tissues and indirectly, by stimulating the production and release of IGF-1, a mediator of several of growth hormone's effects at target tissues. IGF-1 is a small peptide (about 7.5 kDa) structurally related to proinsulin that mediates several of the anabolic and mitogenic effects of GH in peripheral tissues (see Figure 3–6). The most important physiologic effect of GH is stimulation of postnatal longitudinal growth. GH also plays a role in regulation of substrate metabolism, adipocyte differentiation; maintenance and development of the immune system; and regulation of brain and cardiac function.

GH receptor—In the peripheral tissues, GH binds to specific cell surface receptors belonging to the class 1 cytokine receptor superfamily (see Figures 1–6 and 3–4). This family of receptors includes those for prolactin, erythropoietin, leptin, interferons, granulocyte colony-stimulating factor, and interleukins. GH receptors are present in many biologic tissues and cell types, including liver, bone, kidney, adipose tissue, muscle, eye, brain, heart, and cells of the immune system. The GH molecule exhibits 2 binding sites for the GH receptor, resulting in dimerization of the receptor, a step that is required for biologic activity of the hormone. Receptor dimerization is followed by activation of a receptor-associated kinase, Janus-kinase 2. This kinase acts via special signal transducers and activators of transcription proteins (STATs), which dimerize and translocate to the nucleus, transmitting signals to specific regulatory DNA response elements.

GH Effects at Target Organs

Bone—GH stimulates longitudinal growth by increasing the formation of new bone and cartilage. The growth effects of GH are not critical during the gestational period, but begin gradually during the first and second years of life and peak at the time of puberty. Before the epiphyses in long bones have fused, GH stimulates chondrogenesis and widening of the cartilaginous epiphysial plates, followed by bone matrix deposition. In addition to its effects on linear growth stimulation, GH plays a role in regulating the normal physiology of bone formation in the adult by increasing bone turnover, with increases in bone formation and, to a lesser extent, bone resorption. The effects of GH at the epiphysial growth plate are thought to be mediated directly through stimulation of chondrocyte precursor differentiation and indirectly through enhancement of the local production of and responsiveness to IGF-1, which, in turn, acting in an autocrine or paracrine fashion, stimulates clonal expansion of differentiating chondrocytes (see Figure 3–6).

Adipose tissue—GH stimulates release and oxidation of free fatty acids, particularly during fasting. These effects are mediated by a reduction in the activity of lipoprotein lipase, the enzyme involved in clearing triglyceride-rich chylomicrons and very low-density lipoprotein particles from the bloodstream. Thus, GH favors the availability of free fatty acids for adipose tissue storage and skeletal muscle oxidation.

Skeletal muscle—GH has anabolic actions on skeletal muscle tissue. GH stimulates amino acid uptake and incorporation into protein, cell proliferation, and suppression of protein degradation.

Liver—GH stimulates hepatic IGF-1 production and release. GH stimulates hepatic glucose production.

Immune system—GH affects multiple aspects of the immune response, including B-cell responses and antibody production, natural killer cell activity, macrophage activity, and T-lymphocyte function.

GH also has central nervous system effects by modulating mood and behavior. Overall, GH counteracts the action of insulin on lipid and glucose metabolism, by decreasing skeletal muscle glucose utilization, increasing lipolysis, and stimulating hepatic glucose production.

Key aspects of GH physiology can be summarized as follows:

- GH is produced and stored in somatotrophs in the anterior pituitary.
- The production of GH is pulsatile, mainly nocturnal, and is controlled mainly by GHRH and somatostatin.
- Circulating levels of GH increase during childhood, peak during puberty, and fall with aging.
- GH stimulates lipolysis, amino acid transport into cells, and protein synthesis.
- GH stimulates the production of IGF-1, which is responsible for many of the activities attributed to GH.

INSULIN-LIKE GROWTH FACTORS

Many of the growth and metabolic effects of GH are mediated by the insulin-like growth factors (IGFs), or somatomedins. These small peptide hormones are members of a family of insulin-related peptides including relaxin, insulin, IGF-1, and IGF-2.

Regulation of IGF-1 production—IGF-1 is produced primarily in the liver in response to GH stimulation. IGF-1 is transported to other tissues, acting as an endocrine hormone. IGF-1 secreted by extrahepatic tissues, including cartilaginous cells, acts locally as a paracrine hormone. GH, parathyroid hormone, and sex steroids regulate the production of IGF-1 in bone, whereas sex steroids are the main regulators of local production of IGF-1 in the reproductive system. The binding proteins regulate the biologic actions of the IGFs.

Unlike insulin, IGF-1 retains the C peptide and circulates at higher concentrations than insulin either free (half-life is approximately 15–20 minutes) or bound to one of several specific binding proteins that prolong the half-life of the peptide. These binding proteins, like the IGFs, are synthesized primarily in the liver and are produced locally by several tissues, where they act in an autocrine or paracrine manner.

Insulin-like growth factor-binding proteins (IGFBPs)—Six IGFBPs have been identified and constitute an elaborate system for regulating IGF-1 activity. IGFBPs regulate the availability of IGF-1 to its receptor in target tissues. IGFBPs generally inhibit IGF-1 action by binding competitively to it and thereby reducing its bioavailability; however, in some cases, they appear to enhance IGF-1 activity or to act independently of IGF-1. In humans, almost 80% of circulating IGF-1 is carried by IGFBP-3, a ternary complex consisting of 1 molecule of IGF-1, 1 molecule of IGFBP-3, and 1 molecule of a protein named *acid-labile subunit* (ALS). In this form, IGFBP-3 sequesters IGF-1 in the vascular system, increasing its half-life and providing an IGF-1 reservoir at the same time that it prevents excess IGF-1 binding to the insulin receptor. Other IGFBPs form binary complexes with IGF-1 that may cross the capillary boundary, allowing selective transport of IGF-1 to various tissues. The interaction between IGFBPs and IGFs is controlled by 2 different mechanisms: (1) proteolytic cleavage by a family of specific serine proteases, which decreases IGF binding affinity; and (2) binding to the extracellular matrix, which potentiates IGF actions. Cleavage of IGFBPs by their specific proteases also influences IGF-1 bioavailability by reducing the amount of bioavailable IGFBPs. Overall IGF-1 bioactivity in vivo, therefore, represents the combined effect of interactions involving endocrine, autocrine, and paracrine sources of IGF-1, IGFBPs, and IGFBP proteases.

The IGFBPs are produced by a variety of different tissues. Hepatic IGFBP-3 and production of its acid-labile subunit are under stimulation by GH. Insulin is the primary regulator of hepatic IGFBP-1 production. Relatively little is known about the principal regulatory mechanisms that control the expression of IGFBP-2, IGFBP-4, IGFBP-5, and IGFBP-6.

Physiologic effects of IGF-1—IGF-1 exerts its physiologic effects by binding to specific cell surface receptors. Although IGF-1 binds primarily to the IGF-1 receptor, some effects may be mediated through the IGF-2 and insulin receptors. The similarity in structure to insulin explains the ability of IGF-1 to bind (with low affinity) to the insulin receptor. The main effects of IGF-1 are regulation of somatic growth, cell proliferation, transformation, and apoptosis.

IGF-1 mediates the anabolic and linear growth-promoting effects of pituitary GH. IGF-1 stimulates bone formation, protein synthesis, glucose uptake in muscle, neuronal survival, and myelin synthesis. In cartilage cells, IGF-1 has synergistic effects with GH. IGF-1 increases replication of cells of the osteoblastic lineage, enhances osteoblastic collagen synthesis and matrix apposition rates, and decreases collagen degradation in calvariae. IGF-1 is also thought to stimulate bone resorption by enhanced osteoclastic recruitment, thus acting on both bone formation and resorption, possibly coupling the 2 processes. IGF-1 also reverses negative nitrogen balance during food deprivation and inhibits protein degradation in muscle. The importance of this hormone in linear growth is clearly demonstrated by the severe growth failure in children with congenital IGF-1 deficiency.

IGFs act as mitogens, stimulating DNA, RNA, and protein synthesis. Both of the IGFs are essential to embryonic development, and nanomolar concentrations of both persist in the circulation into adult life. After birth, however, IGF-1 appears to have the predominant role in regulating growth, whereas the physiologic postnatal role of IGF-2 is unknown. IGF-1 concentrations are low at birth, increase substantially during childhood and puberty, and begin to decline in the third decade, paralleling the secretion of GH. In adults, IGF-2 occurs in quantities 3-fold higher than those of IGF-1, is minimally GH dependent, and decreases modestly with age.

IGF receptor—The IGF receptors are heterotetramers that belong to the same family of receptors as insulin. IGF-1 and IGF-2 bind specifically to 2 high-affinity membrane-associated receptors that are ligand-activated receptor kinases that become autophosphorylated on hormone binding. The receptor for IGF is composed of 2 extracellular spanning α-subunits and transmembrane β-subunits. The α-subunits have binding sites for IGF-1 and are linked by disulfide bonds. The β-subunit has a short extracellular domain, a transmembrane domain, and an intracellular domain. The intracellular part contains a tyrosine kinase domain, which constitutes the signal transduction mechanism. Ligand binding results in autophosphorylation of the receptor, increasing the kinase activity and allowing it to phosphorylate multiple substrate proteins, such as insulin receptor substrate 1 (IRS1). This produces a continued cascade of enzyme activation via phosphatidylinositol-3 kinase, Grb2 (growth factor receptor-bound protein 2), Syp (a phosphotyrosine phosphatase), Nck (an oncogenic protein), and Shc (src homology domain protein), in association with Grb2. This signaling cascade leads to activation of protein kinases including Raf, mitogen-activated protein kinase, 5 G kinase, and others involved in mediating growth and metabolic responses. A third receptor, the IGF-2 mannose-6-phosphate receptor, binds IGF-2 but has no known intracellular signaling actions.

The insulin and IGF-1 receptors, although similar in structure and function, play different physiologic roles in vivo. In healthy individuals, the insulin receptor is primarily involved in metabolic functions, whereas the IGF-1 receptor mediates growth and differentiation. The separation of these functions is controlled by several factors, including the tissue distribution of the respective receptors, the binding with high affinity of each ligand to its respective receptor, and the binding of IGF to IGFBPs.

PROLACTIN

Prolactin is a polypeptide hormone synthesized and secreted by lactotrophs in the anterior pituitary gland. The lactotrophs account for approximately 15%–20% of the cell population of the anterior pituitary gland. However, this percentage increases dramatically in response to elevated estrogen levels, particularly during pregnancy. Prolactin levels are higher in females than in males, and the role of prolactin in male physiology is not completely understood. Plasma concentrations of prolactin are highest during sleep and lowest during the waking hours in humans.

Regulation of prolactin release—Prolactin release is predominantly under tonic inhibition by dopamine derived from hypothalamic dopaminergic neurons. In addition, prolactin release is also under inhibitory control by somatostatin (SST), and γ-aminobutyric acid (GABA). However, the overall regulation of prolactin release is complex and involves not only inhibition by dopamine, but also stimulation by serotoninergic and opioidergic pathways, GnRH, and possibly galanin.

Dopaminergic inhibition of lactotroph release of prolactin is mediated by dopaminergic (D_2) G_i protein–coupled receptors, resulting in inhibition of adenylate cyclase and inositol phosphate metabolism (see Figure 3–4). In addition, activation of the D_2 receptor modifies at least 5 different ion channels. In particular, dopamine activates potassium current that induces plasma membrane hyperpolarization while decreasing voltage-activated calcium currents. Therefore, dopamine-induced inhibition of prolactin secretion is a function of the inhibition of adenylate cyclase activity, activation of voltage-sensitive potassium channels, and inhibition of voltage- sensitive calcium channels.

Prolactin release is affected by a large variety of stimuli provided by the environment and the internal milieu, the most important being sucking, and increased levels of ovarian steroid hormones, primarily estrogen (Figure 3–7). The release of

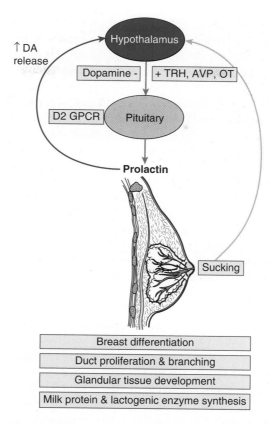

Figure 3–7. Physiologic effects of prolactin. Prolactin plays an important role in the normal development of mammary tissue and in milk production. Prolactin release is predominantly under negative control by hypothalamic dopamine. Sucking stimulates the release of prolactin. Prolactin inhibits its own release by stimulating dopamine release from the hypothalamus. AVP, arginine vasopressin; DA, dopamine; GPCR, G protein–coupled receptor; OT, oxytocin; TRH, thyrotropin-releasing hormone.

prolactin in response to sucking is a classical neuroendocrine reflex also referred to as a stimulus-secretion reflex. This surge in prolactin release in response to a sucking stimulus is mediated by a decrease in the amount of dopamine released at the median eminence, relieving the lactotroph from tonic inhibition. The growth of lactotrophs and the expression of prolactin gene are increased by high estrogen concentrations, such as those that occur during pregnancy.

Several neuropeptides have been identified as prolactin releasing factors. These include TRH, oxytocin, vasoactive intestinal peptide, and neurotensin. These releasing factors fall into two categories of peptides: those which are active in the presence of the physiologic inhibitory tone of dopamine and those that have an effect only when dopamine inhibitory tone has been removed. TRH belongs to the first category and is a potent stimulus for the release of prolactin through stimulation of TRH receptors on the lactotroph cell membrane. However, the physiologic role of TRH-induced prolactin release is unclear. Although exogenous administration of TRH can elevate levels of prolactin; it is important to note that release of TSH and prolactin do not always occur hand in hand under physiologic conditions.

Prolactin regulates its own secretion through a short-loop feedback mechanism by binding to prolactin receptors located in neuroendocrine dopaminergic neurons; resulting in increased hypothalamic dopamine synthesis (see Figure 3–7). When the concentration of dopamine in the hypothalamo-hypophysial portal blood rises, the release of prolactin from the lactotrophs is suppressed.

Physiologic effects of prolactin—The physiologic effects of prolactin are mediated by the prolactin receptor; a single membrane-bound protein that belongs to class 1 of the cytokine receptor superfamily (see Figure 3–4). Prolactin receptors are found in the mammary gland and the ovary, 2 of the best-characterized sites of prolactin actions in mammals, as well as in various regions of the brain. Activation of the prolactin receptor involves ligand-induced sequential receptor dimerization. Prolactin-mediated activation of prolactin receptor results in tyrosine phosphorylation of numerous cellular proteins, including the receptor itself.

The main physiologic effects of prolactin are stimulation of growth and development of the mammary gland, synthesis of milk, and maintenance of milk secretion (see Figure 3–7 and Chapter 9). Prolactin stimulates glucose and amino acid uptake and synthesis of the milk proteins β-casein and α-lactalbumin, the milk sugar lactose, and milk fats by the mammary epithelial cells. During pregnancy, prolactin prepares the breast for lactation. The production and secretion of milk is prevented during pregnancy by the high progesterone levels. Additional effects of prolactin include inhibition of GnRH release, progesterone biosynthesis, and luteal cell hypertrophy during pregnancy. Prolactin also modulates reproductive and parental behavior.

DISEASES OF THE ANTERIOR PITUITARY

As with most endocrine organs, alterations in function of the anterior pituitary can be caused by excess or deficient production of pituitary hormones or to altered responsiveness to hormone effects at the target organ.

Hormone-Producing Pituitary Adenomas

The most common cause of excess production of pituitary hormones is a hormone-producing pituitary adenoma. Prolactinomas are the most common (40%–45%) pituitary tumors, followed by somatotroph (20%), corticotroph (10%–12%), gonadotroph (15%), and rarely thyrotroph (1%–2%) adenomas. Small pituitary adenomas can cause manifestations of excess tropic hormone production, whereas larger tumors can produce neurologic symptoms by mass effect in the sellar area. Patients with a prolactinoma present with elevated levels of prolactin (hyperprolactinemia), milk secretion (galactorrhea), and reproductive dysfunction (infertility). In most cases, dopamine agonists are extremely effective in lowering serum prolactin levels, restoring gonadal function, decreasing tumor size, and improving visual fields. Hyperprolactinemia can also be caused by drug-induced inhibition of dopamine release. GH-secreting adenomas can be associated with acromegaly or bone and soft-tissue overgrowth in adults, and with gigantism in children. Corticotropin-releasing adenomas are associated with excess cortisol production or Cushing syndrome; patients present with central obesity, proximal myopathy, hypertension, mood changes, dorsocervical fat pads, and hyperglycemia, among other clinical signs and symptoms. Gonadotroph pituitary adenomas are frequently inefficient in hormone production. Thyrotropin-secreting tumors are rare and are frequently large when diagnosed.

Hypopituitarism

Hypopituitarism, or deficiency of anterior pituitary hormones, can be congenital or acquired. Isolated GH and gonadotropin deficiencies are the most common. The most frequent cause of pituitary insufficiency is traumatic injury, such as that associated with surgery, penetrating injury, or automobile accidents. Severe blood loss and hypoperfusion of the pituitary can also lead to pituitary insufficiency. Ischemic damage to the pituitary gland or hypothalamic-pituitary stalk during the peripartum period (due to excessive blood loss) leads to Sheehan syndrome, manifested as hypothyroidism, adrenal insufficiency, hypogonadism, GH deficiency, and hypoprolactinemia.

GH deficiency and retarded growth may result from impaired release of GH from the pituitary gland because of diseases of the hypothalamus or pituitary gland or genetic predisposition. Alternatively, mutations in the gene for the GH receptor can cause insensitivity to GH and growth retardation with low serum IGF-1 concentrations.

Growth Hormone Insensitivity

Growth failure can be the result of decreased GH release, decreased GH action, or GH insensitivity syndrome, also known as *Laron syndrome*. The syndrome is characterized by deletions or mutations in the GH receptor gene, resulting in failure to generate IGF-1 and IGFBP-3. The typical manifestation is short stature or dwarfism, which can be prevented by IGF-1 treatment. The study of these patients has provided much of our understanding of the differential effects of GH and IGF-1.

Evaluation of Anterior Pituitary Function

Measurements of anterior pituitary hormone concentrations and of the respective target gland hormone levels are used to assess the functional status of the system (Table 3–4). For example, paired measures of TSH and thyroid hormone, FSH and estradiol, and ACTH and cortisol are used to evaluate the integrity of the respective systems. In addition, stimulation and inhibition tests can be used to assess the functional status of the pituitary gland. These tests are based on the normal physiologic feedback mechanisms that control tropic hormone release as discussed in Chapter 1.

Table 3–4. Pituitary tropic hormone and target organ hormone pairs

Pituitary tropic hormone	Target organ hormone
ACTH (8:00 AM)	Cortisol (8:00 AM)
<80 pg/mL (<80 pmol/L)	140–690 nmol/L (5–25 µg/dL)
GH	IGF-1
2–6 ng/mL (<5 µg/L)	140–400 ng/mL
LH (adult, premenopausal)	Estradiol
Female: 5–25 IU/L (3–35 mIU/mL)	Female: 70–220 pmol/L (20–60 pg/mL)
Male: 5–20 IU/L (5–20 mIU/mL)	Male: <180 pmol/L (50 pg/mL)
FSH	Progesterone
Female: 5–20 IU/L (20–50 mIU/mL)	Female: luteal peak >16 nmol/L (75 ng/mL)
Male: 5–20 IU/L (20–50 mIU/mL)	Male: <6 nmol/L (<2 ng/mL) Testosterone female: <3.5 nmol/L (<1 ng/mL) Male: 10–35 nmol/L (3–10 ng/mL)
TSH	Thyroxine
0.4–5 mU/L (0.4–5 µU/mL)	64–154 nmol/L (5–12 µg/dL) Triiodothyronine 1.1–2.9 nmol/L (70–190 ng/dL)

ACTH, adrenocorticotropic hormone; FSH, follicle-stimulating hormone; GH, growth hormone; IGF-1, insulinlike growth factor 1; LH, luteinizing hormone; TSH, thyroid-stimulating hormone.

KEY CONCEPTS

Anterior pituitary function is regulated by the hypothalamus.

Anterior pituitary hormone release is under feedback regulation by peripheral hormone levels.

Pulsatile release of hypothalamic, pituitary, and target organ hormones plays an important role in endocrine function.

Growth hormone exerts direct and indirect (IGF-1) effects on linear growth and metabolism.

With the exception of prolactin, adenohypophysial hormones are under stimulatory hypothalamic control.

3–1. A 40-year-old truck driver has had difficulty using his side mirrors to see traffic behind him. He has never had any major medical problems in the past. He visits an optometrist, who determines that he has bilateral lateral visual field deficits, but his vision is 20/20. A head computed tomography scan reveals slight enlargement of the sella turcica. He complains of decreased libido for the past 6–9 months. Which of the following hormones is most likely being secreted in excessive amounts in this man?

   a. Antidiuretic hormone

   b. Prolactin

   c. ACTH

   d. Growth hormone

   e. Luteinizing hormone

3–2. A 30-year-old woman, who has 2 healthy children ages 3 and 4, notes that she has had no menstrual periods for the past 6 months. A pregnancy test is negative, and she is not taking any medications. She also complains of headaches for the past 3 months and has had problems with her lateral vision. On physical examination, she is afebrile and normotensive. Laboratory values are within normal ranges for glucose, Na, K. A magnetic resonance imaging study reveals a pituitary mass. Which of the following is most likely to be present in this woman?

   a. Increased serum cortisol

   b. Increased serum alkaline phosphatase

   c. Hyperprolactinemia

   d. Abnormal glucose tolerance test

   e. Decreased serum AVP

3–3. Laceration of the median eminence during traumatic injury sustained while kickboxing, resulting in the disruption of the hypothalamo-hypophysial portal circulation would result in which of the following alterations (↑ increase, ↓ decrease, or ↔ no change)in circulating levels of hormones?

	Insulinlike growth factor I	Prolactin	PTH	Growth hormone releasing hormone
A	↔	↑	↓	↔
B	↓	↑	↔	↑
C	↑	↓	↓	↑
D	↑	↔	↔	↓
E	↔	↓	↑	↓

3–4. Which of the following abnormalities would be most likely to occur as a result of impaired growth hormone action?

   a. Low birth weight and failure to thrive

   b. Failure to double birth weight at 6 months

   c. Short stature in a 12-year-old boy

   d. Fasting hyperglycemia and impaired glucose tolerance

   e. Deepening of the voice and increased facial hair

3.5.   A hybrid glycoprotein consisting of the α-subunit of follicle-stimulating hormone (FSH) and the β-subunit of thyrotropin (TSH) is injected into a 35-year-old patient at the National Institutes for Health Clinical Research Unit to investigate her endocrine responsiveness. Which of the following responses is expected following this injection?

	Na^+/I^- symporter activity	Luteolysis	Thyroglobulin synthesis	Ovulation	T_4 release
A	↔	↓	↔	↓	↓
B	↑	↓	↑	↓	↑
C	↑	↔	↓	↔	↔
D	↓	↓	↑	↑	↓
E	↑	↔	↑	↔	↑

SUGGESTED READINGS

Freeman ME, Kanyicska B, Lerant A, Nagy G. Prolactin: structure, function, and regulation of secretion. *Physiol Rev.* 2000;80:1523.

Goldenberg N, Barkan A. Factors regulating GH secretion in humans. *Endocrinol Metab Clin North Am.* 2007; 36:37–55.

Laron Z. Insulin-like growth factor 1 (IGF-1): a growth hormone. *Mol Pathol.* 2001;54:311.

LeRoith D. Seminars in medicine of the Beth Israel Deaconess Medical Center: insulin-like growth factors. *N Engl J Med.* 1997;336:633.

LeRoith D, McGuinness M, Shemer J, et al. Insulin-like growth factors. *Biol Signals.* 1992;1:173.

Müller EE, Locatelli V, Cocchi D. Neuroendocrine control of growth hormone secretion. *Physiol Rev.* 1999;79:511.

Ohlsson C, Bengtsson B, Isaksson OGP, Andreassen TT, Slootweg MC. Growth hormone and bone. *Endocr Rev.* 1998;19:55–79.

Pritchard LE, Turnbull AV, White A. Pro-opiomelanocortin (POMC) processing in the hypothalamus: impact on melanocortin signalling and obesity. *J Endocrinol.* 2002;172:411.

Samson WK, Taylor MM, Baker JR. Prolactin-releasing peptides. *Regul Pept.* 2003;114:1.

Tsatmali M, Ancans J, Thody AJ. Melanocyte function and its control by melanocortin peptides. *J Histochem Cytochem.* 2002;50:125.

Woodhouse LJ, Mukherjee A, Shalet SM, Ezzat S. The influence of growth hormone status on physical impairments functional limitations and health-related quality of life in adults. *Endocr Rev.* 2006; 27(3):287–317.

Thyroid Gland

OBJECTIVES

▶ Identify the steps and control factors of thyroid hormone biosynthesis, storage, and release.

▶ Describe the distribution of iodine and the metabolic pathway involved in thyroid hormone synthesis.

▶ Explain the importance of thyroid hormone binding in blood for free and total thyroid hormone levels.

▶ Understand the significance of the conversion of tetraiodothyronine (T_4) to triiodothyronine (T_3) and reverse T_3 (rT_3) in extrathyroidal tissues.

▶ Understand how thyroid hormones produce their cellular effects.

▶ Describe their effects on development and metabolism.

▶ Understand the causes and consequences of excess and deficiency of thyroid hormones.

Thyroid hormones play important roles in maintaining energy homeostasis and regulating energy expenditure. Their physiologic effects, mediated at multiple target organs, are primarily to stimulate cell metabolism and activity. The vital roles of these hormones, particularly in development, differentiation, and maturation, are underscored by the severe mental retardation observed in infants with deficient thyroid hormone function during gestation. Thyroid hormones are derived from the amino acid tyrosine and are produced by the thyroid gland in response to stimulation by thyroid-stimulating hormone (TSH) produced by the anterior pituitary. TSH, in turn, is regulated by the hypophysiotropic peptide thyrotropin-releasing hormone (TRH) (Figure 4–1). Thyroid hormone production is also under regulation by dietary iodine.

FUNCTIONAL ANATOMY

The thyroid gland is a highly vascular, ductless alveolar (acinar) gland located in the anterior neck in front of the trachea. The gland weighs 10–25 g and consists of a right and left lobe connected by the isthmus. The cellular composition of the thyroid gland is diverse, including the following:

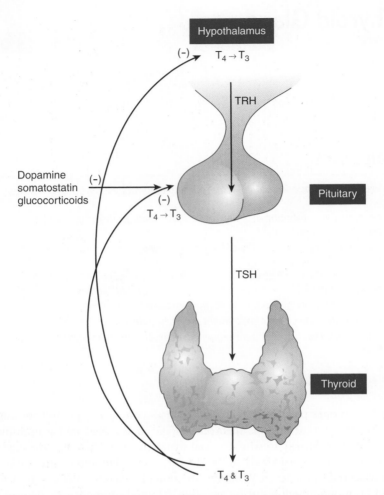

Figure 4–1. The hypothalamic-pituitary-thyroid axis. Thyrotropin-releasing hormone (TRH) is synthesized in parvicellular neurons of the paraventricular nucleus of the hypothalamus and released from nerve terminals in the median eminence, from where it is transported via the portal capillary plexus to the anterior pituitary. TRH binds to a G protein–coupled receptor in the anterior pituitary, leading to an increase in intracellular Ca^{2+} concentration, which in turn results in stimulation of exocytosis and release of thyroid-stimulating hormone (TSH) into the systemic circulation. TSH stimulates the thyroid gland to increase the synthesis and secretion of tetraiodothyronine (T_4) and triiodothyronine (T_3) into the circulation. T_4 and T_3 inhibit the secretion of thyrotropin both directly and indirectly by inhibiting the secretion of TRH. Additional factors that inhibit TSH release are glucocorticoids, somatostatin, and dopamine.

- Follicular (epithelial) cells, involved in thyroid hormone synthesis
- Endothelial cells lining the capillaries that provide the blood supply to the follicles
- Parafollicular or C cells, involved in the production of calcitonin, a hormone involved in calcium metabolism
- Fibroblasts, lymphocytes, and adipocytes

Thyroid Follicle

The main function of the thyroid gland is the synthesis and storage of thyroid hormone. The secretory or functional unit of the thyroid gland is the thyroid follicle, consisting of a layer of thyroid epithelial cells arranged around a large central cavity filled with colloid. Colloid makes up approximately 30% of the thyroid gland mass and contains a protein called **thyroglobulin (Tg)**. Tg plays a central role in the synthesis and storage of thyroid hormone, as discussed later. The thyroid epithelial cells are morphologically and functionally polarized. That is, each side or compartment of the cell has specific functions pertaining to the synthesis of thyroid hormones and their release. The apical surface of the follicular cell faces the follicular lumen, where colloid is stored. The basolateral surface faces the interstitium and is therefore exposed to the bloodstream.

The polarity of the thyroid follicular cells is important in the overall function of the cell. Thyroid hormone synthesis requires the iodination of tyrosine residues on the protein Tg, which is stored in the colloid. This process occurs in the colloid at the apical plasma membrane, yet iodine is obtained from the circulation. Whereas thyroid hormone synthesis occurs on the apical side of the thyroid epithelial cell, hormone release occurs at the basolateral side of the cell. Thus, the polarity of the thyroid epithelial cells is critical for maintaining basolaterally located iodide uptake and T_4 (tetraiodothyronine) deiodination, and apically located iodide efflux and iodination mechanisms.

The parafollicular cells surrounding the follicles synthesize and secrete the hormone **calcitonin**, and therefore they are frequently referred to as **C cells**. They are preferentially located in central regions of the thyroid gland lobes, where follicular cell activity is the greatest. Parafollicular cells secrete regulatory factors other than calcitonin that modulate follicular cell activity in a paracrine fashion.

Blood and Nerve Supply

The thyroid gland is highly vascularized with arterial blood derived from the superior and inferior thyroid arteries. The veins draining the thyroid gland form a plexus on the surface of the gland and on the front of the trachea and give rise to the superior, middle, and inferior thyroid veins, which drain into the internal jugular and innominate veins. The lymphatic vessels end in the thoracic and right lymphatic trunks. Innervation to the thyroid gland is provided through the middle and inferior cervical ganglia of the sympathetic nervous system.

REGULATION OF BIOSYNTHESIS, STORAGE, AND SECRETION OF THYROID HORMONES

Hypothalamic Regulation of Thyroid-Stimulating Hormone Release

Thyroid hormone synthesis and release are under negative feedback regulation by the **hypothalamic-pituitary-thyroid axis** (see Figure 4–1). TRH is a tripeptide synthesized in the hypothalamus and released from nerve terminals in the median eminence from where it is transported through the portal capillary plexus to the anterior pituitary. TRH binds to cell membrane $G_{q/11}$ receptors on thyrotrophs of the anterior pituitary gland, where it activates phospholipase C, resulting in the hydrolysis of phosphatidylinositol bisphosphate and the generation of inositol triphosphate and diacylglycerol. This process leads to an increase in the intracellular Ca^{2+} concentration, resulting in stimulation of exocytosis and release of TSH into the systemic circulation.

TSH is transported in the bloodstream to the thyroid gland, where it binds to the TSH receptor located on the basolateral membrane of thyroid follicular epithelial cells. The TSH receptor is a cell membrane G protein–coupled receptor. Adequate function of the TSH receptor is critical in the development, growth, and function of the thyroid gland. Binding of TSH to its receptor initiates signaling through cyclic 3′,5′-adenosine monophosphate (cAMP), phospholipase C, and the protein kinase A signal transduction systems. Activation of adenylate cyclase, formation of cAMP, and activation of protein kinase A regulate iodide uptake and transcription of Tg, thyroid peroxidase (TPO), and the activity of the sodium-iodide (Na^+/I^-) symporter. Signaling through phospholipase C and intracellular Ca^{2+} regulate iodide efflux, H_2O_2 production, and Tg iodination. The TSH receptor is an important antigenic site involved in thyroid autoimmune disease. Autoantibodies to the receptor may act as agonists mimicking the actions of TSH in the case of Graves disease; or antagonists in the case of autoimmune hypothyroidism (Hashimoto thyroiditis).

TSH receptor activation results in stimulation of all of the steps involved in thyroid hormone synthesis, including iodine uptake and organification, production and release of iodothyronines from the gland, and promotion of thyroid growth. As part of this process, TSH regulates thyroidal uptake of nutrients as well as intracellular transport of specific proteins involved in thyroid hormone synthesis, storage, and release. These cellular events involve regulation of cellular metabolic processes, morphologic differentiation, cell proliferation, and protection from apoptosis. Specifically, the biologic effects of TSH include stimulation of gene transcription of the following:

- Na^+/I^- symporter, the protein involved in transporting and concentrating iodide in the thyroid epithelial cell

- Tg, the glycoprotein that serves as a scaffold for tyrosine iodination and thyroid hormone synthesis, as well as storage of thyroid hormone

- TPO, the enzyme involved in catalyzing the oxidation of iodide and its incorporation into tyrosine residues of Tg

- Thyroid hormones T_4 and T_3 (triiodothyronine)

As mentioned earlier, both growth and function of the thyroid are stimulated by the rise in cAMP produced by TSH stimulation. Therefore, continued stimulation of the cAMP pathway by binding to the TSH receptor causes hyperthyroidism and thyroid hyperplasia.

Thyroid Hormone Regulation of Thyroid-Stimulating Hormone Release

The production and release of thyroid hormones are under negative feedback regulation by the hypothalamic-pituitary-thyroid axis. The release of TSH is inhibited mainly by T_3, produced by conversion of T_4 to T_3 in the hypothalamus, and in the anterior pituitary by type II deiodinase. The contribution of this intracellularly derived T_3 in producing the negative feedback inhibition of TSH release is greater than that of T_3 derived from the circulation. Other neuroendocrine mediators that inhibit TSH release include dopamine, somatostatin, and glucocorticoids at high levels, which produce partial suppression of TSH release (see Chapter 10).

Thyroid Hormone Synthesis

Thyroglobulin, plays an important role in the synthesis and storage of thyroid hormone (Figure 4–2). Tg is a glycoprotein containing multiple tyrosine residues. It is synthesized in the thyroid follicular epithelial cells and secreted through the apical membrane into the follicular lumen, where it is stored in the colloid. A small amount of noniodinated Tg is also secreted through the basolateral membrane into the circulation. Although circulating levels of Tg can be detected under normal conditions, levels are elevated in diseases such as thyroiditis and Graves disease.

Tg can be considered a scaffold upon which thyroid hormone synthesis takes place. Once Tg is secreted into the follicular lumen, it undergoes major post-translational modification during the production of thyroid hormones. At the apical surface of the thyroid follicular epithelial cells, multiple tyrosine residues of Tg are iodinated, followed by coupling of some of the iodotyrosine residues to form T_3 and T_4.

The iodide required for thyroid hormone synthesis is readily absorbed from dietary sources, primarily from iodized salt, but also from seafood and plants grown in soil that is rich in iodine. Following its absorption, iodide is confined to the extracellular fluid, from which it is removed primarily by the thyroid (20%) and the kidneys (80%). The total excretion of iodide by the kidneys is approximately equal to daily intake. The balance between dietary intake and renal excretion preserves the total extracellular pool of iodide.

Regulation of Iodine Metabolism in the Thyroid Follicular Cell

Iodide is concentrated in thyroid epithelial cells by an active, saturable, energy-dependent process mediated by a Na^+/I^- symporter located in the basolateral plasma membrane of the follicular cell (Figure 4–3). Additional tissues that express the Na^+/I^- symporter include the salivary glands, the gastric

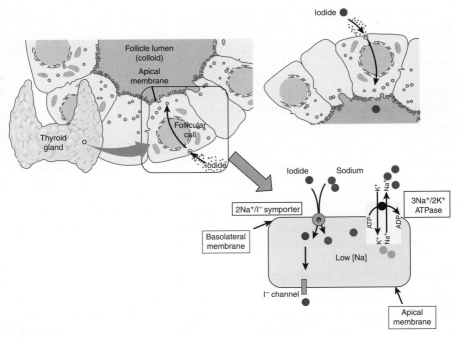

Figure 4–2. Mechanism of iodide concentration by the thyroid gland. Iodide is transported into the cytosol of the follicular cell by a sodium-iodide (Na$^+$/I$^-$) symporter. Two Na$^+$ ions are transported inside the thyroid follicular cell with each iodide molecule. Na$^+$ moves down its concentration gradient, which is maintained by a Na$^+$/K$^+$-ATPase that constantly pumps Na$^+$ out of the cytoplasm of the thyroid follicular epithelial cell maintaining the low intracytoplasmic Na$^+$ concentrations. Iodide must reach the colloid space, where it is used for organification of thyroglobulin. This process is achieved by efflux through the iodide channel. One of the early effects of thyroid-stimulating hormone (TSH) binding to its receptor is the opening of these channels facilitating the leak of iodide into the extracellular space. This transcellular transport of iodide relies on the functional and morphological polarization of the thyroid follicular epithelial cell.

mucosa, the placenta, and the mammary glands. However, transport of iodine in these tissues is not under TSH regulation.

The iodination of Tg residues is a process that occurs at the apical membrane. Thus, once inside the cell, iodide must leave the follicular cell through apical efflux by an iodide-permeating mechanism consisting of a chloride-iodide transporting protein (iodide channel) located in the apical membrane of the thyroid follicular cell. The uptake, concentration, and efflux of iodide through the iodide channel are all a function of TSH-stimulated transepithelial transport of iodide. As already mentioned, this transcellular transport of iodide is possible because of the morphologic and functional polarization of the thyroid epithelial cell.

Thyroid hormone synthesis

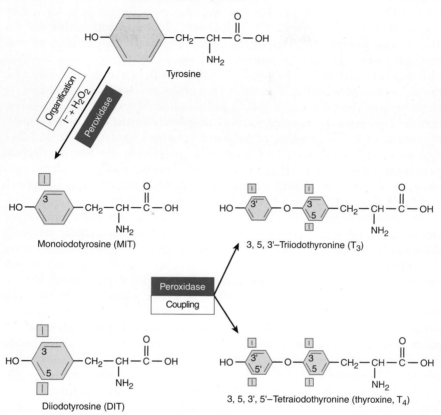

Figure 4–3. Biochemistry of thyroid hormone synthesis. In the follicular lumen, tyrosine residues within the thyroglobulin matrix are iodinated by iodine (I^+; formed by oxidation of I^- by thyroid peroxidase). Iodine bonds to carbon 3 or to carbon 5 of the tyrosine residues of thyroglobulin in a process referred to as the organification of iodine. This iodination of specific tyrosines located on thyroglobulin yields monoiodinated tyrosine (MIT) and diiodinated tyrosine (DIT) residues that are enzymatically coupled to form triiodothyronine (T_3) or tetraiodothyronine (T_4). The coupling of iodinated tyrosine residues, either of 2 diiodotyrosines or of 1 monoiodotyrosine and 1 diiodotyrosine residue, is catalyzed by the enzyme thyroid peroxidase.

The transport of iodine through the Na^+/I^- symporter can be substituted by other substances including perchlorate and pertechnetate. Radiolabeled pertechnetate ($^{99m}TcO_4$) can be used for imaging of the thyroid gland. Moreover, the ability of the thyroid gland to accumulate iodine allows therapeutic administration of radioactive iodine leading to ablation of thyroid tissue, which is important in the treatment of thyroid malignancies. In the follicular lumen, tyrosine residues of Tg are iodinated by iodine (I^+; formed by oxidation of I^- by TPO) (see Figure 4–2). This reaction requires hydrogen peroxide, which is generated by a flavoprotein Ca^{++}-dependent reduced nicotinamide adenine dinucleotide phosphate oxidase at the apical cell surface and serves as an electron acceptor in the reaction process. As shown in the figure, iodine bonds to carbon 3 or to carbon 5 of the tyrosine residues on Tg in a process referred to as the *organification of iodine*. This iodination of specific tyrosines located on Tg yields monoiodinated tyrosine (MIT) and diiodinated tyrosine (DIT) residues that are enzymatically coupled to form **triiodothyronine** (T_3) or **tetraiodothyronine** (T_4). The coupling of iodinated tyrosine residues, either of 2 DIT residues or of 1 MIT and 1 DIT residue, is catalyzed by the enzyme **thyroid peroxidase**. Because not all of the iodinated tyrosine residues undergo coupling, Tg stored in the follicular lumen contains MIT and DIT residues as well as formed T_3 and T_4 (Figure 4–4).

As mentioned previously, TSH controls the energy-dependent uptake and concentration of iodide by the thyroid gland and its transcellular transport through the follicular epithelial cell. However, iodine metabolism within the thyroid can also be regulated independently of TSH. This mechanism is important when plasma iodide levels are elevated (15–20-fold above normal) because this elevation inhibits the organic binding of iodine within the thyroid. This autoregulatory phenomenon consisting of inhibition of the organification of iodine by elevated circulating levels of iodide is known as the **Wolff-Chaikoff effect**. This effect lasts for a few days and is followed by the so-called escape phenomenon, at which point the organification of intra-thyroidal iodine resumes and the normal synthesis of T_4 and T_3 returns. The escape phenomenon results from a decrease in the inorganic iodine concentration inside the thyroid gland from downregulation of the Na^+/I^- symporter. This relative decrease in intra-thyroidal inorganic iodine allows the $TPO–H_2O_2$ system to resume normal activity. The mechanisms responsible for the acute Wolff-Chaikoff effect have not been elucidated but may be caused by the formation of organic iodocompounds within the thyroid.

Regulation of Thyroid Hormone Release

The preceding sections have described the steps involved in the synthesis of thyroid hormone, TSH regulation of the iodination of tyrosine residues on Tg, and coupling of the iodinated residues for the formation of thyroid hormones (see Figure 4–4). TSH also regulates the release of thyroid hormones from the thyroid gland. The synthesis of thyroid hormone takes place in the colloid space. As mentioned previously, the apical surface of the follicular epithelial cell faces the colloid and not the interstitial space, and thus has no access to the bloodstream. Therefore, thyroid hormone release involves endocytosis of vesicles containing Tg from the apical surface of the follicular cell. The vesicles fuse with follicular epithelial phagolysosomes, leading to proteolytic digestion and cleavage of Tg. In addition to the thyroid hormones T_4 and T_3, the products of this reaction include iodinated tyrosine residues (MIT and DIT). MIT and DIT are deiodinated intracellularly,

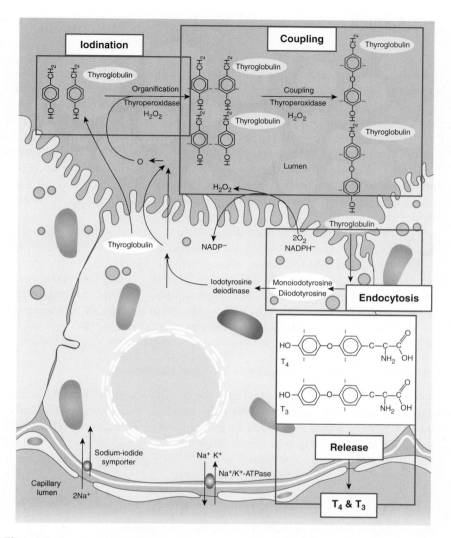

Figure 4–4. Overview of the process of thyroid hormone synthesis in the thyroid follicular epithelial cell. Thyroid hormone synthesis involves concentration of iodide by the Na$^+$/I$^-$ symporter and the transport of iodide through the epithelial cell and into the extracellular compartment within the follicular cells where it is oxidized to iodine by thyroid peroxidase and is then used in the iodination of thyroglobulin (Tg). Iodine organification is an extracellular process that takes place inside the thyroid follicles at the apical membrane surface facing the follicular lumen. Secretion of the hormone involves the endocytosis of colloid containing thyroglobulin followed by degradation of thyroglobulin and release of tetraiodothyronine (T$_4$) and triiodothyronine (T$_3$). Some of the T$_4$ produced is deiodinated in the thyroid follicle to T$_3$, which is then released into the bloodstream. In addition, intracellular deiodination provides a mechanism for recycling of iodide to participate in the synthesis of new TH at the apical cell surface. A small fraction of Tg is released from the follicular epithelial cell into the circulation. A fraction of T$_4$ produced is deiodinated to T$_3$ prior to release from the thyroid. TSHR, thyroid-stimulating hormone receptor. (Reproduced with permission from Kopp PA. Reduce, recycle, reuse-iodotyrosine deiodinase in thyroid iodide metabolism. *N Engl J Med.* 2008;358(17):1856–1859. Copyright © Massachusetts Medical Society. All rights reserved.)

and iodide is transported by apical efflux into the follicular colloid space, where it is reused in thyroid hormone synthesis. T_4 and T_3 are released from the basolateral membrane into the circulation. The thyroid gland releases greater amounts of T_4 than T_3, so plasma concentrations of T_4 are 40-fold higher than those of T_3 (90 vs 2 nM). Most of the circulating T_3 is formed peripherally by deiodination of T_4, a process that involves the removal of iodine from carbon 5 on the outer ring of T_4. Thus, T_4 acts as a prohormone for T_3. Although this deiodination occurs predominantly in the liver, some occurs in the thyroid follicular epithelial cell itself. This intrathyroidal deiodination of T_4 is the result of TSH stimulation of the type I deiodinase.

Two additional facts regarding thyroid hormone activity and storage should be noted. First, at physiologic levels, T_4 is relatively inactive because it possesses 100-fold lower affinity than T_3 for binding to the thyroid receptor and does not enter the cell nucleus at high enough concentrations to occupy the ligand-binding site of the thyroid hormone receptor. Second, in contrast to most endocrine glands, which do not have storage capacity for their product, the thyroid gland is able to store 2–3 months' supply of thyroid hormones in the Tg pool. Key features of thyroid regulation and function are listed in Table 4–1.

Transport and Tissue Delivery of Thyroid Hormones

Once thyroid hormones are released into the circulation, most of them circulate bound to protein. Approximately 70% of T_4 and T_3 is bound to thyroid-binding globulin. Other proteins involved in thyroid binding include transthyretin, which binds 10% of T_4, and albumin, which binds 15% of T_4 and 25% of T_3. A small fraction of each hormone (0.03% of T_4 and 0.3% of T_3) circulates in its free form.

Table 4–1. Key features of thyroid regulation and function

	Key features
TSH	Binds to G_s protein–coupled receptor on thyroid cells Main second-messenger system is cAMP Stimulates all steps involved in thyroid hormone synthesis: iodine uptake and organification, production and release of thyroid hormone, and promotion of thyroid growth
Thyroid gland	Can store 2- to 3-mo supply of thyroid hormones in the thyroglobulin pool (colloid) Produces more T_4 than T_3
Thyroid hormone	Synthesis and release are under negative feedback regulation by the hypothalamic-pituitary-thyroid axis T_4 is converted to T_3 in peripheral tissues Biologic activity of T_3 is greater than that of T_4 Binds to nuclear receptors and modulates gene transcription

cAMP, cyclic adenosine monophosphate; T_3, triiodothyronine; T_4, tetraiodothyronine; TSH, thyroid-stimulating hormone.

This fraction of the circulating hormone pool is bioavailable and can enter the cell to bind to the thyroid receptor. Of the 2 thyroid hormones, T_4 binds more tightly to binding proteins than T_3 and thus has a lower metabolic clearance rate and a longer half-life (7 days) than T_3 (1 day). The kidneys readily excrete free T_4 and T_3. Binding of thyroid hormones to plasma proteins ensures a circulating reserve and delays their clearance.

The release of hormone from its protein-bound form is in a dynamic equilibrium. Although the role of binding proteins in delivery of hormone to specific tissues remains to be fully understood, it is known that drugs such as salicylate may affect thyroid hormone binding to plasma proteins. The binding-hormone capacity of the individual can also be altered by disease or hormonal changes. For example, liver disease is associated with a decrease in the synthesis of binding proteins, whereas high estrogen levels (eg, during pregnancy) increase binding-protein synthesis. These changes in the total amount of plasma proteins available to bind thyroid hormone will impact the total amount of circulating thyroid hormone because of a constant homeostatic adjustment to changes in free hormone levels. As in a classic feedback system, the hypothalamic-pituitary-thyroid axis is controlled by the amount of free hormone available. Thus, a decrease in free thyroid hormone because of an increase in plasma-binding proteins will stimulate the release of TSH from the anterior pituitary, which will in turn stimulate the synthesis and release of thyroid hormone from the thyroid gland. In contrast, a decrease in binding-protein levels, with a resulting rise in free thyroid hormone levels, will suppress TSH release and decrease thyroid hormone synthesis and release. These dynamic changes occur throughout the life of the individual, whether in health or disease. Disruption in these feedback mechanisms will result in manifestations of excess or deficient thyroid hormone function.

Thyroid Hormone Metabolism

As already mentioned, the thyroid releases mostly T_4 and very small amounts of T_3, yet T_3 has greater thyroid activity than T_4. The main source of circulating T_3 is peripheral deiodination of T_4 by **deiodinases** (Figure 4–5). Approximately 80% of T_4 produced by the thyroid undergoes deiodination in the periphery. Approximately 40% of T_4 is deiodinated at carbon 5 in the outer ring to yield the more active T_3, principally in liver and kidney. In approximately 33% of T_4, iodine is removed from carbon 5 in the inner ring to yield **reverse T_3 (rT_3)**. Reverse T_3 has little or no biologic activity, has a higher metabolic clearance rate than T_3, and has a lower serum concentration than T_3. Following conversion of T_4 to T_3 or rT_3, these are converted to T_2, a biologically inactive hormone. Therefore, thyroid hormone peripheral metabolism is a sequential deiodination process, leading first to a more active form of thyroid hormone (T_3) and finally to complete inactivation of the hormone. Thus, loss of a single iodine from the outer ring of T_4 produces the active hormone T_3, which may either exit the cell (in deiodinase type I–containing cells), enter the nucleus directly (in deiodinase type II–containing cells), or possibly even both (eg, in human skeletal muscle). Thyroid hormones can be excreted following hepatic sulfo- and glucuronide conjugation and biliary excretion.

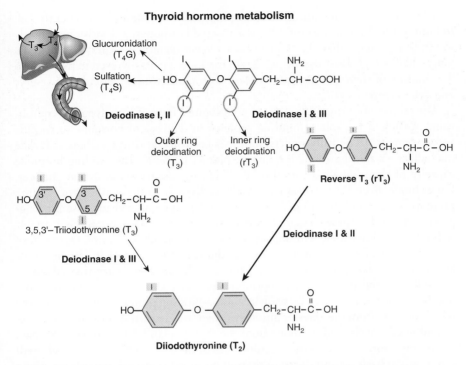

Figure 4–5. Peripheral metabolism of thyroid hormone involves the sequential removal of iodine molecules converting tetraiodothyronine (T_4) into a more active triiodothyronine (T_3) as well as inactivating thyroid hormone prior to their excretion. In addition, thyroid hormone can undergo conjugation in the liver, which increases their solubility and facilitates their biliary excretion. The type I iodothyronine deiodinase is expressed predominantly in liver, kidney, and thyroid. It catalyzes both outer and inner ring deiodination of thyroid hormone. It is the primary site for clearance of plasma reverse triiodothyronine (rT_3) and a major source of circulating T_3. Type II deiodinase is expressed primarily in the human brain, anterior pituitary, and thyroid. It only has outer-ring deiodination activity and plays an important role in the local production of T_3 in tissues expressing this enzyme. The type III deiodinase is located predominantly in human brain, placenta, and fetal tissues. It only has inner-ring activity and catalyzes the inactivation of T_3 more effectively than that of T_4, thereby regulating intracellular T_3 levels.

This extrathyroidal progressive deiodination of thyroid hormones catalyzed by deiodinases plays a significant role in thyroid hormone metabolism and requires the trace element selenocysteine for optimal enzymatic activity. Three types of deiodinases have been identified, which differ in their tissue distribution, catalytic profiles, substrate specificities, physiologic functions, and regulation.

TYPE I DEIODINASE

Type I deiodinase catalyzes outer- and inner-ring deiodination of T_4 and rT_3. It is found predominantly in the liver, kidney, and thyroid. It is considered the primary deiodinase responsible for T_4 to T_3 conversion in hyperthyroid patients in the periphery. This enzyme also converts T_3 to T_2. The activity of type I deiodinase expressed in the thyroid gland is increased by TSH-stimulated cAMP production and has a significant influence on the amount of T_3 released by the thyroid. Propylthiouracil and iodinated x-ray contrast agents such as iopanoic acid inhibit the activity of this enzyme and consequently the thyroidal production of T_3.

TYPE II DEIODINASE

Type II deiodinase is expressed in the brain, pituitary gland, brown adipose tissue, thyroid, placenta, and skeletal and cardiac muscle. Type II deiodinase has only outer-ring activity and converts T_4 to T_3. This enzyme is thought to be the major source of T_3 in the euthyroid state. This enzyme plays an important role in tissues that produce a relatively high proportion of the receptor-bound T_3 themselves, rather than deriving T_3 from plasma. In these tissues, type II deiodinases are an important source of intracellular T_3 and provide more than 50% of the nuclear receptor-bound T_3. The critical role of the type II deiodinases is underscored by the fact that T_3 formed in the anterior pituitary is necessary for negative feedback inhibition of TSH secretion.

TYPE III DEIODINASE

Type III deiodinase is expressed in the brain, placenta, and skin. Type III deiodinase has inner-ring activity and converts T_4 to rT_3, and T_3 to T_2, thus inactivating T_4 and T_3. This process is an important feature in placental protection of the fetus. The placental conversion of T_4 to rT_3 and of T_3 to T_2 reduces the flow of T_3 (the most active thyroid hormone) from mother to fetus. Small amounts of maternal T_4 are transferred to the fetus and converted to T_3, which increases the T_3 concentration in the fetal brain, preventing hypothyroidism. In the adult brain, the expression of type III deiodinases is enhanced by thyroid hormone excess, serving as a protective mechanism against high thyroid hormone concentrations.

Biologic Effects of Thyroid Hormones

Thyroid hormone receptors are expressed in virtually all tissues and affect multiple cellular events. Their effects are mediated primarily by the transcriptional regulation of target genes, and are thus known as **genomic effects**. Recently, it has become evident that thyroid hormones also exert **nongenomic effects**, which do not require modification of gene transcription. Some of these effects include stimulation of activity of Ca^{2+}-adenosine triphosphatase (ATPase) at the plasma membrane and sarcoplasmic reticulum, rapid stimulation of the Na^+/H^+ antiporter, and increases in oxygen consumption (see Chapter 10). The nature of the receptors that mediate these effects and the signaling pathways involved are not yet completely elucidated. However, T_3 exerts rapid effects on ion fluxes and electrophysiologic events, predominantly in the cardiovascular system.

 Thyroid hormones enter cells by a carrier-mediated energy-, temperature-, and Na^+-dependent process (Figure 4–6). Several transporters have been identified to be involved in their entry into the cell, including

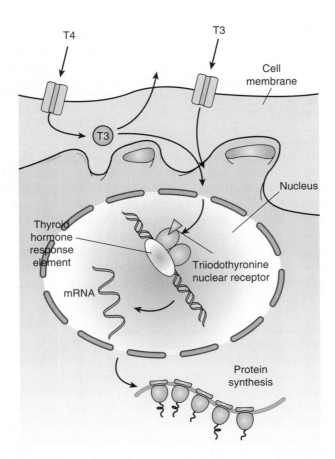

Figure 4–6. Cellular effects of thyroid hormones. Thyroid hormones (T$_3$ and T$_4$) enter the cell and bind to their receptors located in the nucleus. The affinity for T$_3$ is greater than for T$_4$. The thyroid nuclear receptors function as ligand-activated transcription factors that influence transcription from target genes. Nuclear receptors bind enhancer elements on DNA called *hormone response elements* to regulate transcription from genes. Binding of thyroid hormone, leads to recruitment of specific coactivators leading to gene activation and ultimately protein synthesis.

those belonging to the sodium taurocholate cotransporting polypeptide (NTCP), the sodium-independent organic anion transporting polypeptide (OATP), L- and T-type amino acid transporters, and members of the monocarboxylate transporter family. Two transporters have been demonstrated to have particular specificity for thyroid hormone transport, the OATP1C1, which shows preference for T$_4$ and the MCT8 which shows preference for T$_3$. Mutations or deletions in the *MCT8* gene have been linked to psychomotor retardation and thyroid hormone resistance, indicating their contribution to optimal thyroid hormone function.

Thyroid Hormone Receptors

The cellular actions of thyroid hormones are mediated by multiple thyroid hormone receptor isoforms derived from 2 distinct genes (α and β) encoding thyroid hormone receptors. The functional significance of the different isoforms has not yet been elucidated. Thyroid hormone receptors are nuclear receptors intimately associated with chromatin (see Figure 4–6). Thyroid hormone receptors are DNA-binding transcription factors that function as molecular switches in response to hormone binding. The hormone receptor can activate or repress gene transcription, depending on the promoter context and ligand-binding status. Unoccupied thyroid hormone receptors are bound to DNA thyroid hormone response elements and are associated with a complex of proteins containing corepressor proteins. Hormone binding to the receptor promotes corepressor dissociation and binding of a coactivator, leading to modulation of gene transcription. Thyroid hormone receptors bind the hormone with high affinity and specificity. They have low capacity but high affinity for T_3. The majority (85%) of nuclear-bound thyroid hormone is T_3, and approximately 15% is T_4.

Because thyroid hormone receptors are present in virtually all tissues, thyroid hormones play a vital role in cellular metabolism. The cellular events that they mediate include the following:

- Transcription of cell membrane Na^+/K^+-ATPase, leading to an increase in oxygen consumption
- Transcription of uncoupling protein, enhancing fatty acid oxidation and heat generation without production of adenosine triphosphate
- Protein synthesis and degradation, contributing to growth and differentiation
- Epinephrine-induced glycogenolysis, and insulin-induced glycogen synthesis and glucose utilization
- Cholesterol synthesis and low-density lipoprotein receptor regulation

Organ-Specific Effects of Thyroid Hormone

Thyroid hormones are essential for normal growth and development; they control the rate of metabolism and hence the function of practically every organ in the body. Their specific biologic effects vary from one tissue to another. The following are some examples of the specific effects of thyroid hormone.

Bone—Thyroid hormone is essential for bone growth and development through activation of osteoclast and osteoblast activities. Deficiency during childhood affects growth. In adults, excess thyroid hormone levels are associated with increased risk of osteoporosis.

Cardiovascular system—Thyroid hormone has cardiac inotropic and chronotropic effects, increases cardiac output and blood volume, and decreases systemic vascular resistance. These responses are mediated through thyroid hormone changes in gene transcription of several proteins including Ca^{2+}-ATPase, phospholamban, myosin, β-adrenergic receptors, adenylyl cyclase, guanine-nucleotide–binding proteins, Na^+/Ca^{2+} exchanger, Na^+/K^+-ATPase, and voltage-gated potassium channels.

Fat—Thyroid hormone induces white adipose tissue differentiation, lipogenic enzymes, and intracellular lipid accumulation; stimulates adipocyte cell proliferation; stimulates uncoupling proteins; and uncouples oxidative phosphorylation. Hyperthyroidism enhances and hypothyroidism decreases lipolysis through different mechanisms. The induction of catecholamine-mediated lipolysis by thyroid hormones results from an increased β-adrenoceptor number and a decrease in phosphodiesterase activity resulting in an increase in cAMP level and hormone-sensitive lipase activity.

Liver—Thyroid hormone regulates triglyceride and cholesterol metabolism, as well as lipoprotein homeostasis. Thyroid hormone also modulates cell proliferation and mitochondrial respiration.

Pituitary—Thyroid hormone regulates the synthesis of pituitary hormones, stimulates growth hormone production, and inhibits TSH.

Brain—Thyroid hormone controls expression of genes involved in myelination, cell differentiation, migration, and signaling. Thyroid hormone is necessary for axonal growth and development.

DISEASES OF THYROID HORMONE OVERPRODUCTION AND UNDERSECRETION

The widespread distribution of thyroid hormone receptors and the multitude of physiologic effects that they exert are highlighted in cases of abnormal thyroid function (Table 4–2). Dysfunction can result from 3 factors: (1) alterations in the circulating levels of thyroid hormones, (2) impaired metabolism of thyroid hormones in the periphery, and (3) resistance to thyroid hormone actions at the tissue level.

An individual whose thyroid function is normal is said to be in a euthyroid state. The clinical state resulting from an alteration in thyroid function is classified as either **hypothyroidism** (low thyroid function) or **hyperthyroidism** (excessive thyroid function). As with most endocrine abnormalities, altered thyroid function may be genetic or acquired, and its duration may be transient or permanent. Autoimmune diseases play an important role in thyroid disease. Abnormal immune responses directed to thyroid-related proteins result in 2 opposite pathogenic processes: thyroid enlargement (hyperplasia) in **Graves disease** and thyroid destruction in **Hashimoto thyroiditis**.

The most common presentations of thyroid hormone abnormalities are summarized as follows (see Table 4–2).

Hypothyroidism

Hypothyroidism is the condition resulting from insufficient thyroid hormone action. It has an incidence of 2% in adult women and is less common in men. Two main types are distinguished, primary and secondary hypothyroidism, with primary being the most common. Alternatively, patients may present with signs and symptoms of hypothyroidism but without a decrease in circulating thyroid hormone levels. This condition, known as **thyroid hormone resistance**, is a rare dominant inherited condition in which the responsiveness of target tissues to thyroid

Table 4-2. Clinical and laboratory manifestations of excess or deficient thyroid hormone function

Hypothyroidism		Hyperthyroidism	
Clinical presentation	**Laboratory values**	**Clinical presentation**	**Laboratory values**
In utero:	Primary:	Palpitations, exercise impairment, widened pulse pressure, tachycardia at rest and during exercise, increase in blood volume, palpable enlarged thyroid gland, infiltrative ophthalmopathy, nervousness, irritability, hyperactivity, emotional instability, tenseness, pounding of the heart, heat intolerance, weight loss despite increased food intake, decreased or absent menstrual flow, increased number of bowel movements, warm moist skin or velvety texture, proximal muscle weakness, fine hair, fine tremor, excessive sweating, moist skin	Primary:
Cretinism, mental and growth retardation, short limbs	Low free T_4; low or sometimes normal T_3; high TSH		Low TSH below limit of detection (0.1 μU/mL); high T_4 (2-fold) and T_3 (3–4-fold). In Graves disease, elevated anti-TSH receptor antibody titers.
Adult onset:	Secondary:		Secondary:
Tiredness, lethargy, constipation, decreased appetite, cold intolerance, abnormal menstrual flow, hair loss, brittle nails, dry coarse skin, hoarse voice	Low T_4, T_3, and TSH		High TSH, T_4, and T_3
Chronic:			
Myxedema, thickened features, periorbital edema, swelling of hands and feet without indentation, delayed muscle contraction and relaxation, delayed tendon reflexes, reduced stroke volume and heart rate, decreased cardiac output, enlarged heart, pericardial effusion, pleural and peritoneal fluid accumulation, slowing of mental function, impaired memory, slow speech, decreased initiative, somnolence, hypothermia			

T_3, triiodothyronine; T_4, thyroxine; TSH, thyroid-stimulating hormone.

hormone is reduced. It occurs in 1 per 50,000 live births. The low incidence is probably caused by the reduced survival of these embryos. The thyroid-resistant state associated with mutations in the thyroid receptor gene is characterized by elevated circulating levels of free thyroid hormone and normal or elevated levels of TSH. Patients usually present with enlargement of the thyroid gland (**goiter**) and either normal (**euthyroid**) or mildly decreased (**hypothyroid**) metabolic state. The T_3, T_4, and TSH levels may be high in what appears to be a compensatory mechanism to ensure maintenance of euthyroid and eumetabolic states.

Primary Hypothyroidism

The most frequent cause of hypothyroidism (95% of cases) is disease of the thyroid gland. When the decrease in thyroid function occurs in utero, the result is severe mental retardation or cretinism, underscoring the vital role that thyroid hormone plays in development and growth. Hypothyroidism in adult patients may be associated with either a decrease or an increase in thyroid gland size. The decrease in thyroid tissue is usually caused by autoimmune disease, leading to the destruction of thyroid parenchyma, but it can also be the result of surgery or radioactive iodine treatment. Hypothyroidism may also be associated with thyroid enlargement (goiter), resulting from lymphocytic infiltration as in Hashimoto disease or dietary iodine deficiency.

Secondary Hypothyroidism

Secondary hypothyroidism is characterized by decreased TSH secretion and subsequently decreased thyroid hormone release. It is the result of disorders of the anterior pituitary or hypothalamus and can sometimes occur in association with other abnormalities of anterior pituitary hormones. Secondary hypothyroidism is not because of alterations at the level of the thyroid gland itself and is strictly caused by a lack of stimulation of the TSH receptor because of impaired TSH release.

Hyperthyroidism

Hyperthyroidism is excessive functional activity of the thyroid gland, characterized by increased basal metabolism and disturbances in the autonomic nervous system as a result of excess thyroid hormone production. The incidence is higher in women (2%) than in men (0.02%). Several conditions can lead to hyperthyroidism: diffuse toxic goiter or Graves disease, toxic nodular goiter, toxic adenoma, therapy-induced hyperthyroidism (eg, excess T_4 or T_3 substitution), excess iodine intake, thyroiditis, follicular carcinoma, and TSH-producing tumor of the pituitary. However, the most common cause of hyperthyroidism in adults is diffuse toxic goiter or Graves disease.

Graves Disease

Graves disease is an autoimmune condition leading to autonomous excess thyroid hormone secretion because of TSH receptor stimulation by immunoglobulin G. The continuous stimulation of TSH receptor by TSH-like antibodies results in excess T_4 and T_3 production. The incidence of Graves disease peaks in the third to fourth decades and is 8 times more common in women than in men.

Clinically, approximately 40%–50% of patients with hyperthyroidism present with protruding eyes (exophthalmos) as a result of lymphocyte and fibroblast infiltration of the extraocular tissues and muscles, and accumulation of hyaluronate, a glycosaminoglycan produced by fibroblasts in the tissues and muscles. The expression of TSH receptors in the periocular fibroblasts contributes to the pathogenesis of exophthalmos. The majority (90%) of patients with thyroid ophthalmopathy have Graves hyperthyroidism.

THYROID-STIMULATING HORMONE–SECRETING ADENOMAS

Secondary hyperthyroidism is caused by increased thyroid hormone release by the thyroid gland in response to elevated TSH levels derived from TSH-secreting pituitary adenomas. TSH-secreting adenomas represent a small fraction (1%–2%) of all pituitary adenomas and result in a syndrome of excess secretion of TSH. The hormonal profile is characterized by the inability to suppress TSH despite elevated levels of free thyroid hormones (T_3 and T_4).

Euthyroid Sick Syndrome

Euthyroid sick syndrome is a clinical condition in which patients suffering from nonthyroid diseases show biochemical evidence of altered thyroid function, but appear euthyroid when examined clinically. These patients present with normal or decreased T_4 concentration, decreased T_4 binding to thyroid-binding globulin, decreased T_3 concentration, increased rT_3 concentration, normal TSH, and normal scintigraphic imaging. This condition can be precipitated by stresses such as fasting, starvation, anorexia nervosa, protein malnutrition, surgical trauma, myocardial infarction, chronic renal failure, diabetic ketosis, cirrhosis, sepsis, and hyperthermia (see Chapter 10). The alteration in thyroid hormone profile is because of an increase in type III deiodinase activity. Euthyroid sick syndrome may also be because of impaired conversion of T_4 to T_3, as occurs with pharmacologic agents such as propranolol and amiodarone.

Abnormalities in Iodine Metabolism

Iodine is an essential component of thyroid hormone, but both low and high iodine intake may lead to disease. The daily requirement of iodine for thyroid hormone synthesis is 150 μg. As already described, the thyroid gland has intrinsic mechanisms that maintain normal thyroid function even in the presence of iodine excess. The thyroid also tries to compensate when dietary sources of iodine are limited. Several drugs can interfere with the ability of the thyroid gland to concentrate iodide. Perchlorate is a contaminant that can be found in drinking and ground water, and occasionally in cow's milk. Ingestion of high levels, as with consumption of well water can lead to inhibition of iodine transport into the follicular cells. Methimazole, the active form of carbimazole, inhibits iodide uptake and organification of iodine. Thiouracil and propylthio-uracil inhibit iodine organification; the latter also inhibits the peripheral conversion of T_4 to T_3.

Abnormalities in the metabolism or supply of iodine have particular importance in fetal development. Severe iodine deficiency of the mother may lead to insufficient thyroid hormone synthesis in both mother and fetus, resulting in developmental brain injury. Iodine deficiency is the leading cause of preventable mental retardation. Conversely, excess iodine given to the mother (eg, use of amiodarone or excess iodine supplementation) may inhibit fetal thyroid function, leading to hypothyroidism and goiter, or may precipitate hyperthyroidism (iodine toxicity).

A rare familial disorder may lead to a defect in iodide transport. This defect is caused by the genetic absence or derangement of the Na^+/I^- symporter protein, which is involved in the active transport and concentration of iodide in the thyroid follicular cells. This condition can present in neonates as goiter with or without cretinism. In these individuals, T_3 and T_4 levels tend to be low and the TSH level is high. The diagnosis is confirmed by demonstrating poor thyroid uptake of radiolabeled iodine (I^{131}) or sodium pertechnetate ($Na^{99m}TcO_4$).

Thyroiditis

Thyroiditis, or inflammation of the thyroid gland, may lead to abnormalities in thyroid hormone state. This condition may be acute, subacute, or chronic.

ACUTE THYROIDITIS

Patients with **acute thyroiditis** present with a painful thyroid; chills and fever; a hot, enlarged, and palpable gland; and initially with hyperthyroidism. This condition is rare and infectious. Levels of T_3, T_4, and TSH are usually normal, and rT_3 is increased.

CHRONIC THYROIDITIS

Chronic thyroiditis (Hashimoto thyroiditis, chronic lymphocytic thyroiditis, autoimmune thyroiditis) is an autoimmune disease of the thyroid gland characterized by lymphocyte infiltration and circulating autoimmune antibodies. These antibodies inhibit the Na^+/I^- symporter, preventing iodide uptake and consequently thyroid hormone synthesis. Hashimoto thyroiditis is the most common cause of adult hypothyroidism. It is more prevalent in women than in men (ratio 8:1) and peaks at the age of 30–50 years. Individuals presenting with Hashimoto thyroiditis frequently have a family history of thyroid disorders. Hashimoto thyroiditis is also more common in persons with chromosomal disorders, such as Turner, Down, or Klinefelter syndromes, and in some cases is associated with autoimmune conditions such as Addison disease, hypoparathyroidism, and diabetes. Hashimoto thyroiditis may present early on with variable T_4, T_3, and TSH concentrations and antibody titers to TPO and Tg. As the disease progresses, some patients develop hypothyroidism with low T_4 and T_3 levels; high TSH levels and specific antibodies are usually no longer detectable.

EVALUATION OF THE HYPOTHALAMIC-PITUITARY-THYROID AXIS

The previous section provided a brief description of some of the diseases resulting from abnormalities in thyroid function. Tests of thyroid function allow the clinician to diagnose the disease and provide the follow-up necessary once therapy has been instituted. Although the most important keys to diagnosis are a thorough interview and physical examination of the patient, an understanding of the normal physiology of thyroid function allows proper interpretation of the diverse laboratory approaches for measuring function. Some of the most useful approaches are described as follows.

Thyroid-Stimulating Hormone and Thyroid Hormone Levels

Normal TSH values average 0.4–4.5 µU/mL and can be measured in plasma by immunometric assays. TSH levels are useful in evaluation of the patient because small changes in free thyroid hormone levels lead to greater changes in TSH levels. Serum TSH concentrations are considered the single most reliable test to diagnose all common forms of hypothyroidism and hyperthyroidism, particularly in the ambulatory setting. Overt hyperthyroidism is accompanied by low serum TSH concentrations, typically less than 0.1 mIU/L. Interpretation of TSH levels is best done with simultaneous measures of thyroid hormone levels.

Total T_4 and T_3 levels are measured by competitive immunoassay methods, and normal ranges are 5–12 µg/dL and 60–180 ng/dL, respectively. Total T_4 includes both bound and free hormone. As described earlier, only the free hormone (0.05% of the total) is biologically active; thus, changes in the levels of thyroid-binding globulin, albumin, or thyroid-binding prealbumin will affect total T_4 but not the free hormone. The same applies for measures of total T_3. T_3 levels are increased in almost all cases of hyperthyroidism, usually earlier than T_4, making it a more sensitive indicator of hyperthyroidism than total T_4. In hypothyroidism, T_3 is often normal even when T_4 is low. T_3 is decreased during acute illness and starvation and is affected by several medications, including propranolol, steroids, and amiodarone.

Free Triiodothyronine and Tetraiodothyronine

The amount of free hormone depends on how much is bound to proteins. Estrogens and acute liver disease increase thyroid hormone-binding protein synthesis, whereas androgens, steroids, chronic liver disease, and severe illness can decrease it.

Reverse Triiodothyronine

Critical illness is associated with reduced TSH and thyroid hormone secretion, and with changes in peripheral thyroid hormone metabolism, resulting in low serum T_3 and high rT_3. As a result of altered peripheral thyroid hormone metabolism, decreased serum levels of T_3 are associated with increased concentrations of rT_3, an inactive form of thyroid hormone.

Antibody Levels

Determination of antithyroid antibodies is important in establishing the cause of thyroid disease. The antibodies of greatest clinical importance are the anti-thyroid microsomal (antiperoxidase) antibodies, the anti-Tg antibodies, and the thyroid-stimulating immunoglobulins (TSIs). In general, the antithyroid microsomal antibodies are usually elevated in patients with autoimmune thyroiditis (Hashimoto thyroiditis). Less frequently and to a lesser degree, the anti-Tg antibodies may be elevated in patients with autoimmune thyroiditis. Elevation of TSI is associated with Graves disease and is the likely cause of the hyperthyroidism seen in this condition.

Thyroid Nodule

The management of patients with thyroid masses or nodules involves utilization of several diagnostic techniques, which are briefly presented here.

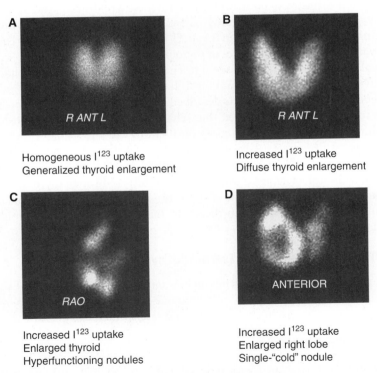

A.
R ANT L
Homogeneous I^{123} uptake
Generalized thyroid enlargement

B.
R ANT L
Increased I^{123} uptake
Diffuse thyroid enlargement

C.
RAO
Increased I^{123} uptake
Enlarged thyroid
Hyperfunctioning nodules

D.
ANTERIOR
Increased I^{123} uptake
Enlarged right lobe
Single-"cold" nodule

Figure 4–7. Radioactive thyroid scans. **A.** Normal to increased thyroid uptake of I^{123}. **B.** Thyroid with a marked decrease in ^{125}I uptake in a large palpable mass. **C.** Increased I^{123} uptake isolated to a single nodule, the "hot nodule." **D.** Decreased thyroid I^{123} uptake in an isolated region, the "cold nodule." (Images courtesy of Richard Kuebler, MD. LSUHSC University Hospital, New Orleans, LA.)

Thyroid ultrasound—Ultrasonography of a thyroid mass allows determination of size, composition (solid, cystic, mixed, or complex), calcifications, and presence of additional nodules.

Fine needle aspiration—Performed by palpation or guided by an ultrasound, this technique allows for cytologic analysis of the fluid and cells obtained through percutaneous needle aspiration of thyroid nodules.

Thyroid scan—The Na^+/I^- symporter of the thyroid follicular epithelial cell does not discriminate between dietary iodide and radioactive isotopes such as iodine-123 or technetium-99. Therefore, these isotopes are used to visualize the functional anatomy of the thyroid. Regions of the thyroid that are functioning and actively incorporating the isotope are detected with a counter. The image of the thyroid reflects the ability of specific regions of the thyroid to take up the isotope and therefore to function normally (Figure 4–7). Areas that do not take up the radiolabeled iodine are referred to as nonfunctional or "cold." Because most malignant tumors do not express the Na^+/I^- symporter, they often present as cold nodules. Areas that accumulate iodide in excess of that of the surrounding tissues are referred to as "hot nodules."

KEY CONCEPTS

The thyroid gland is regulated by the hypothalamic-pituitary-thyroid axis.

Dietary iodine is required for thyroid hormone synthesis.

The thyroid gland produces thyroid hormones by a process of concentration of iodine in the thyroid, iodination of tyrosine residues of Tg in the colloid space of the follicle, and endocytosis of colloid followed by proteolytic release of thyroid hormones (T_4 and T_3).

Thyroid hormones undergo metabolism in peripheral tissues, leading to the production of the more active T_3 and deactivation of thyroid hormones.

The presence of deiodinases and their substrate specificity play a central role in thyroid hormone function in target tissues.

Thyroid hormones are transported into the cell where they bind to hormone receptors that bind DNA and alter gene transcription.

Thyroid hormone actions are systemic and vital for development, growth, and metabolism.

STUDY QUESTIONS

4–1. A 55-year-old woman seeks doctor's advice following a 6-month-long period of restlessness, nervousness, and insomnia. Her physical examination reveals heart rate of 120 beats per minute, tremors, warm moist hands, and an enlarged thyroid gland. Which of the following laboratory values would you expect to find?

	TSH (0.4–4.7 μIU/mL)	T_3(45–137 ng/dL)	rT_3 (10–40 ng/dL)
A	0.15	21	5
B	0.4	50	75
C	0.02	185	38
D	3.75	89	110

4–2. A radioactive iodine scan revealed greater concentration of radioiodine when compared to that of other asymptomatic individuals. Subsequent laboratory values came back positive for serum titers of thyroid-stimulating immunoglobulin (TSI). The physiopathology of disease in this patient involves:

    a. Increased deiodination of T_4 to T_3 in the liver

    b. Decreased thyroid hormone-binding levels

    c. Increased cAMP formation in the thyroid follicular cell

    d. Downregulation of the Na^+/I^- symporter

4–3. A 50-year-old male patient presents to a rural clinic complaining of fatigue, constipation, lethargy, and intolerance to cold. Other than being on conservative treatment (low salt diet) for mild hypertension, he has no outstanding history of prior illness or family disease. He is a farmer and consumes a predominantly vegetarian diet, with water derived from a local well. On physical examination, you notice an enlarged mass in the anterior part of his neck, which he has noticed has been slowly growing. His vital signs are: heart rate, 60 beats per minute; blood pressure, 110/70 mm Hg; temperature, 37.8°C (100°F). Which of the following would you expect to be an underlying mechanism in the pathophysiology in this case?

    a. Decreased thyroid peroxidase activity

    b. Increased deiodinase type III activity

    c. Decreased hepatic thyroid-binding globulin synthesis

    d. Decreased follicular cell iodine concentration

4–4. A 55-year-old woman seeks doctor's advice following a 6-month-long period of restlessness, nervousness, and insomnia. Her physical examination reveals heart rate of 120 beats per minute, tremors, warm moist hands, and an enlarged thyroid gland. Which of the following laboratory values would you expect to find?

	TSH (0.4–4.7 µIU/mL)	T_3 (45–137 ng/dL)	rT_3 (10–40 ng/dL)	Thyroid-stimulating Ig (Negative titers)
A	<0.1	21	5	—
B	0.4	50	75	++
C	<0.1	185	38	++
D	3.75	89	110	++

SUGGESTED READINGS

Davies T, Marians R, Latif R. The TSH receptor reveals itself. *J Clin Invest.* 2002;110:161–164.

Gereben B, Zeöld A, Dentice M, Salvatore D, Bianco AC. Activation and inactivation of thyroid hormone by deiodinases: local action with general consequences. *Cell Mol Life Sci.* 2008;65(4):570–590.

Klein I, Ojamaa K. Mechanisms of disease: thyroid hormone and the cardiovascular system. *N Engl J Med.* 2001;344:501.

Laurberg P, Vestergaard H, Nielsen S, et al. Sources of circulating 3,5,3′-triiodothyronine in hyperthyroidism estimated after blocking of type 1 and type 2 iodothyronine deiodinases. *J Clin Invest.* 2007;92(6):2149–2156.

Nilsson M. Iodide handling by the thyroid epithelial cell. *Exp Clin Endocrinol Diabetes.* 2001;109:13.

Silva JE, Bianco SD. Thyroid-adrenergic interactions: physiological and clinical implications. *Thyroid.* 2008;18(2):157–165.

Visser WE, Friesema EC, Jansen J, Visser TJ. Thyroid hormone transport in and out of cells. *Trends Endocrinol Metab.* 2008;19(2):50–56.

Yen PM. Physiological and molecular basis of thyroid hormone action. *Physiol Rev.* 2001;81:1097.

Parathyroid Gland and Ca²⁺ and PO₄⁻ Regulation

Parathyroid Gland and Ca^{2+} and PO$_4^-$ Regulation

5

OBJECTIVES

▶ *Identify the origin, target organs and cell types, and physiologic effects of parathyroid hormone.*

▶ *Describe the functions of osteoblasts and osteoclasts in bone remodeling and the factors that regulate their activities.*

▶ *Describe the regulation of parathyroid hormone secretion and the role of the calcium-sensing receptor.*

▶ *Identify the sources of vitamin D and describe the biosynthetic pathway involved in modifying it to its biologically active form.*

▶ *Identify the target organs and cellular mechanisms of action of vitamin D.*

▶ *Describe the negative feedback relationship between parathyroid hormone and the biologically active form of vitamin D.*

▶ *Describe the causes and consequences of excess or deficiency of parathyroid hormone and of vitamin D.*

▶ *Describe the regulation of calcitonin release and the cell of origin and target organs for calcitonin action.*

The regulation of plasma Ca^{2+} levels is critical for normal cell function, neural transmission, membrane stability, bone structure, blood coagulation, and intracellular signaling. This regulation relies on the interactions among **parathyroid hormone (PTH)** from the parathyroid glands, dietary **vitamin D**, and **calcitonin** from the thyroid gland (Figure 5–1). PTH stimulates bone resorption and the release of Ca^{2+} into the circulation. In the kidney, PTH promotes Ca^{2+} reabsorption and inorganic phosphate excretion in the urine. In addition, PTH stimulates the hydroxylation of 25-hydroxyvitamin D at the 1-position, leading to the formation of the active form of vitamin D (calcitriol). Vitamin D increases intestinal absorption of dietary Ca^{2+} and facilitates renal reabsorption of filtered Ca^{2+}. In bone, vitamin D increases bone resorption with a resulting increase in the release of Ca^{2+} into the circulation. Calcitonin counteracts the effects of PTH by inhibiting bone resorption and increasing renal Ca^{2+} excretion. The overall result of the interactions among PTH, vitamin D, and calcitonin is the maintenance of normal plasma Ca^{2+} concentrations.

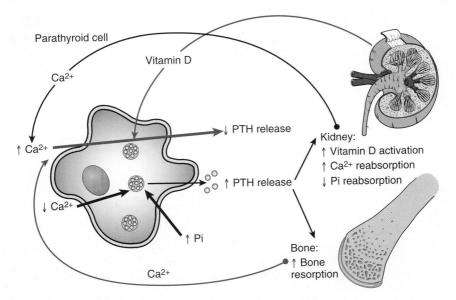

Figure 5–1. Negative feedback regulation of parathyroid hormone (PTH) release. A sudden decrease in Ca^{2+} stimulates the release of PTH from the parathyroid gland. PTH increases the activity of 1α-hydroxylase in the kidney, leading to increased activation of vitamin D. In addition, PTH increases the reabsorption of Ca^{2+} and decreases the reabsorption of inorganic phosphate (Pi). In bone, PTH stimulates bone resorption, increasing the plasma Ca^{2+} levels. The elevations in vitamin D and plasma Ca^{2+} levels exert negative feedback inhibition of PTH release. Elevations in plasma Pi levels stimulate the release of PTH.

FUNCTIONAL ANATOMY

The parathyroid glands are pea-sized glands located at the top and bottom posterior borders of the lateral lobes of the thyroid gland. The glands are richly vascularized and consist primarily of chief cells, with a thin capsule of connective tissue that divides the gland into lobules. The chief cells synthesize and secrete PTH, a polypeptide hormone that plays a major role in bone remodeling and calcium homeostasis. In addition to its central role in the regulation of Ca^{2+} levels and bone mass, PTH participates in the renal excretion of phosphate and in the activation of vitamin D. Because of the central role of PTH in calcium homeostasis, its physiologic effects are described in the context of its interaction with the other major regulators of calcium: calcitonin, the hormone synthesized in the C cells of the thyroid gland; and calcitriol, the active form of vitamin D.

PARATHYROID HORMONE BIOSYNTHESIS AND TRANSPORT

PTH is synthesized as a prepropeptide that is rapidly cleaved to yield pro-PTH and subsequently the mature form of PTH. Mature and intact PTH consists of 84 amino acids. PTH synthesis and release is continuous, with about 6–7 superimposed pulses each hour. PTH is degraded by the kidney and the liver to amino-terminal (PTH 1-34) and carboxy-terminal fragments. The amino-terminal fragments constitute approximately 10% of circulating PTH fragments. They are biologically active but have a short half-life (4–20 minutes). In contrast, the carboxy-terminal fragments, which constitute 80% of the circulating PTH fragments, have no biologic activity and have a longer half-life; they are therefore easier to measure in the plasma. Overall, the intact hormone accounts for 10% of the circulating PTH-related peptides. Because multiple peptide products of PTH breakdown are present in the circulation, determination of the intact molecule is the only reliable index of PTH levels.

Regulation of Parathyroid Hormone Release

The release of PTH is controlled in a tight feedback system by plasma Ca^{2+} concentrations. High calcium suppresses PTH secretion and low calcium stimulates hormone release. Small changes in plasma Ca^{2+} levels are detected by the parathyroid Ca^{2+}-sensing receptor (Figure 5–2). An acute decrease in circulating calcium levels (hypocalcemia) elicits a biphasic wave of PTH release. Preformed PTH is released within seconds, followed by a reduction in intracellular degradation of PTH and increase in PTH release minutes to hours later. Thus, for a given Ca^{2+} level, there is an optimal PTH level in the circulation. The tight regulation of PTH release by circulating calcium levels is another example of the negative feedback regulation of hormone release. In addition the active form of vitamin D [1,25(OH)$_2$D] also contributes to modulation of PTH levels by reducing PTH gene transcription. Phosphate levels also modulate PTH release, with increased phosphate-stimulating PTH release. Magnesium concentrations also modulate PTH release. Table 5–1 lists the factors that regulate PTH release.

Parathyroid Ca^{2+} Receptor

The Ca^{2+} sensor is a G protein (G$_{q/11}$ and G$_i$)–coupled receptor located on the plasma membrane of the parathyroid chief cells; it is also found in kidney tubule cells and thyroid C cells. The release of PTH is inhibited in response to elevations in plasma Ca^{2+} concentrations and activation of the Ca^{2+} receptor (see Figure 5–2). Activation of the Ca^{2+} receptor initiates a signaling cascade involving phospholipases C, D, and A$_2$. The phosphorylation and activation of phospholipase A$_2$ activate the arachidonic acid cascade and increase leukotriene synthesis. The active leukotriene metabolites inhibit PTH secretion. The inhibition of PTH secretion by elevated Ca^{2+} levels is the result of increased degradation of preformed hormone stored in secretory granules. The granules are under regulatory control by plasma Ca^{2+} levels; persistent hypercalcemia leads to rapid degradation of most (90%) of the mature PTH in the cell. This process results in the formation of inactive carboxy-terminal PTH fragments, which are either released into the circulation or further degraded in the parathyroid. The amino acids released during degradation of the formed PTH inside the parathyroid cells are reused in the synthesis of other proteins. In contrast, vitamin D [1,25(OH)$_2$D] inhibits PTH release by decreasing PTH gene expression.

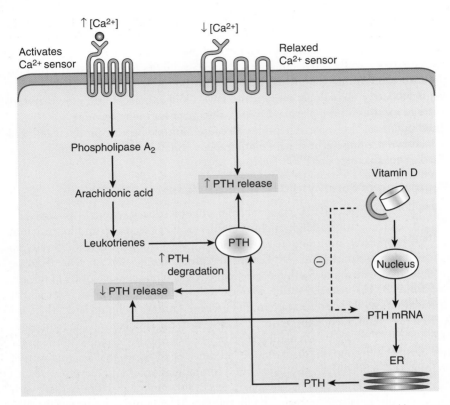

Figure 5–2. Parathyroid Ca^{2+}-sensing receptor and regulation of parathyroid hormone (PTH) release. Increased Ca^{2+} levels activate the Ca^{2+} sensor on parathyroid cells. The calcium sensor is a G protein–coupled receptor that activates phosphatidylinositol–phospholipase C (PI-PLC), leading to intracellular Ca^{2+} mobilization, protein kinase C (PKC) activation, and downstream activation of phospholipase A_2, resulting in activation of the arachidonic acid cascade and the production of biologically active leukotrienes. The leukotrienes trigger the degradation of preformed PTH molecules and decrease the release of intact PTH. The inhibition of PTH release by elevated vitamin D levels is mediated by decreasing the stability of PTH mRNA and consequently the synthesis of PTH. During hypocalcemia, the Ca^{2+} sensor is in a relaxed conformation and does not activate the second messengers involved in the breakdown of preformed PTH. Acute decreases in plasma calcium cause immediate release of preformed PTH and stimulation of new hormone synthesis. ER, endoplasmic reticulum.

Table 5–1. Regulation of parathyroid hormone release

PTH release is increased by	PTH release is suppressed by
Hypocalcemia	Hypercalcemia
Hyperphosphatemia	Vitamin D
Catecholamines	Severe hypomagnesemia

PTH, parathyroid hormone.

During hypocalcemia, the parathyroid Ca^{2+} receptor is relaxed, and PTH secretion is not restrained. The rapid secretion of preformed PTH elicited by acute hypocalcemia is rapidly followed by increased stability of PTH mRNA and the synthesis of new hormone.

Additional Factors That Regulate Parathyroid Hormone Release

PTH release is also under regulatory control by phosphate and magnesium levels. Elevations in plasma phosphate levels increase PTH secretion by decreasing phospholipase A$_2$ activity and arachidonic acid formation, thus removing the inhibitory effect on PTH secretion. Elevations in phosphate levels can also affect PTH release indirectly by decreasing plasma Ca^{2+} levels and vitamin D activation. In contrast, hypophosphatemia markedly decreases PTH mRNA and plasma PTH. The role of phosphate in PTH release is critical in patients with impaired renal function. If not controlled, the increasing levels of phosphate in these individuals result in abnormal elevations in PTH release. As the disease progresses, the negative feedback regulation of PTH release by Ca^{2+} and vitamin D is also impaired, contributing to the elevation in PTH release. As explained in the following section, chronic elevation of PTH results in excess bone resorption and loss of bone mass.

Plasma Mg^{2+} concentrations also regulate PTH secretion in a similar manner to that of calcium. PTH release can be stimulated by a moderate decrease in plasma Mg^{2+}. However, very low serum concentrations of Mg^{2+} induce a paradoxical block in PTH release. The mechanism for this effect has been suggested to be the result of activation of the α-subunits of the calcium-sensing receptor G-proteins, mimicking the activation of the receptor and thus inhibiting PTH secretion.

Plasma magnesium levels reflect those of calcium most of the time. The balance of magnesium is closely linked to that of calcium. Magnesium depletion or deficiency is frequently associated with hypocalcemia. This combined decrease in Mg^{2+} and Ca^{2+} leads to impairment in the individual's ability to secrete PTH. Moreover, severe hypomagnesemia impairs not only the release of PTH from the parathyroid gland in response to hypocalcemia, but it also prevents the responsiveness of bone to PTH-mediated bone resorption. Adrenergic agonists have been shown to increase PTH release through β-adrenergic receptors on parathyroid cells.

PARATHYROID HORMONE TARGET ORGANS AND PHYSIOLOGIC EFFECTS

The primary target organs for the physiologic effects of PTH are kidney and bone. The main physiologic response elicited by PTH is to increase plasma calcium levels by increasing Ca^{2+} renal reabsorption, Ca^{2+} mobilization from bone, and intestinal absorption (indirectly via vitamin D$_3$ activation). PTH also increases 1α-hydroxylase activity and renal phosphate excretion. As with other peptide hormones, the effects of PTH are mediated by binding to a cell membrane receptor in target organs. Three types of PTH receptors have been identified (PTHR1, PTHR2, PTHR3), all of which are G protein–coupled receptors. The important physiologic effects of PTH are mediated by PTHR1; the physiologic importance of PTHR2 and PTHR3 is not clear.

Parathyroid Hormone Receptor 1

PTHR1 is expressed in bone osteoblasts and kidney, where it binds PTH and PTH-related protein (PTHrP). PTHrP differs from PTH in structure, sharing only 13 amino acids with the amino-terminal of the hormone, and is a product of a separate gene. PTHrP is important because it mimics the physiologic effects of PTH in the bone and kidney. The identification of PTHrP followed a long search for the factor responsible for the hypercalcemia of malignancy. Because PTHrP is expressed in multiple tissues, it does not mediate its effects in an endocrine fashion, but rather behaves in a paracrine and autocrine manner. PTHrP binds to the PTHR1 in bone and kidney, resulting in elevated plasma Ca^{2+} levels. Therefore, PTHR1 not only mediates the physiologic effects of PTH, but also plays an important role in the pathophysiologic effects of PTHrP.

PTH binding to the G protein–coupled PTHR1 initiates a cascade of intracellular processes primarily by signaling through the α-subunit of the stimulatory G-protein (Gαs) leading to an increased synthesis of cyclic 3',5'-adenosine monophosphate (cAMP) and activation of protein kinase A and phosphorylation of target proteins at serine residues. The result is the activation of preformed proteins, as well as the induction of gene transcription. In addition, activation of the PTHR1 can use additional signaling pathways through Gαq leading to the activation of phospholipase C, increased intracellular inositol 1, 4, 5-trisphosphate and calcium concentrations.

Cellular Effects of Parathyroid Hormone

In the kidney, PTH directly stimulates Ca^{2+} reabsorption, phosphate excretion, and the activity of 1α-hydroxylase, the enzyme responsible for formation of the active form of vitamin D [$1,25(OH)_2D$]. The site of PTH regulation of Ca^{2+} reabsorption is the distal tubules. Ca^{2+} reabsorption by the proximal tubules occurs primarily through a paracellular pathway that is not regulated by hormones or drugs (Figure 5–3). In the thick ascending limbs, Ca^{2+} is absorbed through a combination of transcellular and paracellular routes. PTH regulates the active, transcellular component, whereas the passive, paracellular route is determined by the extent of concomitant sodium absorption. In the distal tubule, Ca^{2+} absorption is entirely transcellular and is regulated by PTH, vitamin D, and calcitonin; it can also be affected by Ca^{2+}-sparing drugs such as thiazide diuretics. PTH stimulates the insertion and opening of the apical Ca^{2+} channel, facilitating the entry of Ca^{2+} into the cell. These epithelial cells, like the thyroid follicular epithelial cells described in Chapter 4, are polarized; that is, they permit unidirectional flux of the ion from the apical to the basolateral membrane.

Inside the tubular epithelial cell, Ca^{2+} binds to calbindin-D_{28K} and then diffuses out through the basolateral membrane (see Figure 5–3). Calbindin-D_{28K} is a vitamin D–dependent calcium-binding protein that is present in the cytosol of cells lining the distal part of the nephron. Calbindin facilitates the cytosolic diffusion of Ca^{2+} from the apical influx to the basolateral efflux sites. It is thought to act as either a transport protein or a buffer to prevent excess elevation of cytosolic

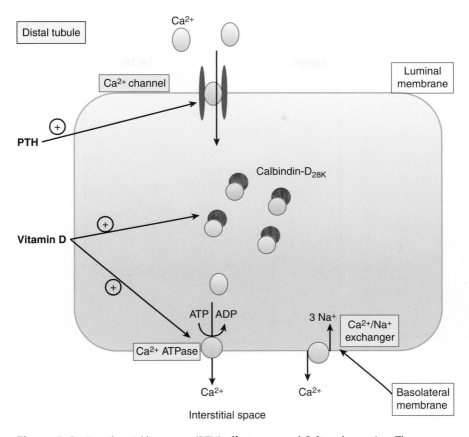

Figure 5–3. Parathyroid hormone (PTH) effects on renal Ca^{2+} reabsorption. The transcellular reabsorption of Ca^{2+} by the distal tubule is regulated by PTH, 1,25(OH)$_2$D, and calcitonin, and by calcium-sparing drugs such as thiazide diuretics. PTH increases the insertion of calcium channels in the apical membrane and facilitates the entry of Ca^{2+}. Inside the cell, Ca^{2+} binds to calbindin-D$_{28K}$, a vitamin D-dependent calcium-binding protein that facilitates the cytosolic diffusion of Ca^{2+} from the apical influx to the basolateral efflux sites. Ca^{2+} transport out of the cell through the basolateral membrane into the interstitial space is mediated by a Na$^+$/Ca^{2+} exchanger and a Ca^{2+}- adenosine triphosphatase (ATPase). Vitamin D contributes to the enhanced calcium reabsorption by stimulating the synthesis of calbindin and the activity of Ca^{2+}-ATPase. ADP, adenosine diphosphate; ATP, adenosine triphosphate.

Ca^{2+} levels. Transport of Ca^{2+} out of the cell into the interstitial space is mediated by a Na$^+$/Ca^{2+} exchanger and a Ca^{2+}-adenosine triphosphatase (ATPase). A similar mechanism to aid in Ca^{2+} absorption is found in intestinal epithelial cells.

PTH decreases the renal (and intestinal) reabsorption of phosphate by decreasing the expression of the type II Na$^+$/PO$_4^{2-}$ cotransporter (Figure 5–4). In the kidney, PTH acutely (in minutes to hours) decreases

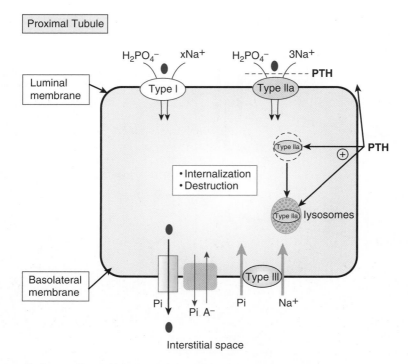

Figure 5–4. Parathyroid hormone (PTH) effects on renal inorganic phosphate reabsorption. Renal reabsorption of phosphate occurs through apical sodium (Na⁺)–inorganic phosphate (Pi) cotransport. Three different Na⁺/Pi cotransporters have been identified: types I, II, and III. Type I and type II cotransporters are located in the apical membrane. Type II cotransporters are expressed in the renal proximal tubule (type IIa) and in the small intestine (type IIb). Type IIa cotransporters are the major target for PTH regulation and contribute to most (up to 70%) of proximal tubular Pi reabsorption. PTH acutely stimulates internalization of the type IIa cotransporters, directing them to the lysosomes for destruction. Type III cotransporters are most likely located at the basolateral membrane and play a general "housekeeping" role in ensuring basolateral P_i influx if apical P_i entry is insufficient to satisfy cellular requirements. Basolateral exit, which is necessary to complete transcellular P_i reabsorption, is not well defined. Several P_i transport pathways have been suggested including Na-P_i cotransport, anion exchange, and even an "unspecific" P_i channel.

the expression of the Na^+/PO_4^{2-} cotransporter by stimulating their internalization via coated vesicles. PTH binding to its receptor initiates signaling pathways (that are still not well understood) leading to membrane retrieval followed by lysosomal degradation of this transporter. The decreased expression of the transporter, results in decreased phosphate reabsorption. Thus, unlike other transporters such as aquaporin 2 (discussed in Chapter 2), once the Na^+/PO_4^{2-} cotransporter is internalized, it is degraded; thus this is an irreversible internalization. Phosphate reabsorption in the proximal tubule can also be decreased by fibroblast growth factor 23 (FGF23), a peptide produced in osteoblasts and osteocytes. FGF23 suppresses 1α-hydroxylase activity and renal and intestinal Na^+/PO_4^{2-} cotransporter expression (discussed in Chapter 10).

In bone, PTH releases calcium from stores that are readily available and in equilibrium with the extracellular fluid (ECF). Subsequently, PTH stimulates release of calcium (and also phosphate) by activation of bone resorption. Thus, PTH is a major mediator of bone remodeling. PTH binds to receptors found in osteoblasts resulting in a cascade of events culminating in osteoclast activation and leading to a rapid release of Ca^{2+} from the bone matrix into the extracellular compartment, where it enters the systemic circulation. These receptor-mediated effects of PTH in osteoblasts are mediated through the synthesis or activity of several proteins, including **osteoclast-differentiating factor (ODF)**, also known as receptor activator of nuclear factor-κB ligand (**RANKL**) or osteoprotegerin ligand (Figure 5–5). PTH-mediated effects in bone involve osteoblast activation and stimulation of genes vital to the processes of degradation of the extracellular matrix and bone remodeling (collagenase-3), production of growth factors (insulin-like growth factor 1), and stimulation and recruitment of osteoclasts (RANKL and interleukin 6). PTH also increases the number of osteoblasts, by decreasing their apoptosis and increasing their proliferation. Although chronic elevations of PTH result in bone resorption, intermittent administration of PTH stimulates bone formation more than bone resorption.

Parathyroid Hormone Mobilization of Bone Ca²⁺

To understand how PTH mobilizes calcium from bone, it is important to have a basic idea of bone structure and of the cells involved in mediating the responses to PTH (see Figure 5–5). Bone consists of an extracellular matrix, the organic phase, which is composed of type I collagen, proteoglycans, and noncollagenous proteins. This extracellular bone matrix also contains growth factors and cytokines that have an important regulatory role in bone remodeling, or formation of new bone. The inorganic phase of bone matrix is composed mainly of calcium hydroxyapatite, which functions as a reservoir of calcium and phosphate ions and plays a major role in the homeostasis of these minerals. Most of the skeleton (80%) is composed of **cortical bone**, found mainly in the shafts of long bones and the surfaces of flat bones. Cortical bone consists of compact bone surrounding central canals (haversian systems) that contain blood vessels, lymphatic tissue, nerves, and connective tissue. **Trabecular bone**, found mainly at the ends of long bones and within flat bones, consists of interconnecting plates and bars, inside which lies hematopoietic or fatty bone marrow. Three cell types are involved in bone metabolism.

Osteoblasts—Osteoblasts express PTH receptors and are responsible for bone formation and mineralization. They are derived from pluripotent mesenchymal stem cells, which can also differentiate into chondrocytes, adipocytes, myoblasts, and fibroblasts. Several hormonal and nonhormonal molecules stimulate the differentiation of osteoblasts from stem cell precursors.

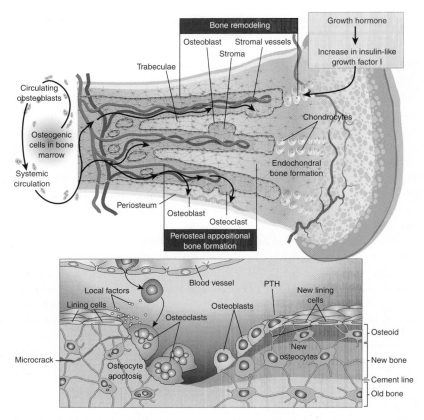

Figure 5–5. Bone remodeling involves bone formation by osteoblasts and bone resorption by osteoclasts. Parathyroid hormone (PTH) stimulates both aspects of the process. Bone remodeling ensures bone repair and is necessary to maintain calcium homeostasis. (Reproduced with permission from Canalis E, Giustina A, Bilezikian JP. Mechanisms of anabolic therapies for osteoporosis. *N Engl J Med.* 2007;357:905–916. Copyright © Massachusetts Medical Society. All rights reserved.)

Osteoclasts—Osteoclasts are large multinucleated bone-resorbing cells derived from hematopoietic precursors of the monocyte-macrophage lineage. They are formed by the fusion of mononuclear cells and are characterized by a ruffled border, which consists of an infolding of the plasma membrane, and a prominent cytoskeleton. Osteoclasts are rich in lysosomal enzymes.

Osteocytes—Osteocytes, the most numerous cells in bone, are small, flattened cells within the bone matrix. They are connected to one another and to osteoblastic cells on the bone surface by an extensive canalicular network that contains the bone's ECF. These cells are terminally differentiated from osteoblasts and ultimately undergo apoptosis or phagocytosis during osteoclastic resorption. Their function and their contribution to osteoclastic bone resorption are not completely understood.

Mechanism of Bone Resorption

Bone remodeling involves the continuous removal of bone (bone resorption) followed by synthesis of new bone matrix and subsequent mineralization (bone formation). This coupling of the functions of osteoblasts and osteoclasts is central not only for the hormonal regulation of bone turnover, but also for the evaluation of their altered function, as discussed later. During skeletal development and throughout life, cells from the osteoblast lineage synthesize and secrete molecules that in turn initiate and control osteoclast differentiation. Osteoclasts are stimulated hormonally and locally by growth factors and cytokines. Osteoclastic activity induced by PTH is indirectly mediated through osteoblast activation. Osteoclastic bone resorption consists of multiple steps, including recruitment and differentiation of osteoclast precursors into mononuclear osteoclasts (preosteoclasts) and fusion of preosteoclasts to form multinucleated functional osteoclasts (Figure 5–6).

The initial event in bone degradation is the attachment of osteoclasts to the bone surface following their recruitment. PTH binding to osteoblasts triggers the synthesis of ODF, also known as RANKL or osteoprotegerin ligand. PTH stimulates the expression of this cell membrane protein in osteoblastic cells. This ligand binds to the ODF receptor (receptor activator of nuclear factor-κB [**RANK**]) expressed on the hemopoietic osteoclastic precursors and stimulates their differentiation into functional osteoclasts. These 2 cell surface proteins, RANK expressed on osteoclast precursor cells and its partner RANKL expressed on osteoblasts, are the key regulators of osteoclast formation and function (see Figures 5–5 and 5–6).

Activation by RANKL increases the expression of specific genes leading to osteoclast maturation. When an osteoclast precursor encounters an osteoblast, the resulting interaction between RANK and RANKL stimulates the osteoclast precursor to mature into a fully differentiated, bone-resorbing osteoclast. Additional proteins play important roles in the regulation of this mechanism. **Osteoprotegerin** is a protein member of the tumor necrosis factor (TNF) receptor superfamily, secreted by osteoblasts which acts as a natural antagonist of RANKL and thus contributes to the regulation of bone resorption. Osteoprotegerin functions as an osteoclastogenesis inhibitory factor. It works as a soluble "decoy" protein that binds to RANKL, preventing it from binding to RANK and thereby effectively inhibiting RANKL-mediated osteoclast maturation. The regulation of osteoprotegerin production is not completely understood. However, it is known that PTH and glucocorticoids decrease the production of osteoprotegerin, whereas estrogens increase its expression.

Osteoclastic bone resorption involves the attachment of osteoclasts by proteins called β-integrins to the bone surface, generating an isolated extracellular microenvironment between osteoclasts and the bone surface that in effect functions as a lysosome. Acidic intracellular vesicles fuse to the ruffled border of the cell membrane facing the bone matrix—the hallmark of the resorbing surface—under which bone resorption takes place. Acidification of this extracellular microenvironment is mediated by H⁺-ATPases recruited into the cell's ruffled membrane. During bone resorption, hydrogen ions generated by carbonic anhydrase II are delivered across the plasma membrane by a proton pump to dissolve bone mineral.

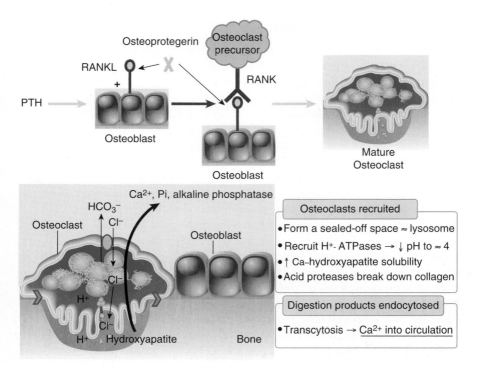

Figure 5–6. PTH effects on bone. PTH binds to osteoblast parathyroid hormone receptor 1 (PTHR1), stimulating the cell surface expression of RANKL, which binds to RANK, a cell surface protein on osteoclast precursors. Binding of RANKL to RANK activates osteoclast gene transcription and the differentiation into a mature osteoclast, characterized by the ruffled membrane under which bone resorption occurs. Osteoclasts attach to the bone surface through β-integrins generating an isolated extracellular microenvironment. Acidic intracellular vesicles fuse to the cell membrane facing the bone matrix forming the scalloped or ruffled border. Hydrogen ions generated by carbonic anhydrase II are delivered across the plasma membrane by H+-ATPases recruited into the cell's ruffled membrane. The acidification of this isolated extracellular microenvironment to a pH of approximately 4 favors the dissolving of hydroxyapatite and provides optimal conditions for the action of the lysosomal proteases including collagenase and cathepsins to dissolve bone mineral. The products of bone degradation are endocytosed by the osteoclast and transported to and released at the cell's antiresorptive surface providing ionized Ca++, inorganic phosphate, and alkaline phosphatases, into circulation. Osteoprotegerin, secreted by osteoblasts serves as a decoy ligand for RANKL, preventing binding of RANKL to RANK, thereby inhibiting the process of osteoclastic bone resorption. Production of osteoprotegerin is increased by estrogen and decreased by glucocorticoids and PTH. ATPase, adenosine triphosphatase; PTH, parathyroid hormone; RANK, receptor activator of nuclear factor-κB; RANKL, receptor activator of nuclear factor-κB ligand.

The decrease in pH (pH 4) in the sealed compartment favors the dissolving of hydroxyapatite bone mineral and provides optimal conditions for the action of the lysosomal proteases, including collagenase and cathepsins secreted by osteoclasts. The products of bone degradation (including Ca^2 and phosphate), are endocytosed by the osteoclast and released at the cell's antiresorptive surface by a process called *transcytosis* (transit across the cell), from where they then reach the systemic circulation. During bone degradation, intracellular enzymes such as alkaline phosphatase are also released into the interstitial space to enter the circulation. An increase in circulating levels of alkaline phosphatase can be used clinically as a marker of increased osteoclastic activity.

CALCIUM HOMEOSTASIS

The human body contains approximately 1100 g of calcium, 99% of which is deposited in bones and teeth. The small amount found in plasma is divided into 3 fractions: ionized calcium (50%), protein-bound calcium (40%), and calcium complexed to citrate and phosphate forming soluble complexes (10%) (Figure 5–7). The complexed and ionized Ca^{2+} fractions (approximately 60% of plasma Ca^{2+}) can cross the plasma membrane. The majority (80%–90%) of protein-bound Ca^{2+} is bound to albumin, and this interaction is sensitive to changes in blood pH.

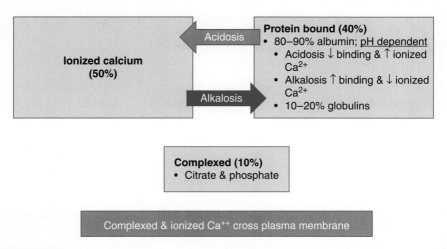

Figure 5–7. Distribution of plasma calcium. Three fractions are identified for circulating calcium—ionized (50%), protein-bound (40%), and complexed—forming soluble complexes (10%). The complexed and ionized Ca^{2+} fractions (approximately 60% of plasma Ca^{2+}) can cross the plasma membrane. The majority of protein-bound Ca^{2+} is bound to albumin, and this interaction is sensitive to changes in blood pH. Acidosis increases "free" or ionized Ca^{2+} in the plasma. Alkalosis decreases ionized Ca^{2+} in the plasma. Hyperventilation resulting in respiratory alkalosis results in neuromuscular hyperexcitability manifested by numbness and carpal spasm caused by reduced neuronal threshold for the action potential firing.

Acidosis leads to a decrease in protein binding of Ca^{2+} and an increase in "free" or ionized Ca^{2+} in the plasma. Alkalosis results in increased Ca^{2+} binding and a decrease in ionized Ca^{2+} in the plasma. A smaller fraction (10%–20%) of protein-bound Ca^{2+} is bound to globulins.

The resting intracellular (cytosolic) calcium concentration is approximately 100 nM, but this can increase to 1 μM by the release of Ca^{2+} from intracellular stores or by uptake of extracellular Ca^{2+} in response to cellular activation. In contrast, the extracellular ionized calcium concentration is approximately 10,000-fold higher than the intracellular calcium concentration and remains virtually constant at approximately 1 mM. Multiple physiologic functions involve calcium ions. Ca^{2+} is a key intracellular messenger and cofactor for various enzymes. Ca^{2+} also has diverse extracellular functions (eg, in the clotting of blood, maintenance of skeletal integrity, and modulation of neuromuscular excitability). Therefore, stable Ca^{2+} levels are critical for normal physiologic function. For example, Na^+ channel voltage-gating is dependent on the extracellular Ca^{2+} concentration. Decreased plasma Ca^{2+} concentrations reduce the voltage threshold for the action potential firing, resulting in neuromuscular hyperexcitability. This can result in numbness and tingling of fingertips, toes, and the perioral region or muscle cramps. Clinically, neuromuscular irritability can be demonstrated by mechanical stimulation of the hyperexcitable nerve leading to tetanic-like muscle contraction by eliciting Chvostek (ipsilateral contraction of facial muscles elicited by tapping the skin over the facial nerve) or Trousseau (carpal spasm induced by inflation of the blood pressure cuff to 20 mm Hg above the patient's systolic blood pressure for 3–5 minutes) sign.

Interaction of Bone, Kidney and Intestine in Maintaining Calcium Homeostasis

Normal plasma concentrations of Ca^{2+} range between 8.5 and 10.5 mg/dL and are mainly regulated by the actions of PTH, vitamin D, and calcitonin on 3 tissues: bone, kidney, and intestine.

Bone—Calcium in bone is distributed in a readily exchangeable pool and a stable pool. The readily exchangeable pool is involved in maintaining Ca^{2+} plasma levels by the daily exchange of 550 mg of calcium between the bone and ECF. The stable Ca^{2+} pool is involved in bone remodeling. Bone is metabolically active throughout life. After skeletal growth is complete, remodeling of both cortical and trabecular bone continues with an annual turnover rate of approximately 10% of the adult skeleton.

Kidney—In the kidney, virtually all filtered Ca^{2+} is reabsorbed. Approximately 40% of the Ca^{2+} that is reabsorbed is under hormonal regulation by PTH. Most filtered Ca^{2+} is reabsorbed in the proximal tubules, mainly by passive transport processes independent of hormonal regulation. Ca^{2+} absorption in the cortical thick ascending limbs is mediated by a combination of active and passive absorption. Ca^{2+} absorption in the distal convoluted tubules is mediated by active cellular absorption, which is stimulated by PTH binding to PTHR1. Transcellular transport of Ca^{2+} is facilitated by vitamin D through the increase in the Ca^{2+}-binding protein calbindin-D_{28K} and in the expression of Ca^{2+} transporters in the basolateral membrane.

Intestine—The availability of dietary calcium is a critical determinant of calcium homeostasis. Dietary intake of calcium averages 1000 mg/d, of which only 30% is absorbed in the intestinal tract (Figure 5–8). This percentage of dietary Ca^{2+} that is absorbed is significantly enhanced by vitamin D during growth, pregnancy, and lactation. During growth, there is a net bone accretion. After completion of the growth phase in the young and healthy individual, there is no net gain or loss of Ca^{2+} from bone despite a continuous turnover of bone mass; the amount of Ca^{2+} lost in urine is approximately equal to net Ca^{2+} absorption.

Intestinal absorption of Ca^{2+} occurs by a saturable, transcellular process and a nonsaturable, paracellular pathway. The paracellular pathway predominates when dietary Ca^{2+} is abundant. The active transcellular pathway is vitamin D–dependent and plays a major role in absorption when the Ca^{2+} supply is limited. Intestinal transepithelial Ca^{2+} transport, similar to that in the distal tubule, is a 3-step process consisting of passive entry across the apical membrane, cytosolic diffusion facilitated by vitamin D–dependent calcium-binding proteins (calbindins), and active extrusion of Ca^{2+} across the opposing basolateral membrane mediated by a high-affinity Ca^{2+}-ATPase and Na$^+$/Ca^{2+} exchanger.

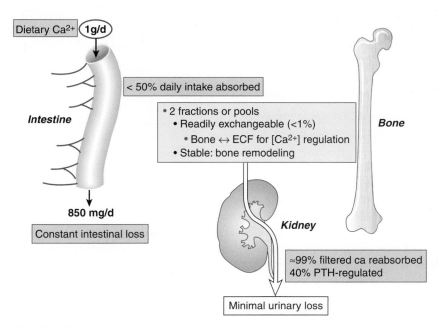

Figure 5–8. Calcium balance. Dietary intake of calcium averages 1 g/d and is a critical determinant of calcium homeostasis. A small fraction is absorbed in the intestinal tract, and this is significantly enhanced by vitamin D. Calcium in bone is distributed in a readily exchangeable pool and a stable pool. The readily exchangeable pool is involved in maintaining Ca^{2+} plasma levels. The stable Ca^{2+} pool is involved in bone remodeling. Virtually all filtered Ca^{2+} is reabsorbed, and approximately 40% of the Ca^{2+} that is reabsorbed is under hormonal regulation by PTH. ECF, extracellular fluid; PTH, parathyroid hormone.

Hormonal Regulation of Calcium Homeostasis

As explained previously, a slight decrease in the free ionized Ca^{2+} level is sensed through the Ca^{2+} sensor in parathyroid chief cells, resulting in an increased release of PTH. PTH binds to receptors in osteoblasts leading to the recruitment of pre-osteoclasts and their maturation to active osteoclasts, which are responsible for increased bone resorption and release Ca^{2+} and inorganic phosphate (Pi) into the circulation. In the kidney, PTH promotes Ca^{2+} reabsorption and Pi excretion in urine. In addition, PTH stimulates the hydroxylation of 25-hydroxyvitamin D_3 at the 1-position, leading to the formation of the active form of vitamin D (calcitriol). Vitamin D increases intestinal absorption of dietary Ca^{2+} and renal reabsorption of filtered Ca^{2+}. In bone, vitamin D increases the number of osteoclasts and stimulates bone resorption, with a resulting increase in the release of Ca^{2+} into the circulation. An increase in free ionized Ca^{2+} levels decreases the release of PTH from the para-thyroid gland, decreases the activation of vitamin D in the kidney, and stimulates parafollicular cells of the thyroid gland to release the hormone calcitonin.

Calcitonin counteracts the effects of PTH. Calcitonin inhibits osteoclast activity, decreasing bone resorption and increases renal Ca^{2+} excretion; the result is a decrease in free ionized Ca^{2+} levels. Overall, PTH, calcitriol, and calcitonin work together to maintain plasma Ca^{2+} levels within a normal range. The previous section described in detail the physiologic effects of PTH. The following section discusses the contributions of vitamin D and calcitonin to the regulation of Ca^{2+} homeostasis.

Role of Vitamin D in Calcium Homeostasis

Synthesis and Activation of Vitamin D

Vitamin D is a lipid-soluble vitamin that can be synthesized from plant-derived precursors or through the action of sunlight from cholesterol-derived precursors found in the skin (see Figure 5–7) or obtained from dietary intake of fortified milk, fatty fish, cod-liver oil, and, to a lesser extent, eggs. Active vitamin D (calcitriol) is the product of 2 consecutive hydroxylation steps, (first in the liver and then in the kidney) of its precursors, cholecalciferol (derived from skin) and ergocalciferol (derived from diet). Cholecalciferol is produced in the skin by ultraviolet radiation from 7-dehydrocholesterol, an inert precursor. This previtamin D_3 (cho-lecalciferol) is isomerized to vitamin D_3 and is transported in the circulation bound to vitamin D-binding protein; the major plasma carrier protein of vitamin D and its metabolites. Cholecalciferol (vitamin D_3) and vitamin D_2 (ergocalciferol from plants) are transported to the liver, where they undergo the first step in bioactivation, the hydroxylation at C-25 to 25-hydroxyvitamin D [25(OH)D]. The resulting prehor-mone, 25-hydroxyvitamin D, is the major circulating form of vitamin D (15–60 ng/mL). 25-hydroxyvitamin D is the principle storage form of vitamin D, has a half-life of 15 days, is in equilibrium with the storage pool in muscle and fat, and is the value measured by most clinical laboratories to assess levels of vitamin D in individuals.

25-hydroxyvitamin D circulates bound to vitamin D–binding protein. This protein can be filtered at the glomerulus and enter the proximal tubular facilitating the delivery of the precursor, 25-hydroxyvitamin D, to the 1α-hydroxylase.

Renal 1α-hydroxylase (under regulation by PTH) is the enzyme responsible for the second step in the activation of the prehormone, the hydroxylation at C-1, resulting in the hormonally active vitamin D [$1,25(OH)_2D$], also known as **calcitriol**. Calcitriol is released into the circulation (20–60 pg/mL), where it functions as an endocrine hormone, regulating cellular processes in a host of target tissues. This second hydroxylation step, the production of $1,25(OH)_2D$ by 1α-hydroxylase in the kidney, is a tightly regulated process and is a central factor in the feedback regulation of calcium homeostasis. The production of the active form of vitamin D is under negative feedback regulation by plasma Ca^{2+} levels. An increase in plasma Ca^{2+} levels inhibits the hydroxylation at C-1 and favors hydroxylation at C-24, leading to the synthesis of an inactive metabolite of vitamin D [$24,25(OH)_2D$].

In summary, PTH stimulates the activity of 1α-hydroxylase, favoring an increase in the synthesis of the active form of vitamin D. Vitamin D, as well as high Ca^{2+} levels, suppress the activity of 1α-hydroxylase, decreasing its own synthesis and favoring the synthesis of $24,25(OH_2)D$, the less active form of the hormone (Figure 5–9).

CELLULAR EFFECTS OF VITAMIN D

The principal physiologic effects mediated by vitamin D result from its binding to a vitamin D steroid receptor located in the principal target organs; intestine, bone, kidney, and parathyroid gland (see Figure 5–9). The receptor has high affinity for calcitriol and very low affinity for the metabolites of the hormone. The effects of active vitamin D are primarily to increase intestinal Ca^{2+} absorption, facilitate PTH-mediated calcium reabsorption in the distal renal tubules, and to suppress the synthesis and release of PTH from the parathyroid gland. Vitamin D also plays a role in regulation of bone resorption and formation. Additional tissues including skin, lymphocytes, skeletal and cardiac muscle, breast, and anterior pituitary express receptors for calcitriol. Thus, calcitriol has additional physiologic effects in modulating immune response, reproduction, cardiovascular function, and cellular differentiation and proliferation.

Vitamin D is able to generate biologic effects both by genomic mechanisms (changes in gene transcription) and rapid nongenomic mechanisms. The genomic effects are dependent on the interaction of $1,25(OH)_2D$ with a cytosolic-nuclear receptor protein, followed by interaction of the steroid-receptor complex in the nucleus with selective regions of the promoters of genes that are either activated or repressed. The stimulation of rapid responses by $1,25(OH)_2D$ may result from interaction of the vitamin with a cell membrane receptor for $1,25(OH)_2D$ that activates a variety of signal transduction systems, including protein kinase C, phospholipase C, and adenylate cyclase, and modulates ion (ie, Ca^{2+} or Cl^-) channels.

ABNORMAL VITAMIN D LEVELS

The US recommended daily allowance of vitamin D is 200 U for adults and 400 U for children, pregnant women, and lactating women. Vitamin D belongs to the class of vitamins that are lipid soluble (ie, A, D, E, and K) and can be stored in tissues. Excess vitamin D may lead to problems such as calcinosis (calcification of soft tissues), deposition of Ca^{2+} and PO_4 in the kidney, and increased plasma Ca^{2+} levels, resulting in cardiac arrhythmia.

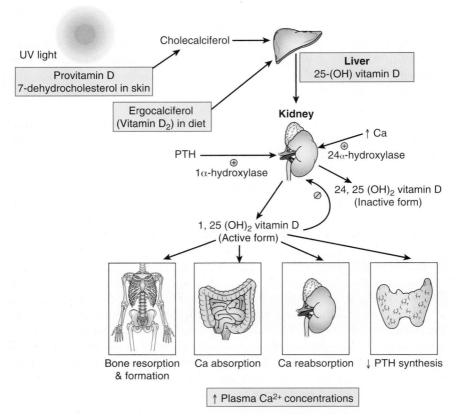

Figure 5–9. Vitamin D metabolism and physiologic effects at target organs. Provitamin D (7-dehydrocholesterol) in the skin is converted to cholecalciferol by ultraviolet (UV) light. Cholecalciferol and ergocalciferol (from plants) are transported to the liver, where they undergo the first step in bioactivation, the hydroxylation at C-25 to 25-hydroxyvitamin D_3 [25(OH)D], the major circulating form of vitamin D. The second hydroxylation step, at C-1, occurs in the kidney and results in the hormonally active vitamin D [1,25(OH)$_2$D], also known as calcitriol. This activation step, mediated by 1α-hydroxylase, is under tight regulation by parathyroid hormone (PTH), Ca^{2+} levels, and vitamin D [1,25(OH)$_2$D]. The activity of 1α-hydroxylase is stimulated by PTH and inhibited by Ca^{2+} and 1,25(OH)$_2$D. Decreased activity of 1α-hydroxylase favors formation of the inactive form of vitamin D by C-24 hydroxylation. Vitamin D increases bone resorption and formation, increases dietary Ca^{2+} absorption, facilitates renal Ca^{2+} reabsorption, and decreases the PTH synthesis by the parathyroid glands. The overall effect of vitamin D is to increase plasma Ca^{2+} concentrations.

Deficiency of vitamin D can be the result of decreased dietary intake or lack of sunlight and the resulting decreased conversion from the inactive precursor in skin to the active form of the vitamin. Vitamin D deficiency results in bone deformities (rickets) when it occurs in children and decreased bone mass (osteomalacia) in adults. Vitamin D deficiency is associated with weakness, bowing of the weight-bearing bones, dental defects, and hypocalcemia. Factors that may contribute to vitamin D deficiency include the use of sunscreen, particularly in the elderly population; lack of sunlight during November through March in certain latitudes (above 40 N and below 40 S); and use of clothing that covers most of the skin. Less frequently, people may have a mutation in 1α-hydroxylase, the enzyme that catalyzes the second and final step in vitamin D activation, or a resistance to vitamin D action in the tissues caused by mutations in the vitamin D receptor.

Role of Calcitonin in Calcium Homeostasis

A third hormone involved in calcium homeostasis, although to a lesser extent than PTH and vitamin D, is calcitonin. Calcitonin is a 32–amino acid peptide hormone derived from procalcitonin, produced by cells of neural crest origin (parafollicular or C cells) in the thyroid gland. Calcitonin belongs to a family of peptides including amylin, calcitonin gene-related peptides (CGRPs) and adrenomedullin. These are distributed in various peripheral tissues as well as in the central nervous system and induce multiple biologic effects including potent vasodilatation (CGRP and adrenomedullin), reduction in nutrient intake (amylin), and decreased bone resorption (calcitonin).

The release of calcitonin is regulated by plasma calcium levels through a Ca^{2+} receptor on the parafollicular cells. Elevations in plasma Ca^{2+} higher than 9 mg/dL stimulate the release of calcitonin. Calcitonin has a half-life of approximately 5 minutes and is metabolized and cleared by the kidney and the liver. The release of calcitonin is also stimulated by gastrin, a gastrointestinal hormone.

CELLULAR EFFECTS OF CALCITONIN

The main physiologic function of calcitonin is to decrease plasma Ca^{2+} and phosphate concentrations, mainly by decreasing bone resorption. The 2 target organs for calcitonin's physiologic effects are bone and kidney. The overall effect of calcitonin in bone is to inhibit bone resorption, predominantly by inhibition of osteoclast motility, differentiation, and ruffled border formation. Calcitonin inhibits osteoclast secretory activity (particularly of tartrate-resistant acid phosphatase), alters Na^+-K^+-ATPase activity, carbonic anhydrase localization, and inhibits H^+-ATPase activity, reducing osteoclast acid secretion. In the kidney, calcitonin increases urinary Ca^{2+} excretion by inhibition of renal tubular calcium reabsorption. The mechanism involved is through opening of low affinity Ca^{2+} channels in the luminal membrane and the stimulation of the Na^+/Ca^{2+} exchanger in the basolateral membrane, both actions depending on the activation of adenylate cyclase. In hypercalcemic patients with metastatic bone disease, the administration of calcitonin induces a rapid decrease in plasma calcium primarily through inhibition of renal tubular reabsorption.

CALCITONIN RECEPTORS

The cellular effects of calcitonin are mediated through G protein (G_s, G_q, or G_i)–coupled receptors from the same receptor family as the PTH, PTHrP, calcitonin, adrenomedullin, secretin receptor superfamily. Several calcitonin receptor subtypes have been identified, and they all bind calcitonin with high affinity.

Calcitonin binding to its receptor stimulates adenylate cyclase, increasing the formation of cAMP and activation of protein kinase A and phospholipase C, resulting in the release of Ca^{2+} from intracellular stores and influx of extracellular Ca^{2+}.

CALCITONIN AND DISEASE

Calcitonin does not appear to be critical for the regulation of calcium homeostasis; in fact, total removal of the thyroid does not produce major alterations in Ca^{2+} homeostasis. In addition, no significant clinical findings have been associated with calcitonin excess or deficiency.

However, calcitonin has been used therapeutically for the prevention of bone loss and for the short-term treatment of hypercalcemia of malignancy. Osteoporosis is a systemic skeletal disease characterized by low bone mass and deterioration of bone tissue, resulting in bone fragility and susceptibility to fracture (discussed in Chapter 10). The ability of calcitonin to inhibit osteoclast-mediated bone resorption has made it a useful agent for the treatment of osteoporosis; it also relieves pain in osteoporotic patients with vertebral crush fractures. Calcitonin is also used in the treatment of Paget disease, which is characterized by an abnormality in bone remodeling, with increased bone resorption and hypercalcemia.

Additional Regulators of Ca^{2+} and Bone Metabolism

Although PTH and vitamin D play central roles in the regulation of bone metabolism, the contribution of other hormones cannot be ignored (Table 5–2). Sex steroids (androgens and estrogens) have been shown to increase 1α-hydroxylase activity, decrease bone resorption, and increase osteoprotegerin synthesis. Estrogen stimulates the proliferation of osteoblasts and the expression of type I

Table 5–2. Factors involved in the regulation of Ca^{2+} and bone metabolism

Regulator	Action
PTH	Increases bone resorption and plasma Ca^{2+}
Vitamin D	Increases intestinal Ca^{2+} absorption, bone resorption, and plasma Ca^{2+}
Calcitonin	Decreases bone resorption and plasma Ca^{2+}
Sex steroids (androgens and estrogens)	Increase 1α-hydroxylase activity, Increase osteoprotegerin synthesis Net decrease in bone loss
Growth hormone and insulinlike growth factor	Stimulate bone synthesis and growth
Thyroid hormone	Increases bone resorption
Prolactin	Increases renal Ca^{2+} reabsorption and 1α-hydroxylase activity
Glucocorticoids	Increase bone resorption, decrease bone synthesis
Inflammatory cytokines	Increase bone resorption

PTH, parathyroid hormone.

collagen and alkaline phosphatase; influences the expression of receptors for vitamin D, growth hormone, and progesterone; and modulates responsiveness of bone to PTH. Estrogen decreases the number and activity of osteoclasts, as well as the synthesis of cytokines affecting bone resorption.

Growth hormone and insulin-like growth factor-1 (IGF-1) both exert effects on bone metabolism. Growth hormone stimulates the proliferation and differentiation of osteoblasts and bone protein synthesis and growth. IGF-1 produced by the liver and locally by osteoblasts, stimulate bone formation by increasing the proliferation of osteoblast precursors and by enhancing the synthesis and inhibiting the degradation of type I collagen. Normal thyroid function is required for physiologic bone remodeling. However, excess thyroid hormone levels result in increased bone resorption. Prolactin increases Ca^{2+} reabsorption and 1α-hydroxylase activity, indirectly modulating bone metabolism. Glucocorticoids play an overall catabolic role in bone metabolism by increasing bone resorption and decreasing bone synthesis, resulting in an increase in the risk of fractures. The mechanisms by which glucocorticoids exert their effects are not fully understood, but inhibition of osteoprotegerin may help stimulate osteoclastic bone resorption. The cytokines tumor necrosis factor, interleukin 1, and interleukin 6 increase the proliferation and differentiation of osteoclast precursors and their osteoclastic activity and are therefore potent stimulators of bone resorption in vitro and in vivo. The overall interaction of these various factors during health and disease plays an important role in maintaining bone mass. Their specific contributions may vary depending on the disease and on the prevailing hormone and cytokine levels in bone.

HORMONAL REGULATION OF BONE METABOLISM

Bone remodeling results from the interactions of multiple elements, including osteoblasts, osteoclasts, hormones, growth factors, and cytokines, the result being a dynamic maintenance of the bone architecture and systemic preservation of calcium homeostasis. Quiescent bone is covered by flat bone-lining cells. During bone resorption, osteoclasts are recruited and activated to remove both organic matrix and mineral content of bone to produce a pit. During bone formation, osteoblasts deposit osteoid in the pit, which is then mineralized under osteoblastic control. Hormones can influence bone remodelling at any stage throughout the remodelling cycle through direct effects on either osteoblasts or osteoclasts to alter either bone resorption or bone formation. It is important to remember that, in vivo, normal bone structure is maintained by complex interactions between osteoblasts and osteoclasts.

In early life, a careful balance exists between bone formation by osteoblasts and bone resorption by osteoclasts. With aging, the process of coupled bone formation-resorption is affected by the reductions in osteoblast differentiation, activity, and life span, which are further potentiated in the perimenopausal years by hormone deprivation (estrogen, testosterone, and adrenal-derived androgens) and an increase in osteoclast activity.

Decreased calcium intake below obligatory calcium loss (through the urine, feces, and skin) mobilizes calcium from the skeleton to maintain the ionized calcium concentration in the ECF, resulting in bone destruction. Vitamin D deficiency lowers the concentration of ionized calcium in the ECF (from loss of the calcemic action of vitamin D on bone), resulting in stimulation of PTH release (secondary hyperparathyroidism), increased phosphate excretion leading to hypophosphatemia, and failure to mineralize new bone as it is being formed. Simple calcium deficiency is associated with compensatory increases in PTH and calcitriol, which together mobilize calcium from bone, potentially decreasing bone mass. True vitamin D deficiency, however, reduces the mineral content of the bony tissue itself and leads to abnormal bone composition. However, these 2 nutritional deficiencies cannot be completely separated because calcium malabsorption is the first manifestation of vitamin D deficiency.

Childhood and puberty—Bone mass increases throughout childhood and adolescence. In girls, the rate of increase in bone mass decreases rapidly after menarche, whereas in boys, gains in bone mass persist up to 17 years of age and are closely linked to pubertal stage and androgen status. By age 17–23 years, the majority of peak bone mass has already been achieved in both sexes. Skeletal growth is achieved primarily through bone modeling and only partially through bone remodeling. These mechanisms involve interaction between osteoblasts and osteoclasts, which work cooperatively under the influence of the mechanical strain placed on bone by skeletal muscle force such as that exerted during exercise. The mechanical loading or strain oscillates within a given range in response to physical activity, leading to bone maintenance without loss or gain. Decreased mechanical strain (such as that associated with prolonged bed rest or immobilization) leads to bone loss, whereas increased mechanical strain (weight-bearing exercise) stimulates osteoblastic activity and bone formation. The loading on the bone cells is exerted primarily by muscles and to a lesser extent by body weight. Muscle force or tension applied on long bones increases the thickness of cortical bone through continuous subperiosteal accretion. This relationship between muscle tension exerted on bones and bone formation is positively affected during exercise.

Peak bone mass is attained in the third decade of life and is maintained until the fifth decade, when age-related bone loss begins both in men and women. Sex steroids play an important role in bone growth and the attainment of peak bone mass. They are also responsible for the sexual dimorphism of the skeleton, which emerges during adolescence and is characterized by larger bone size in males (even when corrected for body height and weight), with both a larger diameter and a greater cortical thickness in the long bones.

Pregnancy and lactation—The uptake and release of calcium from the skeleton are increased during pregnancy, and the rate of calcium mobilization continues to be increased during the early months of lactation, returning to prepregnancy rates during or after weaning. Intestinal calcium absorption and bone mobilization are higher during pregnancy than before conception or after delivery. Urinary calcium excretion is increased during pregnancy, and may be a reflection of the increased glomerular filtration rate, exceeding calcium reabsorption capacity during that period. The increases are evident in early to midpregnancy and precede the increased demand for calcium by the fetus for skeletal growth. The alterations in calcium and bone metabolism during pregnancy are accompanied by increases in vitamin D, but without significant alterations in either intact PTH or calcitonin concentrations. The increase in intestinal calcium absorption is associated with a doubling of 1,25-dihydroxyvitamin D levels and increased intestinal expression of the vitamin D-dependent calcium-binding protein calbindin. Changes in maternal bone mineral content during this period may influence bone mineral status in the long term. After delivery, calcium absorption and urinary calcium excretion return to prepregnancy rates. However, lactating mothers have decreased urinary calcium output and higher bone turnover than at the end of pregnancy. During this period, approximately 5 mmol/d (200 mg/d) of calcium is provided to the infant through breast milk, and this can exceed 10 mmol/d (400 mg/d) in some women. Thus, requirements for calcium are significantly increased during pregnancy and lactation.

Menopause— The acute loss of bone that accompanies menopause involves most of the skeleton but particularly affects the trabecular component. The associated biochemical changes include increases in the complexed fraction of plasma calcium (bicarbonate), increases in plasma alkaline phosphatase and urinary hydroxyproline (representing increased bone resorption followed by a compensatory increase in bone formation), increased obligatory calcium loss in the urine, and a small but significant decline in calcium absorption (Table 5–3). These changes are ameliorated by hormone treatment, calcium supplementation, thiazide administration (which reduces calcium excretion), and restriction of salt intake, which reduces obligatory calcium loss. In some (50%) cases of osteoporosis, calcium absorption is low, and high bone resorption can be suppressed by treatment with vitamin D which in turn leads to improvement in calcium absorption. In males, bone loss begins at approximately the age of 50 years, but it is not associated with an increase in bone resorption markers. Instead, bone loss in men is linked to an age-related decline in gonadal function and is caused by a decrease in bone formation, not so much as an increase in bone resorption.

Estrogen deficiency is a major pathogenic factor in the bone loss associated with menopause and the subsequent development of postmenopausal osteoporosis. Estrogen replacement at or after menopause, whether natural or induced, prevents menopausal bone loss and usually results in an increase in bone mineral density (BMD) during the first 12–18 months of treatment. Estrogen regulates osteoclast activity through effects on osteoclast number, resorptive activity, and life span of the cell. The process of bone loss is progressive, starting at approximately the age of 50 in men and at menopause in women, and loss proceeds at an average rate of 1% per year to the end of life. Bone loss is faster in women than in men and affects some bones more than others; the consequences include decreased BMD and increased risk of fractures.

BONE DENSITY

Bone density determines the degree of osteoporosis and the fracture risk. The main determinants of peak bone density are genetics, calcium intake, and exercise. The most common test for measuring bone density is dual-energy x-ray absorptiometry (DEXA) scanning. Additional approaches include computed tomography, radiologic

Table 5–3. Parameters used for evaluation of parathyroid hormone function, bone metabolism, or Ca^{2+} homeostasis

Parameter	Normal range	Abnormality
Ionized calcium	8.5–10.5 mg/dL	Elevated with ↑ PTH, ↑ vitamin D, ↑ bone resorption
Plasma phosphate	3–4.5 mg/dL	Decreased in hyperparathyroidism, vitamin D deficiency Increased in renal failure, hypoparathyroidism, vitamin D intoxication
Intact plasma PTH levels	10–65 pg/mL	Elevated in hyperparathyroidism; decreased in hypoparathyroidism
Alkaline phosphatase	30–120 U/L	High levels indicate increased osteoblastic activity (bone turnover)
Bone-specific alkaline phosphatase	17–48 U/L	High bone turnover, useful marker of active bone formation
N-telopeptide (NTX)	21–83 nM BCE/ mM creatinine	Reflects collagen breakdown, marker of bone resorption
C-telopeptide (CTX)	60–780 pg/mL	Reflects collagen breakdown, marker of bone resorption
N-terminal propeptide of type I procollagen (PINP)	2.3–6.4 µg/L	By-product of type I collagen deposition, marker of bone formation
Osteocalcin (intact)	<1–23 ng/mL	Reflects activity of osteoblasts, marker for skeletal bone turnover
tartrate-resistant acid phosphatase (TRAP)	<5 ng/mL	Marker for osteoclastic activity (bone resorption)

BCE, bone collagen equivalent; PTH, parathyroid hormone.

techniques (morphometry or densitometry), or bone biopsy. DEXA uses x-rays to measure bone density and provides 2 measures of how dense bone is: the T score and the Z score. The T score compares the person's bone density with the average bone density of 25- to 30-year-olds of the same sex. This age group is used because it is when bone density is at its peak. A T score of 0 means that bone density is the same as the average bone density of 25- to 30-year-olds. A score above 0 (a positive score) means that bones are more dense than the average. A score below 0 (a negative score) means that bones are less dense than the average. The Z score compares a person's bone density with that of people of the same age, sex, and weight, and is less valuable in making predictions of risk of fracture or in making decisions about treatment.

PREVENTION OF OSTEOPOROSIS

Understanding of the hormonal and nutritional regulation of calcium balance has led to the implementation of several measures to reduce bone loss. The principal current approaches are the following.

Estrogen replacement therapy—Estrogen decreases bone loss in postmenopausal women by inhibiting bone resorption, resulting in a 5%–10% increase in BMD over 1–3 years. Estrogen treatment is approved for prevention of osteoporosis. Calcium supplements enhance the effect of estrogen on BMD.

Bisphosphonates—Bisphosphonates have a strong affinity for bone apatite and are potent inhibitors of bone resorption. Bisphosphonates reduce the recruitment and activity of osteoclasts and increase their apoptosis.

Calcitonin—Calcitonin reduces bone resorption by direct inhibition of osteoclast activity. Calcitonin is less effective in prevention of cortical bone loss than cancellous bone loss in postmenopausal women. Calcitonin is approved for treatment of osteoporosis in women who have been postmenopausal for 5 or more years.

Parathyroid hormone—Human recombinant PTH is approved for the treatment of osteoporosis in postmenopausal women and men who are at high risk for fracture. Intermittent PTH administration stimulates new bone formation at the periosteal (outer) and endosteal (inner) bone surfaces and thickening the cortices and existing trabeculae of the skeleton.

Selective estrogen receptor modulators—Selective estrogen receptor modulators (SERMs) are compounds that exert estrogenic effects in specific tissues and antiestrogenic effects in others. Raloxifene, a SERM competitively inhibits the action of estrogen in the breast and the endometrium and acts as an estrogen agonist on bone and lipid metabolism. In early postmenopausal women, raloxifene prevents postmenopausal bone loss at all skeletal sites, reduces markers of bone turnover to premenopausal concentrations, and reduces the serum cholesterol concentration and its low-density lipoprotein fraction without stimulating proliferation in the endometrium. Because raloxifene does not have agonistic effects on the endometrium, unwanted vaginal bleeding and increased risk of endometrial cancer are avoided. Thus, it exerts the beneficial effects of estrogen in the skeleton and cardiovascular system without its adverse effects in the breast and endometrium.

Vitamin D analogs—Vitamin D analogs induce a small increase in BMD that seems to be limited to the spine.

Exercise—Physical activity early in life contributes to high peak bone mass. Various activities, including walking, weight training, and high-impact exercises, induce a small (1%–2%) increase in BMD at some, but not all, skeletal sites. These effects disappear if the exercise program is stopped. Load-bearing exercise is more effective for increasing bone mass than are other types of exercise. Some of the benefits of exercise may be caused by increases in muscle mass and strength, plus a reduction in the risk of falls by approximately 25% in frail elderly individuals.

DISEASES OF PARATHYROID HORMONE PRODUCTION

Primary Hyperparathyroidism

Primary hyperparathyroidism is the result of excess PTH production caused by parathyroid gland hyperplasia, adenoma, or carcinoma. The clinical manifestations include elevated intact PTH levels; increased plasma calcium levels (hypercalcemia); increased urinary calcium excretion (hypercalciuria), which may lead to increased formation of kidney stones (urolithiasis); and decreased plasma phosphate levels. The elevation of PTH results in increased bone resorption and further increases in extracellular calcium concentrations.

Secondary Hyperparathyroidism

Secondary hyperparathyroidism, is the result of alterations outside of the parathyroid gland. Most frequently, it is a complication that occurs in patients with chronic renal failure. In early renal failure, a reduction in plasma vitamin D and moderate decreases in ionized Ca^{2+} contribute to greater synthesis and secretion of PTH. As renal disease progresses, parathyroid expression of vitamin D and Ca^{2+} receptors is reduced, making the parathyroid gland very resistant to both the vitamin D and Ca^{2+} negative feedback regulation of PTH release. Thus, for any increase in plasma Ca^{2+}, the inhibition of PTH secretion is less efficient. As a result, for any particular plasma Ca^{2+} concentration, secretion of PTH is enhanced, resulting in a shift in the Ca^{2+}-PTH set point toward secondary hyperparathyroidism. Hyperphosphatemia (higher than 5 mg/dL in adults), independent of Ca^{2+} and calcitriol levels, further enhances uremia-induced parathyroid gland hyperplasia and PTH synthesis and secretion, the latter by post-transcriptional mechanisms as discussed in Chapter 10.

Hypoparathyroidism

Hypoparathyroidism or low PTH levels may result from surgical removal of the parathyroid glands or can be associated with other endocrine disorders and neoplasias. Because of the important role of PTH in the acute regulation of plasma Ca^{2+} levels, an early manifestation of surgical removal of the parathyroid glands is hypocalcemic tetany. The classic clinical sign is known as the *Chvostek sign*, which is twitching or contraction of the facial muscles in response to tapping the facial nerve at a point anterior to the ear and above the zygomatic bone.

Pseudohypoparathyroidism

Pseudohypoparathyroidism or "not real" hypoparathyroidism is not caused by decreased PTH levels, but by an abnormal response to PTH because of a congenital defect in the G protein associated with the PTHR1. Pseudohypoparathyroidism type Ia is characterized by a generalized hormone resistance to PTH, thyroid-stimulating hormone, luteinizing hormone, and follicle-stimulating hormone and is associated with abnormal physical features including short stature and skeletal anomalies. Pseudohypoparathyroidism type Ib is characterized by renal resistance to PTH and normal appearance. In these patients, the PTHR1 has decreased $G\alpha_s$ activity, and this can be tested by measuring the increase in urinary cAMP in response to PTH administration (which should be low in patients with defective $G\alpha_s$ activity). Patients present with low plasma Ca^{2+} (caused by inability of PTH to increase calcium reabsorption), high phosphate levels (caused by inability to excrete phosphate), and elevated PTH levels (parathyroid gland's attempt to respond to the low calcium and elevated phosphate levels).

Clinical Evaluation of Parathyroid Hormone Abnormalities

Patients' clinical manifestations can be combined with indices of hormone levels (PTH and vitamin D), the metabolites that the hormones regulate (calcium and Pi), and the target tissue effects of excess hormone production (bone densitometry). In addition, magnesium levels, when extremely low can prevent PTH release in response to hypocalcemia, so their determination is also important for overall evaluation. As seen in the brief overview of some of these measures (see Table 5–3 and Appendix), the laboratory values indicate the physiologic regulation of PTH, vitamin D, phosphate, and calcium levels. Plasma PTH levels are determined using radioimmunoassay or more specific and sensitive radioimmunometric assays. Because PTH loses its activity once it is cleaved, only the intact PTH measurement is a reliable indicator of hormone status. Vitamin D levels can be measured, although this test is expensive and time consuming; therefore, the concentrations of the precursor 25-hydroxyvitamin D are used more frequently. Bone density studies using DEXA are used to determine the extent of bone loss. Measurements are usually obtained in the lumbar spine or femur. When there is a possibility of increased bone turnover, as would occur with increased PTHrP production in some malignancies, bone scans are used to assess the rate of incorporation of radiolabeled phosphate. The greater the rate of bone formation, the greater the deposition of labeled phosphate in bone, reflecting an increase in bone turnover. Generalized increases are observed in hyperparathyroidism, whereas focal increases are observed in malignant diseases.

KEY CONCEPTS

1. *PTH release is controlled by circulating Ca^{2+} levels and is under negative feedback regulation by Ca^{2+} and vitamin D.*

2. *The main physiologic effects of PTH are mediated by the PTHR1 expressed in bone and kidney.*

3. *PTHR1 binds PTH and PTHrP, a peptide responsible for the pathophysiologic elevation of Ca^{2+} in some malignancies.*

4. *In the kidney, PTH increases renal Ca^{2+} reabsorption, increases the activity of 1α-hydroxylase (which mediates the final activation step in the synthesis of vitamin D), and decreases Pi reabsorption.*

5. *In bone, PTH increases osteoclast-mediated bone resorption indirectly through stimulation of osteoblast activity.*

Calcitonin decreases bone resorption and lowers plasma Ca^{2+} levels.

Synthesis of active vitamin D involves hydroxylation in the liver (C-25) and kidney (C-1).

Vitamin D increases intestinal Ca^{2+} absorption, facilitates renal Ca^{2+} reabsorption, and bone resorption.

STUDY QUESTIONS

5-1.   A 43-year-old male is admitted to the emergency room for severe pain in his left flank, radiating to the groin. The pain is intermittent and initiated after running a marathon on a hot summer day. The patient is asked for a urine specimen and blood is detected in the urine. He is hydrated, and additional diagnostic procedures are done. Laboratory values show serum Ca^{++} of 12 mg/dL, and PTH values of 130 pg/mL. Which of the following findings would be predictable in this patient?

    a.   Increased serum Pi

    b.   Increased serum alkaline phosphatase

    c.   Increased intestinal Ca loss

    d.   Decreased urinary Ca excretion

5-2.   In the patient described above, the mechanism underlying the abnormalities observed is:

    a.   Increased calcitonin release

    b.   Decreased 25-hydroxylase activity

    c.   Increased osteoclast apoptosis

    d.   Loss of negative feedback regulation of PTH release

5-3.   A 73-year-old woman is admitted to the hospital following a bout of severe vomiting and generalized weakness. Initial laboratory values reveal elevated Ca^{2+} levels. The referring physician tells you that she has breast cancer, and her bone scan indicates metastasis to bone. Which of the following laboratory values would be compatible with this clinical scenario?

    a.   PTH 5 pg/mL, phosphate 6 mg/dL, alkaline phosphatase 600 U/L

    b.   PTH 90 pg/mL, phosphate 6 mg/dL, alkaline phosphatase 30 U/L

    c.   PTH 5 pg/mL, phosphate 2 mg/dL, alkaline phosphatase 20 U/L

    d.   PTH 3 pg/mL, phosphate 2 mg/dL, alkaline phosphatase 100 U/L

5–4. *The most likely cause of hypercalcemia in the patient described in Question 5–3 is:*

    a. Increased PTH production

    b. Increased responsiveness of the PTH receptor 1

    c. Increased PTHrP production

    d. Increased calcitonin release

5–5. *Leading stars of soap operas are prone to enter fits of hysteria associated with hyperventilation. In real life, when that happens it usually leads to muscle cramping (tetanic contractions). What is the physiologic concept that explains what happens in that situation?*

    a. Decreased protein-bound calcium

    b. Hypercalcemia secondary to PTH-mediated bone resorption

    c. Increased dissociation of protein-bound calcium

    d. Decreased ionized plasma calcium levels

    e. Increased renal calcium excretion

5–6. *The physiologic mechanisms affected by medical strategies for the management of osteoporosis include:*

    a. Decreased apoptosis of osteoclasts by bisphosphonates

    b. Increased activation of osteoclast activity by calcitonin

    c. Increased osteoblast differentiation by selective estrogen receptor modulators

    d. Decreased intestinal Ca²⁺ secretion by vitamin D

SUGGESTED READINGS

Brown EM, MacLeod RJ. Extracellular calcium sensing and extracellular calcium signaling. *Physiol Rev.* 2001;81:239.

Canalis E, Giustina A, Bilezikian JP. Mechanisms of anabolic therapies for osteoporosis. *N Engl J Med.* 2007;357:905–916.

Glenville J, Strugnell SA, DeLuca HF. Current understanding of the molecular actions of vitamin D. *Physiol Rev.* 1998;78:1193.

Khosla S. Minireview: the OPG/RANKL/RANK system. *Endocrinology.* 2001;142:5050.

Gensure RC, Gardella TJ, Juppner H. Parathyroid hormone and parathyroid hormone-related peptide, and their receptors. *Biochem Biophys Res Commun.* 2005;328:666.

Manolagas SC, Jilka RL. Bone marrow, cytokines, and bone remodeling: emerging insights into the pathophysiology of osteoporosis. *N Engl J Med.* 1995;332:305.

Marx SJ. Medical progress: hyperparathyroid and hypoparathyroid disorders. *N Engl J Med.* 2000;343:1863.

Murer H, Hernando N, Forster L, Biber J. Molecular mechanisms in proximal tubular and small intestinal phosphate reabsorption. *Mol Membr Biol.* 2001;18:3.

Slatopolsky E, Brown A, Dusso A. Role of phosphorus in the pathogenesis of secondary hyperparathyroidism. *Am J Kidney Dis.* 2001;37:S54.

Teitelbaum SL. Bone resorption by osteoclasts. *Science.* 2000;289:1504.

Adrenal Gland

6

OBJECTIVES

▶ Identify the functional anatomy and zones of the adrenal glands and the principal hormones secreted from each zone.

▶ Describe and contrast the regulation of synthesis and release of the adrenal steroid hormones (glucocorticoids, mineralocorticoids, and androgens) and the consequences of abnormalities in their biosynthetic pathways.

▶ Understand the cellular mechanism of action of adrenal cortical hormones and identify their major physiologic actions, particularly during injury and stress.

▶ Identify the major mineralocorticoids, their biologic actions, and their target organs or tissues.

▶ Describe the regulation of mineralocorticoid secretion and relate this to the regulation of sodium and potassium excretion.

▶ Identify the causes and consequences of oversecretion and undersecretion of glucocorticoids, mineralocorticoids, and adrenal androgens.

▶ Identify the chemical nature of catecholamines and their biosynthesis and metabolic fate.

▶ Describe the biologic consequences of sympatho-adrenal medulla activation and identify the target organs or tissues for catecholamine effects along with the receptor types that mediate their actions.

▶ Describe and integrate the interactions of adrenal medullary and cortical hormones in response to stress.

▶ Identify diseases caused by oversecretion of adrenal catecholamines.

The adrenal glands are important components of the endocrine system. They contribute significantly to maintaining homeostasis particularly through their role in the regulation of the body's adaptive response to stress, in the maintenance of body water, sodium and potassium balance, and in the control of blood pressure. The main hormones produced by the human adrenal glands belong to 2 different families based on their structure; these are the steroid hormones including the glucocorticoids, mineralocorticoids and androgens; and the catecholamines norepinephrine and epinephrine. The adrenal gland, like the pituitary, has 2 different embryologic origins, which as we will discuss, influence the mechanisms that control hormone production by each of the 2 components.

FUNCTIONAL ANATOMY AND ZONATION

The adrenal glands are located above the kidneys. They are small, averaging 3–5 cm in length, and weigh 1.5–2.5 g and as mentioned above, consist of 2 different components; the cortex and the medulla (Figure 6–1), each with a specific embryologic origin. The outer adrenal cortex is derived from mesodermal tissue

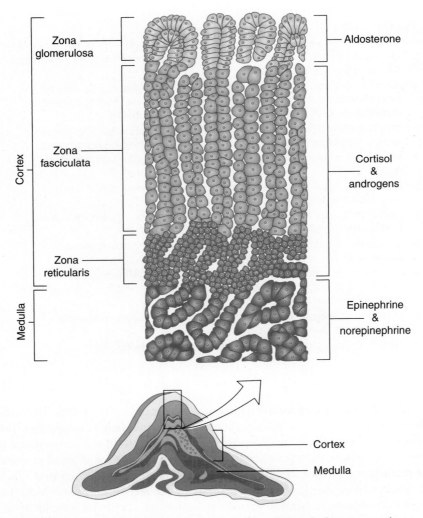

Figure 6–1. Adrenal glands. The adrenal glands are composed of a cortex and a medulla, each derived from a different embryologic origin. The cortex is divided into 3 zones: reticularis, fasciculata, and glomerulosa. The cells that make up the 3 zones have distinct enzymatic capacities, leading to a relative specificity in the products of each of the adrenal cortex zones. The adrenal medulla is made of cells derived from the neural crest.

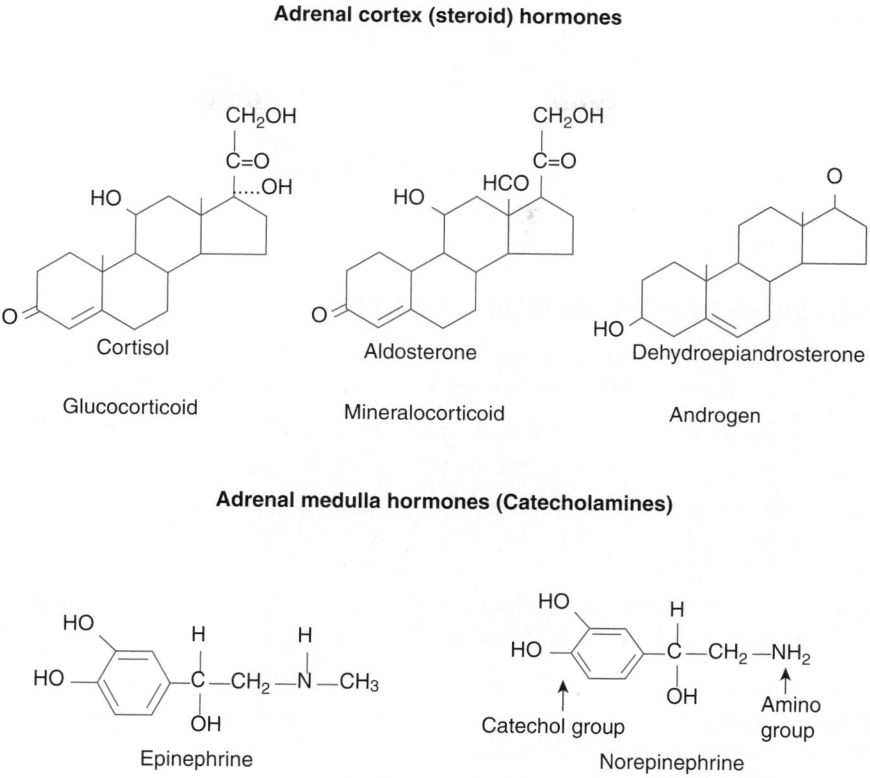

Adrenal cortex (steroid) hormones

| Cortisol | Aldosterone | Dehydroepiandrosterone |
| Glucocorticoid | Mineralocorticoid | Androgen |

Adrenal medulla hormones (Catecholamines)

Epinephrine   Catechol group   Amino group

Norepinephrine

Figure 6–2. Adrenal gland hormones. The principal hormones synthesized and released by the adrenal cortex are the glucocorticoid cortisol, the mineralocorticoid aldosterone, and the androgen dehydroepiandrosterone (DHEA). These steroid hormones are derived from cholesterol. The principal hormones synthesized and released by the adrenal medulla are the catecholamines epinephrine and norepinephrine. These catecholamines are derived from L-tyrosine.

and accounts for approximately 90% of the weight of the adrenals. The cortex synthesizes the adrenal steroid hormones called *glucocorticoids, mineralocorticoids,* and *androgens* (eg, cortisol, aldosterone, and dehydroepiandrosterone [DHEA]) in response to hypothalamic-pituitary-adrenal hormone stimulation (Figure 6–2). The inner medulla is derived from a subpopulation of neural crest cells and makes up the remaining 10% of the mass of the adrenals. The medulla synthesizes catecholamines (eg, epinephrine and norepinephrine) in response to direct sympathetic (sympatho-adrenal) stimulation.

Several features of the adrenal glands contribute to the regulation of steroid hormone and catecholamine synthesis, including the architecture, blood supply, and the enzymatic machinery of the individual cells. Blood supply to the adrenal glands is derived from the superior, middle, and inferior suprarenal arteries.

Branches of these arteries form a capillary network arranged so that blood flows from the outer cortex toward the center area, following a radially oriented sinusoid system. This direction of blood flow controls the access of steroid hormones to the circulation and concentrates the steroid hormones at the core of the adrenals, thus modulating the activities of enzymes involved in catecholamine synthesis. The venous drainage of the adrenal glands involves a single renal vein on each side; the right vein drains into the inferior vena cava and the left vein drains into the left renal artery.

HORMONES OF THE ADRENAL CORTEX

The adrenal cortex consists of 3 zones that vary in both their morphologic and functional features and thus, the steroid hormones they produce (see Figure 6–1).

- The **zona glomerulosa** contains abundant smooth endoplasmic reticulum and is the unique source of the mineralocorticoid aldosterone.

- The **zona fasciculata** contains abundant lipid droplets and produces the gluco-corticoids, cortisol and corticosterone, and the androgens, DHEA and DHEA sulfate (DHEAS).

- The **zona reticularis** develops postnatally and is recognizable at approximately age 3 years; it also produces glucocorticoids and androgens.

The products of the adrenal cortex are classified into 3 general categories: glucocorticoids, mineralocorticoids, and androgens (see Figure 6–2) which reflect the primary effects mediated by these hormones. This will become clear when their individual target organ effects are discussed.

Chemistry and Biosynthesis

Steroid hormones share an initial step in their biosynthesis (steroidogenesis), which is the conversion of cholesterol to pregnenolone (Figure 6–3). Cholesterol used for steroid hormone synthesis can be derived from the plasma membrane or from the steroidogenic cytoplasmic pool of cholesteryl-esters. Free cholesterol is generated by the action of the enzyme cholesterol ester hydrolase. Cholesterol is transported from the outer mitochondrial membrane to the inner mitochondrial membrane, followed by the conversion to pregnenolone by P450scc enzyme; an inner mitochondrial membrane present in all steroidogenic cells. This is considered the **rate-limiting step** in steroid hormone synthesis and requires the STeroid Acute Regulatory (STAR) protein. STAR is critical in mediating cholesterol transfer to the inner mitochondrial membrane and the cholesterol side chain cleavage enzyme system.

This conversion of cholesterol to pregnenolone is the first step in a sequence of multiple enzymatic reactions involved in the synthesis of steroid hormones. Because the cells that constitute the different sections of the adrenal cortex have specific enzymatic features, the synthetic pathway of steroid hormones will result in preferential synthesis of glucocorticoids, mineralocorticoids, or androgens, depending on the region.

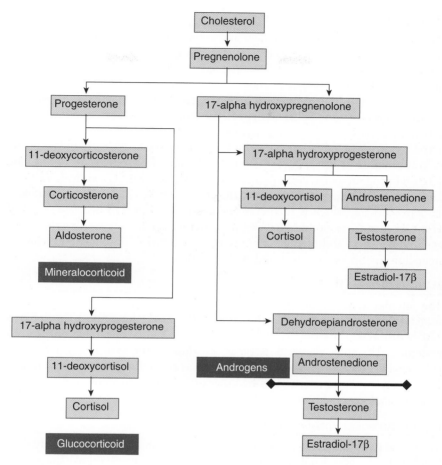

Figure 6–3. Adrenal steroid hormone synthetic pathway. Cholesterol is converted to pregnenolone by the cytochrome P450 side-chain cleavage enzyme. Pregnenolone is converted to progesterone by 3β-hydroxysteroid dehydrogenase or to 17α-OH-pregnenolone by 17α-hydroxylase. Thereafter, 17α-OH-pregnenolone is converted to 17α-OH-progesterone by 3β-hydroxysteroid dehydrogenase, 17α-OH-progesterone is converted to 11-deoxycortisol by the enzyme 21-hydroxylase, and 11-deoxycortisol is converted to cortisol by 11β-hydroxylase. In addition, 17α-OH-progesterone can be converted to androstenedione. Both 17α-OH-pregnenolone and 17α-OH-progesterone can be converted to the androgens dehydroepiandrosterone (DHEA) and androstenedione, respectively. DHEA is converted to androstenedione. Cells in the zona glomerulosa do not have 17α-hydroxylase activity. Therefore, pregnenolone can be converted only into progesterone. The zona glomerulosa possesses aldosterone synthase activity, and this enzyme converts deoxycorticosterone to corticosterone, corticosterone to 18-hydroxycorticosterone, and 18-hydroxycorticosterone to aldosterone, the principal mineralocorticoid produced by the adrenal glands. The line denotes which steps occur outside the adrenal glands.

GLUCOCORTICOID HORMONE SYNTHESIS

Cells of the adrenal zona fasciculata and zona reticularis synthesize and secrete the glucocorticoids cortisol or corticosterone through the following pathway (see Figure 6–3). Pregnenolone exits the mitochondria and is converted to either progesterone or 17α-OH-pregnenolone. Conversion of pregnenolone to progesterone is mediated by **3β-hydroxysteroid dehydrogenase**. Progesterone is converted to 11-deoxycorticosterone by **21-hydroxylase;** then 11-deoxycorticosterone is converted to corticosterone by **11β-hydroxylase**. Conversion of pregnenolone to 17α-OH-pregnenolone is mediated by **17α-hydroxylase**; 17α-OH-pregnenolone is converted to 17α-OH-progesterone by 3β-hydroxysteroid dehydrogenase; 17α-OH-progesterone is converted to either 11-deoxycortisol or androstenedione. The enzyme 21-hydroxylase mediates the conversion of 17α-OH-progesterone to 11-deoxycortisol, which is then converted to cortisol by 11β-hydroxylase. Both 17α-OH-pregnenolone and 17α-OH-progesterone can be converted to the androgens DHEA and androstenedione, respectively. DHEA is converted to androstenedione by 3β-hydroxysteroid dehydrogenase.

MINERALOCORTICOID HORMONE SYNTHESIS

The adrenal zona glomerulosa cells preferentially synthesize and secrete the mineralocorticoid aldosterone. The cells of the zona glomerulosa do not have 17α-hydroxylase activity. Therefore, pregnenolone can be converted only to progesterone. The zona glomerulosa possesses **aldosterone synthase** activity, and this enzyme converts 11-deoxycorticosterone to corticosterone, corticosterone to 18-hydroxycorticosterone, and 18-hydroxycorticosterone to aldosterone, the principal mineralocorticoid produced by the adrenal glands.

ADRENAL ANDROGEN HORMONE SYNTHESIS

The initial steps in the biosynthesis of DHEA from cholesterol are similar to those involved in glucocorticoid and mineralocorticoid hormone synthesis. The product of these initial enzymatic conversions, pregnenolone, undergoes 17α-hydroxylation by microsomal P450c17 and conversion to DHEA. 17α-pregnenolone can also be converted to 17α-OH-progesterone, which in turn can be converted to androstenedione in the zona fasciculata.

Regulation of Adrenal Cortex Hormone Synthesis

As already mentioned, the initial steps in the biosynthetic pathways of steroid hormones are identical regardless of the steroid hormone synthesized. The production of the hormones can be regulated acutely and chronically. Acute regulation results in the rapid production of steroids in response to immediate need and occurs within minutes of the stimulus. The biosynthesis of glucocorticoids to combat stressful situations and the rapid synthesis of aldosterone to rapidly regulate blood pressure are examples of this type of regulation. Chronic stimulation, such as that which occurs during prolonged starvation and chronic disease, involves the synthesis of enzymes involved in steroidogenesis to enhance the synthetic capacity of the cells. Although both glucocorticoids and mineralocorticoids are released in response to stressful conditions, the conditions under which they are stimulated differ, and the cellular mechanisms responsible for stimulating their release are different. Thus, the mechanisms involved in the regulation of their release differ and are specifically controlled as described below.

GLUCOCORTICOID SYNTHESIS AND RELEASE

The pulsatile release of cortisol is under direct stimulation by adrenocorticotropic hormone (ACTH) released from the anterior pituitary. ACTH, or corticotropin, is synthesized in the anterior pituitary as a large precursor, proopiomelanocortin (POMC). POMC is processed post-translationally into several peptides, including corticotropin, β-lipotropin, and β-endorphin, as presented and discussed in Chapter 3 (see Figure 3–4). The release of ACTH is pulsatile with approximately 7–15 episodes per day. The stimulation of cortisol release occurs within 15 minutes of the surge in ACTH. An important feature in the release of cortisol is that in addition to being pulsatile, it follows a circadian rhythm that is exquisitely sensitive to environmental and internal factors such as light, sleep, stress, and disease (see Figure 1–8). Release of cortisol is greatest during the early waking hours, with levels declining as the afternoon progresses. As a result of its pulsatile release, the resulting circulating levels of the hormone vary throughout the day, and this has a direct impact on how cortisol values are interpreted according to the timing of blood sample collection.

ACTH stimulates cortisol release by binding to a $G\alpha_s$ protein–coupled plasma membrane melanocortin 2 receptor on adrenocortical cells, resulting in activation of adenylate cyclase, an increase in cyclic adenosine monophosphate, and activation of protein kinase A (see Figure 3–4). Protein kinase A phosphorylates the enzyme cholesteryl-ester hydrolase, increasing its enzymatic activity; leading to increased cholesterol availability for hormone synthesis. In addition, ACTH activates and increases the synthesis of STAR, the enzyme involved in the transport of cholesterol into the inner mitochondrial membrane. Therefore, ACTH stimulates the 2 initial and rate-limiting steps in steroid hormone synthesis.

The release of ACTH from the anterior pituitary is regulated by the hypothalamic peptide corticotropin-releasing hormone (CRH) discussed in Chapter 3. Cortisol inhibits the biosynthesis and secretion of CRH and ACTH in a classic example of negative feedback regulation by hormones. This closely regulated circuit is referred to as the hypothalamic-pituitary-adrenal (HPA) axis (Figure 6–4).

METABOLISM OF GLUCOCORTICOIDS

Because of their lipophilic nature, free cortisol molecules are mostly insoluble in water. Therefore, cortisol is usually found in biologic fluids either in a conjugated form (eg, as sulfate or glucuronide derivatives) or bound to carrier proteins (noncovalent, reversible binding). The majority of cortisol is bound to glucocorticoid-binding α_2-globulin (transcortin or cortisol-binding globulin [CBG]), a specific carrier of cortisol. Normal levels of CBG average 3–4 mg/dL and are saturated

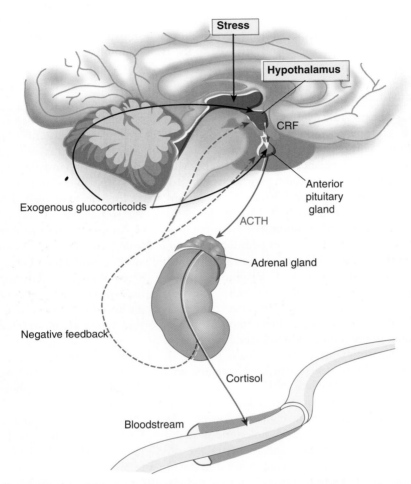

Figure 6–4. Hypothalamic-pituitary-adrenal axis. Corticotropin-releasing factor (CRF), produced by the hypothalamus and released in the median eminence, stimulates the synthesis and processing of proopiomelanocortin, with resulting release of proopiomelanocortin peptides that include adrenocorticotropic hormone (ACTH) from the anterior pituitary. ACTH binds to the melanocortin-2 receptor in the adrenal gland and stimulates the cholesterol-derived synthesis of adrenal steroid hormones. Glucocorticoids released into the systemic circulation exert negative feedback inhibition of corticotropin-releasing factor (CRF) and ACTH release from the hypothalamus and pituitary, respectively, in a classic example of negative feedback hormone regulation. This closely regulated circuit is referred to as the hypothalamic-pituitary-adrenal (HPA) axis.

with cortisol levels of 28 μg/dL. The hepatic synthesis of CBG is stimulated by estrogen and decreased by hepatic disease (cirrhosis). Approximately 20%–50% of bound cortisol is bound nonspecifically to plasma albumin. A small amount (<10%) of total plasma cortisol circulates unbound and is referred to as the free fraction. This is considered to represent the biologically active fraction of the hormone that is directly available for action.

As discussed in Chapter 1, the major role of plasma-binding proteins is to act as a "buffer" or reservoir for active hormones. Protein-bound steroids are released into the plasma in free form as soon as the free hormone concentration decreases. Plasma-binding proteins also protect the hormone from peripheral metabolism (notably by liver enzymes) and increase the half-life of biologically active forms. The half-life of cortisol is 70–90 minutes.

Because of their lipophilic nature, steroid hormones diffuse easily through cell membranes and therefore have a large volume of distribution. In their target tissues, steroid hormones are concentrated by an uptake mechanism that relies on their binding to intracellular receptors.

The liver and kidney are the 2 major sites of hormone inactivation and elimination. Several pathways are involved in this process, including reduction, oxidation, hydroxylation, and conjugation, to form the sulfate and glucuronide derivatives of the steroid hormones. These processes occur in the liver through phase I and phase II biotransformation reactions, leading to generation of a more water-soluble compound for easier excretion. Inactivation of cortisol to cortisone and to tetrahydrocortisol and tetrahydrocortisone is followed by conjugation and renal excretion. These metabolites are referred to as *17-hydroxycorticosteroids*, and their determination in 24-hour urine collections is used to assess the status of adrenal steroid production.

Localized tissue metabolism contributes to modulation of the physiologic effects of glucocorticoids by the isoforms of the enzyme 11β-hydroxysteroid dehydrogenase. Corticosteroid **11β-hydroxysteroid dehydrogenase type I** is a low-affinity nicotinamide adenine dinucleotide phosphate–dependent reductase that converts cortisone back to its active form, cortisol. This enzyme is expressed in liver, adipose tissue, lung, skeletal muscle, vascular smooth muscle, gonads, and the central nervous system. The high expression of this enzyme, particularly in adipose tissue has gained recent attention, as it is thought to contribute to the pathophysiology of metabolic syndrome (see Chapter 10).

The conversion of cortisol to cortisone, its less active metabolite, is mediated by the enzyme **11β-hydroxysteroid dehydrogenase type II**. This high-affinity nicotinamide adenine dinucleotide–dependent dehydrogenase is expressed primarily in the distal convoluted tubules and collecting ducts of the kidney, where it contributes to specificity of mineralocorticoid hormone effects. As discussed below, conversion of cortisol to cortisone is critical in preventing excess mineralocorticoid activity resulting from cortisol binding to the mineralocorticoid receptor. Increased expression and activity of 11β-hydroxysteroid dehydrogenase type I amplifies glucocorticoid action within the cell, whereas increased 11β-hydroxysteroid dehydrogenase type II activity decreases glucocorticoid action.

MINERALOCORTICOID SYNTHESIS AND RELEASE

Aldosterone synthesis and release in the adrenal zona glomerulosa is predominantly regulated by angiotensin II and extracellular K^+ and, to a lesser extent, by ACTH. Aldosterone is part of the **renin-angiotensin-aldosterone** system, which is responsible for preserving circulatory homeostasis in response to a loss of salt and water (eg, with intense and prolonged sweating, vomiting, or diarrhea). The components of the renin-angiotensin-aldosterone system respond quickly to reductions in intravascular volume and renal perfusion. Angiotensin II is the principal stimulator of aldosterone production when intravascular volume is reduced.

Both angiotensin II and K^+ stimulate aldosterone release by increasing intracellular Ca^{2+} concentrations. Angiotensin II receptor-mediated signaling leads to increased intracellular calcium levels, while increased K^+ concentrations depolarize the cell leading to Ca^{2+} influx via voltage-gated L- and T-type Ca^{2+} channels.

The main physiologic stimulus for aldosterone release is a decrease in the effective intravascular blood volume (Figure 6–5). A decline in blood volume leads

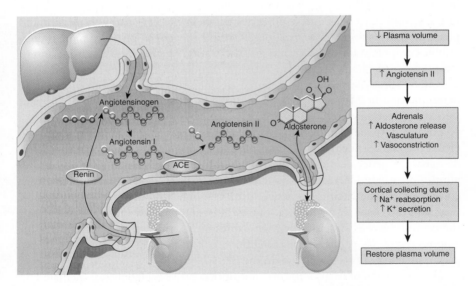

Figure 6–5. Regulation of aldosterone release by the renin-angiotensin-aldosterone system. A decrease in the effective circulating blood volume triggers the release of renin from the juxtaglomerular apparatus in the kidney. Renin cleaves angiotensinogen, the hepatic precursor of angiotensin peptides, to form angiotensin I. Angiotensin I is converted to angiotensin II by angiotensin-converting enzyme (ACE), which is bound to the membrane of vascular endothelial cells. Angiotensin II is a potent vasoconstrictor and stimulates the production of aldosterone in the zona glomerulosa of the adrenal cortex. Aldosterone production is also stimulated by potassium, ACTH, norepinephrine, and endothelins. (Modified, with permission, from Weber KT. Mechanisms of disease: aldosterone in congestive heart failure. *N Engl J Med.* 2001;345:1689. Copyright © Massachusetts Medical Society. All rights reserved.)

to decreased renal perfusion pressure, which is sensed by the juxtaglomerular apparatus (baroreceptor) and triggers the release of renin. Renin release is also regulated by sodium chloride (NaCl) concentration in the macula densa, plasma electrolyte concentrations, angiotensin II levels, and sympathetic tone. Renin catalyzes the conversion of angiotensinogen, a liver-derived protein, to angiotensin I. Circulating angiotensin I is converted to angiotensin II by angiotensin-converting enzyme (ACE), highly expressed in vascular endothelial cells. The increase in circulating angiotensin II produces direct arteriolar vasoconstriction, stimulates adrenocortical cells of the zona glomerulosa to synthesize and release aldosterone, and stimulates arginine vasopressin release from the posterior pituitary (see Chapter 2).

Potassium is also a major physiologic stimulus for aldosterone production, illustrating a classic example of hormone regulation by the ion it controls. Aldosterone is critical in maintaining potassium homeostasis by increasing K^+ excretion in urine, feces, sweat, and saliva, preventing hyperkalemia during periods of high K^+ intake or after K^+ release from skeletal muscle during strenuous exercise. In turn, elevations in circulating K^+ concentrations stimulate the release of aldosterone from the adrenal cortex.

METABOLISM OF MINERALOCORTICOIDS

The total amount of aldosterone released is markedly less than that of glucocorticoids. Plasma aldosterone levels average 0.006–0.010 µg/dL (in contrast to cortisol levels of 13.5 µg/dL). Secretion can be increased 2- to 6-fold by sodium depletion or by a decrease in the effective circulating blood volume, such as occurs with ascites. Binding of aldosterone to plasma proteins is minimal, resulting in a short plasma half-life of approximately 15–20 minutes. This fact is relevant to mineralocorticoid and glucocorticoid receptor-mediated effects, and their specificity as will be discussed below.

Aldosterone is metabolized in the liver to tetrahydroglucuronide derivative and excreted in the urine. A fraction of aldosterone is metabolized to aldosterone 18-glucuronide, which can be hydrolyzed back to free aldosterone under low pH conditions; thus it is an "acid-labile conjugate." Approximately 5% of aldosterone is excreted in the acid-labile form; a small fraction of aldosterone appears intact in the urine (1%) and up to 40% is excreted as tetraglucuronide.

ADRENAL ANDROGEN SYNTHESIS AND RELEASE

The third class of steroid hormones produced by the zona reticularis of the adrenal glands is the adrenal androgens, including DHEA and DHEAS (see Figure 6–3). DHEA is the most abundant circulating hormone in the body and is readily conjugated to its sulfate ester DHEAS. Its production is controlled by ACTH.

METABOLISM OF ADRENAL ANDROGENS

The adrenal androgens are converted into androstenedione and then into potent androgens or estrogens in peripheral tissues. The synthesis of dihydrotestosterone and 17β-estradiol, the most potent androgen and estrogen from DHEA, respectively, involves several enzymes, including 3β-hydroxysteroid dehydrogenase/D5-D4 isomerase, 17β-hydroxysteroid dehydrogenase, and 5β-reductase or aromatase (see Chapters 8 and 9). The importance of the adrenal-derived androgens to the overall production of sex steroid hormones is highlighted by the fact that approximately 50% of total androgens in the prostate of adult men are derived from adrenal steroid precursors.

The control and regulation of the release of adrenal sex steroids are not completely understood. However, it is known that adrenal secretion of DHEA and DHEAS increases in children at the age of 6–8 years, and values of circulating DHEAS peak between the ages of 20 and 30 years. Thereafter, serum levels of DHEA and DHEAS decrease markedly. In fact, at 70 years of age, serum DHEAS levels are at approximately 20% of their peak values and continue to decrease with age. This 70%–95% reduction in the formation of DHEAS by the adrenal glands during the aging process results in a dramatic reduction in the formation of androgens and estrogens in peripheral target tissues. Despite the marked decrease in the release of DHEA as the individual ages, this is not paralleled by a similar decrease in ACTH or cortisol release. The clinical impact of this age-related deficiency in DHEA production is not fully understood but may play an important role in the regulation of immune function and intermediary metabolism, among other aspects of physiology of the aging process.

Steroid Hormone Target Organ Cellular Effects

The physiologic effects of steroid hormones can be divided into genomic and nongenomic effects. Most of the physiologic effects of glucocorticoid and mineralocorticoid hormones are mediated through binding to intracellular receptors that operate as ligand-activated transcription factors to regulate gene expression. Binding of steroid hormones to their specific receptors leads to conformational changes in the receptor, leading to their ability to act as a ligand-dependent transcription factors. The steroid-receptor complex binds to hormone-responsive elements on the chromatin and thereby regulates gene transcription, resulting in the synthesis or repression of proteins, which are ultimately responsible for the physiologic effects of the hormones.

Steroid hormones can also exert their physiologic effects through nongenomic actions. A nongenomic action is any mechanism that does not directly involve gene transcription, such as the rapid steroid effects on the electrical activity of nerve cells or the interaction of steroid hormones with the receptor for γ-aminobutyric acid. In contrast to the genomic effects, nongenomic effects require the continued presence of the hormone and occur more quickly because they do not require the synthesis of proteins. Some of the nongenomic effects may be mediated by specific receptors located on the cell membrane. The nature of these receptors and the signal transduction mechanisms involved are not completely understood and are still under investigation.

Steroid Hormone Receptors

Mineralocorticoid and glucocorticoid receptors share 57% homology in the ligand-binding domain and 94% homology in the DNA-binding domain, and are classified in 2 types of receptors: type I and type II. Type

I receptors are expressed predominantly in the kidney, are specific for mineralo-corticoids, but have a high affinity for glucocorticoids. Type II receptors are expressed in virtually all cells and are specific for glucocorticoids.

As already mentioned, plasma concentrations of glucocorticoid hormones are much higher (100- to 1000-fold) than those of aldosterone. The higher concentration of glucocorticoids coupled with the high affinity of the mineralocorticoid receptor for glucocorticoids raises the issue of ligand-receptor specificity and resulting physiologic action. Given the high levels of cir-culating glucocorticoids (cortisol), one might predict permanent maximal occupancy of the mineralocorticoid receptor by cortisol, leading to sustained maximal sodium reabsorption and precluding any regulatory role of aldosterone. However, several factors are in place to enhance the specificity of the mineralocor-ticoid receptor for aldosterone (Figure 6–6). First, glucocorticoids circulate bound to CBG and albumin, allowing only a small fraction of the unbound hormone to freely cross cell membranes. Second, aldosterone target cells possess enzymatic activity of **11β-hydroxysteroid dehydrogenase type II**. This enzyme converts cortisol into its inactive form (cortisone) which has significantly less affinity for the mineralocorticoid receptor (see Figure 6–6). Third, the mineralocorticoid receptor discriminates between aldosterone and glucocorticoids. Aldosterone dis-sociates from the mineralocorticoid receptor 5 times more slowly than do the glucocorticoids, despite their similar affinity constants. In other words, aldoste-rone is less easily displaced from the mineralocorticoid receptor than is cortisol. Together, these mechanisms ensure that under normal conditions, mineralocorti-coid action is restricted to aldosterone. However, it is important to keep in mind that when production and release of glucocorticoids is excessive, or when the con-version of cortisol to its inactive metabolite cortisone is impaired; the higher cir-culating and tissue cortisol levels may lead to binding and stimulation of mineralocorticoid receptors.

Specific Effects of Adrenal Cortex Hormones

GLUCOCORTICOIDS

Cortisol, the principal glucocorticoid exerts multisystemic effects because virtually all cells express glucocorticoid receptors. Glucocorticoids as their name imply play an important role in regulation of glucose homeo-stasis. Glucocorticoids affect intermediary metabolism, stimulate proteolysis and gluconeogenesis, inhibit muscle protein synthesis, and increase fatty acid mobili-zation. Their hallmark effect is to increase blood glucose concentrations, hence the name "glucocorticoids." In the liver, glucocorticoids increase the expression of gluconeogenic enzymes such as phosphoenolpyruvate carboxykinase, tyrosine aminotransferase, and glucose-6-phosphatase. In muscle, glucocorticoids inter-fere with glucose transporter 4 translocation to the plasma membrane (see Chapter 7). In bone and cartilage, glucocorticoids decrease insulin-like growth factor 1, insulin-like growth factor-binding protein 1, and growth hor-mone expression and action, and affect thyroid hormone interactions. Excessive glucocorticoid levels result in osteoporosis and impair skeletal growth and bone

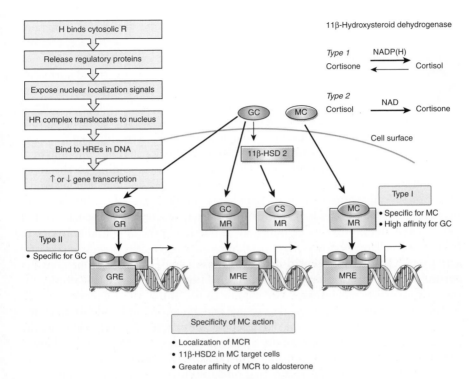

Figure 6–6. Steroid hormone receptors. Mineralocorticoids (MC) (aldosterone) and glucocorticoid (GC) (cortisol) hormones bind to intracellular receptors that share 57% homology in the ligand-binding domain and 94% homology in the DNA-binding domain. Cortisol binds the mineralocorticoid (MR) receptor with high affinity. Once GC and MC bind to intracellular receptors, these dimerize prior to nuclear translocation and binding to DNA GC- or MC-responsive elements increasing or suppressing transcription of specific genes. Cortisol binds with high affinity to the MR and can produce MC-like effects (sodium retention). Cortisol conversion to cortisone (CS) decreases the affinity for the receptor shown in the figure by the ill fit of CS with the MR. Decreased activity of the 11β-HSD2 leads to decreased conversion of cortisol to cortisone and increased MC activity. GR, Glucocorticoid receptor; GRE, glucocorticoid responsive element; H, hormone; HR, hormone–receptor; HRE, Hormone responsive element; HSD, hydroxysteroid dehydrogenase; HSD2, hydroxysteroid dehydrogenase type II; MRE, mineralocorticoid responsive element; NAD, nicotinamide adenine dinucleotide; NADP(H), nicotinamide adenine dinucleotide phosphate; R, receptor.

formation by inhibiting osteoblasts and collagen synthesis. Particularly at high circulating levels, glucocorticoids are catabolic and result in loss of lean body mass including bone and skeletal muscle. Glucocorticoids modulate the immune response by increasing antiinflammatory cytokine synthesis and decreasing proinflammatory cytokine synthesis, exerting an overall anti-inflammatory effect. Their anti-inflammatory effects have been exploited by the use of synthetic analogs of

Table 6-1. Physiologic effects of glucocorticoids

System	Effects
Metabolism	Degrades muscle protein and increases nitrogen excretion
	Increases gluconeogenesis and plasma glucose levels
	Increases hepatic glycogen synthesis
	Decreases glucose utilization (anti-insulin action)
	Decreases amino acid utilization
	Increases fat mobilization
	Redistributes fat
	Permissive effects on glucagon and catecholamine effects
Hemodynamic	Maintains vascular integrity and reactivity
	Maintains responsiveness to catecholamine pressor effects
	Maintains fluid volume
Immune function	Increases antiinflammatory cytokine production
	Decreases proinflammatory cytokine production
	Decreases inflammation by inhibiting prostaglandin and leukotriene production
	Inhibits bradykinin and serotonin inflammatory effects
	Decreases circulating eosinophil, basophil, and lymphocyte counts (redistribution effect)
	Impairs cell-mediated immunity
	Increases neutrophil, platelet, and red blood cell counts
Central nervous system	Modulates perception and emotion
	Decreases CRH and ACTH release

ACTH, adrenocorticotropic hormone; CRH, corticotropin-releasing hormone.

glucocorticoids, such as prednisone, for the treatment of chronic inflammatory diseases. In the vasculature, glucocorticoids modulate reactivity to vasoactive substances, like angiotensin II and norepinephrine. This interaction becomes evident in patients with glucocorticoid deficiency and manifests as hypotension and decreased sensitivity to vasoconstrictor administration. In the central nervous system, they modulate perception and emotion and may produce marked changes in behavior. This should be kept in mind when administering synthetic analogs, particularly in elderly patients. Some of the main physiologic effects of glucocorticoids are summarized in Table 6–1.

MINERALOCORTICOIDS

The principal physiologic function of aldosterone is to regulate mineral (sodium and potassium) balance; specifically renal potassium excretion and sodium reabsorption, hence the name "mineralocorticoid." Aldosterone receptors are expressed in the distal nephron including the distal convoluted tubule and the collecting duct. Within the collecting duct, the principal cells express significantly more mineralocorticoid receptors than do the intercalated cells. Thus, the most relevant physiologic effects of aldosterone are mediated by its binding to the mineralocorticoid receptor in the principal cells of the distal tubule and the collecting duct of the nephron (Figure 6–7). Aldosterone-induced

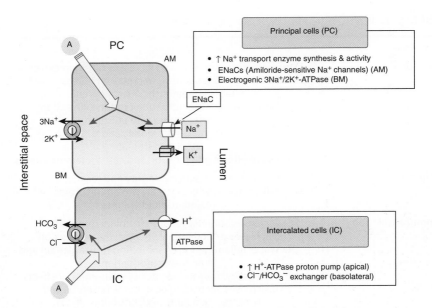

Figure 6–7. Aldosterone renal physiologic effects. Aldosterone diffuses across the plasma membrane and binds to its cytosolic receptor. The receptor-hormone complex is translocated to the nucleus where it interacts with the promoter region of target genes, activating or repressing their transcriptional activity producing an increase in transepithelial Na$^+$ transport. Aldosterone increases Na$^+$ entry at the apical membrane of the cells of the distal nephron through the amiloride-sensitive epithelial Na$^+$ channel (ENaC). Aldosterone promotes potassium excretion through its effects on Na$^+$/K$^+$-adenosine triphosphatase (ATPase) and epithelial Na$^+$ and K$^+$ channels in collecting-duct cells. Additional effects of aldosterone on intercalated cells leads to increased activation of the H-ATPase and Cl/HCO$_3$ exchanger. A, aldosterone; AM, apical membrane; BM, basolateral membrane; ENaC: epithelial sodium channel.

activation of preexisting proteins and stimulation of new proteins mediate an increase in transepithelial sodium transport. The specific effects of aldosterone are to increase the synthesis of Na$^+$ channels in the apical membrane, increase the synthesis and activity of Na$^+$/K$^+$-adenosine triphosphatase (ATPase) in the baso-lateral membrane (which pulls cytosolic Na$^+$ to the interstitium in exchange for K$^+$ transport into the cell), and increase the expression of H$^+$-ATPase in the apical membrane and the Cl$^-$/HCO$_3$ exchanger in the basolateral membrane of interca-lated cells. Intercalated cells express carbonic anhydrase and contribute to the acidification of urine and alkalinization of plasma. Thus, aldosterone increases sodium entry at the apical membrane of the cells of the distal nephron through ‚the amiloride-sensitive epithelial Na$^+$ channel. The Na$^+$/K$^+$-ATPase, located in the basolateral membrane of the cells, maintains the intracellular sodium concentra-tion by extruding the reabsorbed sodium toward the extracellular and blood com-partments creating an electrochemical gradient that facilitates the transfer of intracellular K^+ from tubular cells into the urine. The increase in Na^+ reabsorption leads to increased water reabsorption. When most of the filtered Na^+ is reabsorbed in the proximal tubule, only a small amount of sodium reaches the distal tubule (the site of aldosterone regulation). In this case, no net Na^+ reabsorption occurs even in the presence of elevated levels of aldosterone. As a result, potassium excretion is minimal. In fact, only 2% of filtered sodium is under regulation by aldosterone. The role of aldosterone in regulation of sodium transport is a major factor determining total-body Na^+ levels and thus long-term blood pressure regulation (see Chapter 10).

Mineralocorticoid receptors are not as widely expressed as those for glucocorticoids. Classic aldosterone-sensitive tissues include epithelia with high electrical resistance, such as the distal parts of the nephron, the surface epithelium of the distal colon, and the salivary and sweat gland ducts. More recently, other cells that express mineralocorticoid receptor have been identified, such as epidermal keratinocytes, neurons of the central nervous system, cardiac myocytes, and endothelial and smooth muscle cells of the vasculature (large vessels). Therefore, additional effects of aldosterone include increased sodium reabsorption in salivary and sweat glands, increased K^+ excretion from the colon, and a positive inotropic effect on the heart.

Recent studies indicate that aldosterone may be synthesized in tissues other than the adrenal cortex. Aldosterone synthase activity, messenger RNA, and aldosterone production has been demonstrated in endothelial and vascular smooth muscle cells in the heart and blood vessels. The physiologic importance of locally produced aldosterone (paracrine effects) is not yet clear, but some clinician scientists have proposed that it may contribute to tissue repair after myocardial infarction as well as promote cardiac hypertrophy and fibrosis. In the brain, aldosterone affects neural regulation of blood pressure, salt appetite, volume regulation, and sympathetic outflow. Extra-adrenal sites of aldosterone production, release, and action have become prevalent areas of targeted pharmacologic manipulation.

ANDROGENS

The physiologic effects of DHEA and DHEAS are not completely understood. However, their importance is evident in congenital adrenal hyperplasia associated with deficiencies of either 21-hydroxylase or 11β-hydroxylase, in which pregnenolone is shunted to the androgen biosynthetic pathway as discussed later in this chapter. In females adrenal androgens may contribute to libido. In addition, their contribution to androgen levels in aging males and females is considerable as discussed in Chapters 8 and 9. Current knowledge indicates that low levels of DHEA are associated with cardiovascular disease in men and with an increased risk of premenopausal breast and ovarian cancer in women. In contrast, high levels of DHEA might increase the risk of postmenopausal breast cancer. Exogenous administration of DHEA to the elderly increases several hormone levels, including insulin-like growth factor 1, testosterone, dihydrotestosterone, and estradiol. However, the clinical benefit of these changes and the side effects of long-term use remain to be clearly defined. Furthermore, the specific mechanisms through which DHEA exerts its actions are not completely understood.

Diseases of Overproduction and Undersecretion of Glucocorticoids

ABNORMALITIES IN STEROID HORMONE BIOSYNTHESIS

Any deficiency in the pathway of enzymatic events leading to the synthesis of glucocorticoids, mineralocorticoids, and androgens causes serious pathology. The key enzymes involved in steroid hormone synthesis and the consequences of their deficiency are described in Table 6–2. The severity of enzyme deficiency manifestations ranges from death in utero as in the case of congenital deficiency of cholesterol side chain cleavage enzyme (P450scc, also known as 20,22 desmolase), to abnormalities that become evident in adult life and that are not life-threatening. An enzymatic defect of 21-hydroxylase accounts for 95% of the genetic abnormalities in adrenal steroid hormone synthesis (see Figure 6–8). This enzyme converts progesterone to 11-deoxycorticosterone and 17α-hydroxyprogesterone to 11-deoxycortisol. The second most frequent abnormality in glucocorticoid synthesis is deficiency of the enzyme 11β-hydroxylase, which converts 11-deoxycortisol to cortisol.

Table 6–2. Key enzymes involved in steroid hormone synthesis and metabolism

Enzyme and relevance	Physiologic function	Consequence of deficiency
21-Hydroxylase		
Accounts for 95% of genetic abnormalities in adrenal steroid hormone synthesis	Converts progesterone to 11-deoxycorticosterone and 17α-hydroxyprogesterone to 11-deoxycortisol	Decreased cortisol and aldosterone Hypoglycemia because of low cortisol Loss of sodium because of mineralocorticoid deficiency Virilization because of excess androgen production
11β-Hydroxylase		
Second most frequent abnormality in adrenal steroid hormone synthesis	Converts 11-deoxycorticosterone to corticosterone; 11-deoxycortisol to cortisol	Excess 11-deoxycortisol and 11-deoxycorticosterone Excess mineralocorticoid activity Hypoglycemia because of low cortisol Salt and water retention
11β-Hydroxysteroid dehydrogenase type II		
Inhibited by glycyrrhetinic acid, a compound of licorice	Converts cortisol into corticosterone, which has less affinity for the mineralocorticoid receptor	Decrease in glucocorticoid inactivation in mineralocorticoid-sensitive cells leading to excess mineralocorticoid activity

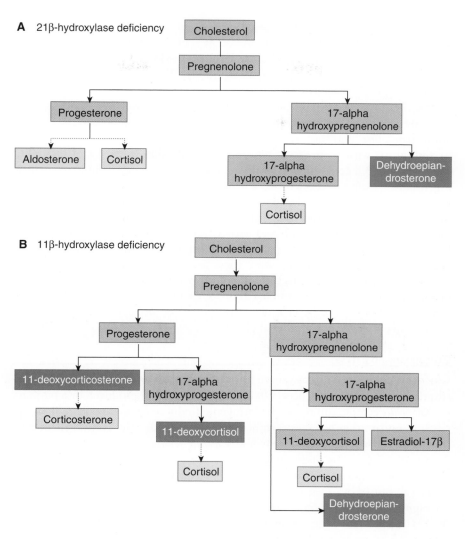

Figure 6–8. Alterations in steroid hormone synthesis. **A.** Deficiency of 21-hydroxylase accounts for 95% of genetic abnormalities in adrenal steroid hormone synthesis. This enzyme converts progesterone to deoxycorticosterone and 17-hydroxyprogesterone to 11-deoxycortisol. Thus, more pregnenolone is shunted to the DHEA-androstenedione pathway (more androgen synthesis), resulting in virilization (presence of masculine traits). In addition, aldosterone deficiency leads to sodium wasting. **B.** Deficiency of 11β-hydroxylase is the second most frequent abnormality in glucocorticoid synthesis. 11β-hydroxylase is the enzyme that converts deoxycortisol to cortisol and 11-deoxycorticosterone to corticosterone. Its deficiency results in excess 11-deoxycortisol and 11-deoxycorticosterone production. Both metabolites have active mineralocorticoid activity. The resulting excess in mineralocorticoid-like activity leads to salt and water retention and may cause hypertension. Metabolites in dark boxes are produced in excess. Dotted lines indicate pathways affected by enzymatic abnormalities.

Deficiencies in these enzymes result in impaired cortisol synthesis, lack of negative feedback inhibition of the release of ACTH, resulting in elevated ACTH levels, and greater stimulation of cholesterol conversion to pregnenolone (initial step shared by adrenal steroid hormone synthesis). The ACTH-mediated increase in steroidogenesis produces increased synthesis of the intermediate metabolites (before the enzymatic step that is deficient). Their buildup leads to a shunting to the alternate enzymatic pathways. Thus, more pregnenolone is shunted to the DHEA-androstenedione pathway and more intermediate metabolites are converted to androgens, with their excess resulting in virilization (presence of masculine traits). Additional consequences of 21-hydroxylase deficiency include hyponatremia resulting from mineralocorticoid deficiency and hypoglycemia resulting from deficient cortisol synthesis. In contrast, patients with 11β-hydroxylase deficiency produce excess 11-deoxycortisol and 11-deoxycorticosterone, both intermediate metabolites with mineralocorticoid activity. Because of the resulting excess in mineralocorticoid-like activity, patients with this deficiency retain salt and water and may present with hypertension. These individuals may also manifest with hypoglycemia because they lack cortisol and with increased virilization because of shunted intermediaries to adrenal androgen synthesis. The sustained elevation of ACTH levels caused by lack of cortisol-mediated negative feedback leads to growth (hyperplasia) of the adrenal gland.

GLUCOCORTICOID EXCESS

Glucocorticoid excess can be caused by overproduction by an adrenal tumor, overstimulation of adrenal glucocorticoid synthesis by ACTH produced by a pituitary tumor or an ectopic tumor, or the iatrogenic (induced by a physician's prescription) administration of excess synthetic glucocorticoids. The clinical manifestation of glucocorticoid excess, known as *Cushing syndrome*, can be separated into 2 categories depending on its etiology.

ACTH-dependent Cushing syndrome is characterized by elevated glucocorticoid levels caused by excess stimulation by ACTH produced by pituitary or ectopic (extrapituitary tissue) tumors. The most frequent source of ectopically produced ACTH is small cell lung carcinoma. Ectopic secretion of ACTH is usually not suppressed by exogenously administered glucocorticoids (dexamethasone), and this feature is helpful in its differential diagnosis. The name "Cushing disease" is reserved for Cushing syndrome caused by excess secretion of ACTH by pituitary tumors and is the most common form of the syndrome.

In ACTH-independent Cushing syndrome, excess cortisol production is caused by abnormal adrenocortical glucocorticoid production regardless of ACTH stimulation. In fact, the elevated circulating cortisol levels suppress CRH and ACTH levels in plasma.

Clinically, the most common presentation of glucocorticoid excess is weight gain, which is usually central but may be general in distribution; thickening of the facial features, giving the typical round face or "moon face"; an enlarged dorsocervical fat pad, or "buffalo hump"; and increased fat that bulges above the supraclavicular fossae. Hypertension, glucose intolerance, decreased or absent menstrual flow in premenopausal women, decreased libido in men, and spontaneous bruising are frequent concomitant findings. Muscle wasting and weakness are manifested by difficulty in climbing stairs or rising from a low chair. In children and young adolescents, glucocorticoid excess causes stunted linear growth and excessive weight gain. Depression and insomnia often accompany the other symptoms. Older patients and those with chronic Cushing syndrome tend to have thinning of the skin and osteoporosis, with low back pain and vertebral collapse caused by increased bone turnover leading to osteoporosis.

GLUCOCORTICOID DEFICIENCY

Glucocorticoid deficiency is less common than diseases caused by excess production of glucocorticoids. Glucocorticoid deficiency can result from adrenal dysfunction (primary deficiency) or from lack of ACTH stimulation of adrenal glucocorticoid production (secondary deficiency). Exogenous administration of synthetic analogs of glucocorticoids in the chronic treatment of some diseases suppresses CRH and ACTH (Figure 6-4). Therefore, the sudden discontinuation of treatment may be manifested as an acute case of adrenal insufficiency, a medical emergency. Thus, it is important to carefully taper the withdrawal of glucocorticoid treatment allowing CRH and ACTH production rhythms to be restored and the endogenous synthesis of cortisol to be normalized.

Most cases of ACTH deficiency involve deficiencies of other pituitary hormones. Because aldosterone is mainly under the regulation of angiotensin II and K^+, individuals may not necessarily manifest with simultaneous mineralocorticoid deficiency when impaired ACTH release is the causative factor. Glucocorticoid deficiency caused by adrenal hypofunction is known as *Addison disease*, which can be the result of autoimmune destruction of the adrenal gland or inborn errors of steroid hormone synthesis (described earlier).

Diseases of Overproduction and Undersecretion of Mineralocorticoids

ALDOSTERONE EXCESS

Excess aldosterone can be classified as primary, secondary, tertiary, or pseudohyperaldosteronism.

Primary hyperaldosteronism, also known as Conn syndrome, is a condition in which autonomous benign tumors of the adrenal glands hypersecrete aldosterone. The excess aldosterone leads to hypertension because of Na^+ and H_2O retention and hypokalemia because of excess K^+ secretion. The release of renin is suppressed.

Secondary hyperaldosteronism is the result of excess aldosterone production in response to increased renin-angiotensin system activity. A decrease in the effective arterial blood volume resulting from other pathologic states, such as ascites or heart failure, leads to continuous stimulation of the renin-angiotensin system which in turn leads to stimulation of aldosterone release.

Tertiary hyperaldosteronism can be caused by rare genetic disorders such as Bartter or Gitelman syndromes. Bartter and Gitelman syndromes result from mutations in ion transporters in the kidney resulting in excess sodium loss. In addition, they may be associated with increased renal prostaglandin E2 production. To compensate for the loss of NaCl in the urine and contracted circulating volume and aided by the excess prostaglandin E2 production; the kidney increases renin release, which in turn stimulates angiotensin II production and aldosterone release.

Pseudohyperaldosteronism is the excess mineralocorticoid activity caused by mineralocorticoid receptor activation by substances other than aldosterone. This condition is known as the syndrome of apparent mineralocorticoid excess. Several factors have been associated with this syndrome:

- Congenital adrenal hyperplasia (11β-hydroxylase deficiency and 17α-hydroxylase deficiency) leading to excess production of 11-deoxycortisone (an active mineralocorticoid).
- Deficiency of 11β-hydroxysteroid dehydrogenase type II, which leads to insufficient conversion of cortisol to its inactive metabolite cortisone in the principal cells of the distal tubule. An example of this alteration occurs with excess consumption of licorice. Glycyrrhetinic acid, a compound of licorice, inhibits the activity of 11β-hydroxysteroid dehydrogenase. Inhibition of this enzyme results in a decrease in the inactivation of glucocorticoids in mineralocorticoid-sensitive cells.
- Primary glucocorticoid resistance, characterized by hypertension, excess androgens, and increased plasma cortisol concentrations.
- Liddle syndrome, caused by activating mutations of the renal epithelial sodium channel (ENaC), leading to salt-sensitive hypertension.
- Mutations in the mineralocorticoid receptor resulting in constitutive mineralocorticoid receptor activity and altered receptor specificity. In this condition, progesterone and other steroids lacking 21-hydroxyl groups become potent agonists of the mineralocorticoid receptor.

In summary, excess mineralocorticoid-like activity can result not only from excess production of aldosterone, but also from other mechanisms, including overproduction of 11-deoxycorticosterone, inadequate conversion of cortisol to cortisone by 11β-hydroxysteroid dehydrogenase type II in target tissues, glucocorticoid receptor deficiency, and constitutive activation of renal sodium channels.

Chronic excess of mineralocorticoids can result in what is known as an **escape phenomenon**. Although sodium retention increases during the initial phase of mineralocorticoid excess, compensatory mechanisms involved in sodium excretion subsequently go into effect, resulting in new sodium equilibrium in the body maintained by higher sodium excretion. The importance of this escape mechanism is that it limits the volume expansion related to Na^+ retention.

ALDOSTERONE DEFICIENCY

Deficient aldosterone activity can be classified as primary, secondary, or pseudohypoaldosteronism.

Primary hypoaldosteronism is the lack of adrenal gland production of aldosterone because of Addison disease (destruction of the adrenal gland because of infection, injury, or autoimmune processes), from genetic disorders affecting the entire gland, or from genetic disorders affecting specific enzymatic conversions required for aldosterone biosynthesis. Two of these genetic diseases, the salt-wasting forms of 21-hydroxylase and 3β-hydroxysteroid dehydrogenase deficiencies, also affect cortisol biosynthesis. In primary aldosterone deficiency, plasma renin activity is elevated, so this condition is also known as *hyperreninemic hypoaldosteronism*.

Secondary hypoaldosteronism is lack of aldosterone production caused by inadequate stimulation by angiotensin II (hyporeninemic hypoaldosteronism) despite normal adrenal function. This condition is usually associated with renal insufficiency.

Pseudohypoaldosteronism is caused by unresponsiveness to mineralocorticoid hormone action and characterized by severe neonatal salt wasting, hyperkalemia, metabolic acidosis. This inherited disease can be caused by a loss-of-function mutation in the mineralocorticoid receptor or, in the more severe recessive form, to a loss-of-function mutation in the ENaC subunits.

Diseases of Overproduction and Undersecretion of Adrenal Androgens

ADRENAL ANDROGEN EXCESS

The most likely cause of excessive androgen secretion is dysregulation of the 17-hydroxylase and 17,20-lyase activities of P450c17, the rate-limiting step in androgen biosynthesis. Congenital adrenal hyperplasia because of 21-hydroxylase deficiency is one of the most common autosomal recessive disorders. As discussed above, impaired cortisol production leads to a lack of negative glucocorticoid feedback resulting in an increase in ACTH release, increased steroid hormone biosynthesis, buildup of cortisol and aldosterone precursors, and increased shunting to the androgen synthetic pathway. The classic form of congenital adrenal hyperplasia presents in infancy and early childhood as signs and symptoms of virilization with or without adrenal insufficiency.

ADRENAL ANDROGEN DEFICIENCY

Similar to the deficiencies of glucocorticoids and mineralocorticoids, adrenal androgen deficiency can be primary or secondary to hypopituitarism. Of greater importance is the continuous decrease in adrenal androgen production that is associated with aging and menopause (discussed in Chapters 8 and 9). Pharmacologic treatment with oral glucocorticoids results in ACTH suppression, which in turn results in reduced adrenal androgen production.

HORMONES OF THE ADRENAL MEDULLA

All of the previous discussion focused on the hormones produced and released from the adrenal cortex. As mentioned at the beginning of this chapter, the adrenal gland is composed of 2 embryologically distinct regions. The medulla can be considered a sympathetic nervous system ganglion, which, in response to preganglionic sympathetic neuron stimulation, release of acetylcholine, and its binding to a cholinergic receptor in chromaffin cells, stimulates the production and release of catecholamines. The medulla is the central part of the adrenal gland (see Figure 6–1). It is extremely vascular and consists of large chromaffin cells arranged in a network. It is made of 2 cell types called *pheochromocytes*, which are epinephrine-producing (more numerous) and norepinephrine-producing cells. These cells synthesize and secrete the catecholamines **epinephrine** (in greater amounts)**, norepinephrine** and, to a lesser extent, **dopamine (see Figure 6–2)**.

Chemistry and Biosynthesis

Catecholamines are amino acid–derived hormones, synthesized from the amino acid tyrosine (Figure 6–9). Tyrosine is actively transported into the cells, where it undergoes 4 enzymatic cytosolic reactions for its conversion to epinephrine. These are as follows:

- Hydroxylation of tyrosine to 3,4-dihydroxyphenylalanine (L-dopa) by the enzyme **tyrosine hydroxylase**. This enzyme is found in the cytosol of catecholamine-producing cells and is the main control point for catecholamine

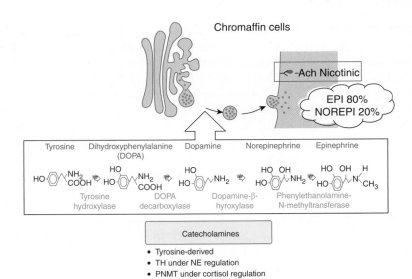

Figure 6–9. The catecholamines epinephrine (Epi) and norepinephrine (Norepi) are synthesized in chromaffin cells in the adrenal medulla in response to acetylcholine (Ach) release from preganglionic neurons of the sympathetic nervous system. Catecholamine synthesis from the precursor L-tyrosine involves 4 enzymatic reactions that take place in the cytosol of chromaffin cells. These are (1) hydroxylation of tyrosine to 3,4-dihydroxyphenylalanine (L-dopa) by **tyrosine hydroxylase (TH)**, (2) decarboxylation of L-dopa to dopamine by **dopa decarboxylase**, (3) hydroxylation of dopamine to norepinephrine by **dopamine β-hydroxylase**, and (4) methylation of norepinephrine to epinephrine by **phenylethanolamine N-methyltransferase (PNMT)**. NE, norepinephrine.

synthesis. The activity of this enzyme is inhibited by norepinephrine, providing feedback control of catecholamine synthesis.

- Decarboxylation of L-dopa to dopamine by the enzyme **dopa decarboxylase** in a reaction that requires pyridoxal phosphate as a cofactor. This end product is packaged into secretory vesicles.

- Hydroxylation of dopamine to norepinephrine by the enzyme **dopamine β-hydroxylase**, a membrane-bound enzyme found in synaptic vesicles that uses vitamin C as a cofactor. This reaction occurs inside the secretory vesicles.

- Methylation of norepinephrine to epinephrine by the enzyme **phenylethanolamine N-methyltransferase**. The activity of this cytosolic enzyme is modulated by adjacent adrenal steroid hormone production, underscoring the importance of radial arterial flow from the cortex to the medulla.

Conversion of norepinephrine to epinephrine occurs in the cytoplasm and thus requires that norepinephrine leave the secretory granules by a passive transport mechanism. The epinephrine produced in the cytoplasm must reenter the secretory vesicles through adenosine triphosphate (ATP)-driven active transport. The transporters involved are the vesicular monoamine transporters, which are expressed exclusively in neuroendocrine cells. Because of the expression of these transporters in sympathomedullary tissues, their function can be used diagnostically (like that of the iodide transporter) for radioimaging and localization of catecholamine-producing tumors (pheochromocytomas). Catecholamines in secretory vesicles exist in a dynamic equilibrium with the surrounding cytoplasm, with catecholamine uptake into the vesicles being balanced by their leakage into the cytoplasm. In the cytoplasm, epinephrine is converted to metanephrine and norepinephrine is converted to normetanephrine by the enzyme catechol-O-methyltransferase (COMT) (Figure 6-10). The catecholamine metabolites then leak out of the cell continuously to become free metanephrines. The synthesis of catecholamines can be regulated by changes in the activity of tyrosine hydroxylase by release from end-product inhibition (acute) or by an increase in enzyme synthesis (chronic).

Release of Catecholamines

The release of catecholamines is a direct response to sympathetic nerve stimulation of the adrenal medulla. Acetylcholine released from the preganglionic sympathetic nerve terminals binds to nicotinic cholinergic receptors (ligand-gated ion channels) in the plasma membrane of the chromaffin cells leading to rapid Na^+ influx and cell membrane depolarization. Depolarization of the cells leads to activation of voltage-gated Ca^{2+} channels, producing an influx of Ca^{2+}. The synaptic vesicles containing the preformed catecholamines are docked beneath the synaptic membrane and are closely associated with voltage-gated Ca^{2+} channels. The influx of Ca^{2+} triggers the exocytosis of secretory granules, which release catecholamines into the interstitial space, from where they are transported in the circulation to their target organs. The physiologic role of the peptides (chromogranins, ATP, adrenomedullin, POMC

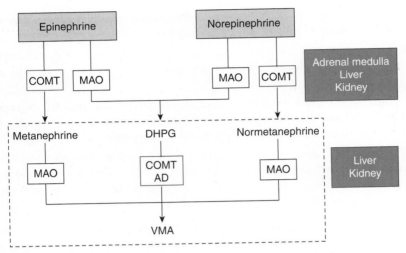

Figure 6–10. Catecholamine metabolism. Catecholamines are metabolized to metanephrines primarily by membrane-bound catecholamine-*O*-methyltransferase (COMT): epinephrine to metanephrine and norepinephrine to normetanephrine in chromaffin cells. Sympathetic neuron cytoplasmic norepinephrine is metabolized to 3,4-dihydroxyphenylglycol (DHPG) by monoamine oxidase (MAO). DHPG leaks from sympathetic neurons and is converted to vanillylmandelic acid (VMA). Extra-adrenal/neuronal catecholamine metabolic pathway is via MAO that converts both epinephrine and norepinephrine to DHPG. DHPG is further metabolized by COMT and aldehyde dehydrogenase (AD) to VMA. Catecholamines and metanephrines also undergo conjugation of with sulfate or glucuronide. Catecholamines, their metabolites, and conjugates are excreted in the urine. Normally, the proportions of urine catecholamines and metabolites are approximately 50% metanephrines, 35% VMA, 10% conjugated catecholamines and other metabolites, and less than 5% free catecholamines.

products, and other peptides) coreleased with the catecholamines has not been fully established and will not be discussed.

Catecholamine Transport and Metabolism

The half-life of circulating catecholamines is short (<2 minutes). Most (>50%) of the catecholamines released circulate bound to albumin with low affinity. Circulating catecholamines can undergo reuptake by extraneuronal sites, degradation at target cells by **catechol-*O*-methyltransferase (COMT)** or **monoamino oxidase (MAO)**, or direct filtration into the urine (Figure 6–10). MAO catalyzes the first step of oxidative deamination of catecholamines. COMT catalyzes conversion of epinephrine and norepinephrine to metanephrine and normetanephrine. The joint action of MAO, COMT, and aldehyde dehydrogenase on norepinephrine and epinephrine; especially in the liver, produces the metabolite **vanillylmandelic acid (VMA)**, the major end product of norepinephrine and epinephrine metabolism. Dopamine metabolized through this pathway yields homovanillic acid (HVA). VMA and HVA are water soluble and have high levels of urinary excretion. Their urinary excretion rate is an important index and useful clinical marker for the detection of tumors, such as pheochromocytomas, that produce excess catecholamines.

Target Organ Cellular Effects

The physiologic effects of catecholamines are mediated by binding to cell membrane G protein–coupled adrenergic receptors distributed widely throughout the body. Because they do not cross the blood-brain barrier easily, catecholamines released from the adrenal medulla exert their effects almost exclusively in peripheral tissues and not in the brain. Catecholamines have differential effects depending on the subtype of G protein to which the receptor is associated with and the signal transduction mechanism linked to that specific G protein (Table 6–3).

The adrenergic receptors are classified as predominantly stimulatory receptors (α) or predominantly inhibitory receptors (β). Understanding the selectivity of the receptors and their tissue distribution is therefore key to predicting the individual's response to their therapeutic use.

ALPHA-ADRENERGIC RECEPTORS

Alpha-adrenergic receptors have greater affinity for epinephrine than for norepinephrine or for isoproterenol, a synthetic agonist. They are subdivided into α_1- and α_2-receptors.

Alpha$_1$-adrenergic receptors are further subdivided into α_{1A}, α_{1B}, and α_{1D}. These are G protein–coupled receptors ($G\alpha_{q/11}$) that activate phospholipase C, resulting in activation of protein kinase C, and an increase in intracellular Ca^{2+} (via inositol 1,4,5-trisphosphate), and phospholipase A_2 (see Table 6–3). The increase in

Table 6–3. Adrenergic receptors and signaling pathways

Adrenergic receptor	G protein	Second messenger
β-Adrenergic receptors β_1, β_2, β_3	$G\alpha_s$ G protein	Activate adenylate cyclase
α_1-Adrenergic receptors α_{1A}, α_{1B}, α_{1D}	Mostly $G_{q/11}$ family of G proteins	Usually activate PLCα (thereby activating PKC via DAG and increasing intracellular Ca^{2+} via IP$_3$) or PLA$_2$
α_2-Adrenergic receptors α_{2A}, α_{2B}, α_{2C}	Mostly varied $G\alpha_i$ and G_0 proteins	May decrease the activity of adenylate cyclase (opposing the effects of β-adrenergic receptors) Activate K channels Inhibit Ca^{2+} channels and activate PLCβ or PLA$_2$ (an effect similar to that of α_1-adrenergic receptors)

DAG, diacylglycerol; IP$_3$, inositol 1,4,5-trisphosphate; PKC, protein kinase C; PLA2, phospholipase A2; PLCβ, phospholipase Cβ.

Table 6–4. Catecholamine physiologic effects

α-Adrenergic mediated	β-Adrenergic mediated
Vasoconstriction	Vasodilation
Iris dilation	Cardioacceleration
Intestinal relaxation	Increased myocardial strength
Intestinal sphincter contraction	Intestinal and bladder wall relaxation
Pilomotor contraction	Uterus relaxation
Bladder sphincter contraction	Bronchodilation
Bronchoconstriction	Calorigenesis
Uterine smooth muscle contraction	Glycogenolysis
Cardiac contractility	Lipolysis
Hepatic glucose production	Increased renin release
Decreased insulin release	Increased glucagon release

intracellular Ca^{2+} calmodulin kinase–mediated phosphorylation of myosin light-chain kinase in smooth muscle produces contraction in vascular, bronchial, and uterine smooth muscle. Alpha$_1$-adrenergic receptors play important roles in the regulation of several physiologic processes, including myocardial contractility and chronotropy and hepatic glucose metabolism (Table 6–4).

Alpha$_2$-adrenergic receptors are also subdivided into 3 groups, including α_{2A}, α_{2B}, and α_{2C}, and have varied second-messenger systems. They may be associated with $G\alpha_i$ and G_0 proteins and may decrease adenylate cyclase activity, activate K^+ channels, inhibit Ca^{2+} channels, and activate phospholipase $C\beta$ or phospholipase A_2 (see Table 6–3). Alpha$_2$-adrenergic receptors were initially characterized as presynaptic receptors involved in a negative feedback loop to regulate the release of norepinephrine. However, they are also involved in postsynaptic functions and play a role in blood pressure homeostasis (see Table 6–4). Some of the physiologic effects mediated by this subtype of receptor involve actions at 2 counteracting α_2-receptor subtypes. For example, stimulation of α_{2A} receptors decreases sympathetic outflow and blood pressure, whereas stimulation of α_{2B} receptors increases blood pressure by direct vasoconstriction. Alpha$_2$-adrenergic receptors are implicated in diverse physiologic functions, particularly in the cardiovascular system and the central nervous system. Alpha$_2$-adrenergic receptor agonists are used clinically in the treatment of hypertension, glaucoma, and attention deficit disorder; in the suppression of opiate withdrawal; and as adjuncts to general anesthesia.

BETA-ADRENERGIC RECEPTORS

Beta-adrenergic receptors have been subclassified as β_1, β_2, and β_3 receptors. They have greater affinity for isoproterenol than for epinephrine or norepinephrine. All 3 receptor subtypes are associated with $G\alpha_s$ proteins, and their stimulation leads to an increase in cyclic adenosine monophosphate (see Table 6–3).

The β_1-adrenergic receptor plays an important role in regulating contraction and relaxation of cardiac myocytes through phosphorylation of sarcolemma L-type Ca^{2+} channels, ryanodine-sensitive Ca^{2+} channels in the sarcoplasmic reticulum, troponin I, and phospholamban (see Table 6–4). The overall physiologic effect is an increase in cardiac contractility. β_1-receptor antagonists are first-line medication for patients with hypertension, coronary heart disease, or chronic heart failure.

The β_2-adrenergic receptor mediates several physiologic responses, including vasodilatation, bronchial smooth muscle relaxation, and lipolysis, in various tissues. Selective agonists for the β_2-adrenergic receptor are used as bronchodilators in the management of asthma.

The β_3-adrenergic receptor plays an important role in mediating catecholamine-stimulated thermogenesis and lipolysis.

Catecholamine Physiologic Effects

Catecholamines are released in response to sympathetic stimulation and are central to the stress response to a physical or psychological insult such as severe blood loss, decrease in blood glucose concentration, traumatic injury, surgical intervention, or a fearful experience. Because catecholamines are part of the "fight or flight" response, their physiologic effects include arousal, papillary dilation, piloerection, sweating, bronchial dilation, tachycardia, inhibition of smooth muscle activity, and constriction of the sphincters in the gastrointestinal tract (see Table 6–4). Most of the events involved in coping with a stressful situation require the expenditure of energy. Catecholamines ensure substrate mobilization from the liver, muscle, and fat by stimulating breakdown of glycogen (glycogenolysis) and fat (lipolysis). Thus, an increase in circulating catecholamines is associated with elevations in plasma glucose, glycerol, and free fatty acid levels. Some of the most important effects of catecholamines are exerted in the cardiovascular system, where they increase heart rate (tachycardia), produce peripheral vasoconstriction, and elevate vascular resistance.

Regulation of Adrenergic Receptors

The release of catecholamines and their effects are of short duration under normal physiologic conditions. However, chronic stimulation leading to sustained elevations in circulating catecholamines and the resulting stimulation of adrenergic receptors can lead to alterations in tissue responsiveness. Similar alterations in responsiveness can be elicited by either endogenously produced agonists or exogenously administered pharmacologic agonists. Examples include β-agonist–promoted desensitization in asthma and α-agonist–stimulated tachyphylaxis in patients receiving sympathomimetic nasal decongestants. Persistent exposure to an agonist of the adrenergic receptor can also result in an actual loss of receptors because of degradation or receptor desensitization. Several mechanisms of desensitization have been described. For example, after only a few minutes of exposure to a β_2-adrenergic agonist, the receptor is phosphorylated. This phosphorylation interferes with receptor coupling to the G protein. Following a more prolonged exposure to adrenergic-receptor agonists, the receptors are internalized below the cell surface. Finally, with chronic exposure to receptor agonists, the number of receptors in the plasma membrane can be reduced because of decreased synthesis of the receptor (downregulation).

Adrenergic receptors can also undergo upregulation because of increased transcription of the gene for the receptor. Two hormones are known to produce this effect: glucocorticoids and thyroid hormone. In addition, glucocorticoids and thyroid hormone can regulate the expression of several types of adrenergic receptors through post-transcriptional events. The various subtypes of adrenergic receptors differ in their susceptibility to these agonist-promoted events. Receptor upregulation by thyroid hormone is critical in hyperthyroid patients because the combined effects of thyroid hormone and catecholamines can exacerbate cardiovascular manifestations of disease.

Diseases of Overproduction and Undersecretion of Adrenal Catecholamines

As mentioned at the beginning of this chapter, the adrenal medulla and ganglia of the sympathetic nervous system are derived from the embryonic neural crest. On the basis of histochemical staining (black-colored staining caused by chromaffin oxidation of catecholamines), the endocrine cells of this sympathoadrenal system are named chromaffin cells, and the tumors arising from these cells are called *pheochromocytomas*. Pheochromocytomas produce catecholamines, and patients present with signs of excess catecholamine effects, such as sustained or paroxysmal hypertension associated with headache, sweating, or palpitations. Elevated plasma and urinary levels of catecholamines, and their metabolites (VMA and metanephrines) are the cornerstone for the diagnosis.

Biochemical Evaluation of Adrenal Function

Several approaches to the evaluation of adrenal function are available for clinical use. All of them involve the physiologic basis of metabolism and regulation of adrenal hormone production. Some of the most prevalent are mentioned here. The simplest approach is the measurement of urinary hormone or degradation products of hormone metabolism. The 24-hour urine collection for these measurements has the advantage of providing an integrated measure of hormone production throughout the 24 hours.

Because of the variability in plasma concentrations of cortisol as a result of its pulsatile release and circadian rhythm, measures of plasma cortisol levels are difficult to interpret. Cortisol hypersecretion is confirmed by measuring urinary cortisol excretion over a 24-hour period; which integrates the changes in cortisol concentrations during the entire day and is a more reliable measure of total cortisol production.

DEXAMETHASONE SUPPRESSION TEST

Administration of low-dose dexamethasone, a synthetic glucocorticoid analog either over 2 days (at a low dose) or overnight (when given at a higher dose), suppresses CRH and ACTH release and thus cortisol production. The basis of this test is that, in most situations, the corticotroph tumor cells in Cushing disease retain some responsiveness to the negative feedback effects of glucocorticoids. In contrast, ectopic ACTH-producing tumors do not. The standard test is performed on 24-hour collections of urine for the measurement of cortisol or its metabolite. Therefore, the dexamethasone-CRH test is used to differentiate between pituitary ACTH-dependent (Cushing disease) and ectopic ACTH-dependent (Cushing syndrome) hypercortisolism.

METYRAPONE STIMULATION TEST

The metyrapone test measures the ability of the HPA axis to respond to an acute reduction in serum cortisol levels. Metyrapone inhibits 11β-hydroxylase preventing the last steps in cortisol synthesis. The decrease in cortisol levels should result in increased ACTH release and adrenal steroidogenesis with an increase in circulating levels of 11-deoxycortisol, the last precursor in the synthesis of cortisol. Patients with adrenal insufficiency do not respond to the increase in ACTH produced by the decreased cortisol levels.

CORTICOTROPIN-RELEASING HORMONE STIMULATION TEST

The CRH stimulation test measures the ability of the pituitary gland to secrete ACTH as well as the ability of the adrenal gland to respond with an increase in cortisol. CRH testing may help differentiate between a pituitary source (ie, Cushing disease) and an ectopic source of ACTH. Patients with Cushing disease respond to CRH administration with a significant (~2-fold) increase in plasma ACTH and cortisol. In contrast, patients with ectopic ACTH-producing tumors rarely respond with an exacerbation of cortisol levels following CRH administration.

KEY CONCEPTS

 Glucocorticoid production and release is under ACTH regulation.

 Mineralocorticoid release is under angiotensin II and K⁺ regulation.

 Steroid hormone receptors produce their effects by binding to hormone-responsive elements in DNA and modulating (increase or decrease) gene transcription.

 Specificity of the mineralocorticoid receptor is conferred by specificity in tissue distribution and localized conversion of glucocorticoids to cortisone by 11β-hydroxysteroid dehydrogenase.

Glucocorticoids facilitate fuel mobilization, decrease glucose utilization, and produce immunosuppression.

 Aldosterone increases renal sodium reabsorption and in exchange stimulates potassium excretion.

 Catecholamine release is under sympathetic nervous system control.

 The response to stress by the host relies on close interaction between the cortisol and catecholamines to ensure adequate fuel mobilization and hemodynamic control.

STUDY QUESTIONS

6–1. A 49-year-old construction worker has a 10-month history of muscle weakness, easy bruising, backache, and headache. Physical examination reveals cutaneous hyperpigmentation, pronounced truncal obesity with a "buffalo hump," and blood pressure of 180/100 mm Hg. Laboratory analyses reveal elevated concentrations of circulating cortisol with an absence of a circadian rhythm. With high-dose administration of a glucocorticoid agonist, you notice that the levels of plasma cortisol are reduced significantly. What is the most likely cause of these symptoms?

 a. Adrenocortical hypersecretion of pituitary origin

 b. Autoimmune destruction of the adrenal cortex

 c. Congenital adrenal hyperplasia

 d. Ectopic ACTH production in the lung

 e. Primary hyperaldosteronism

6–2. A 35-year-old woman has noted a weight gain of 7 kg over the past year. She has normal menstrual periods. On physical examination, her blood pressure is 170/105 mm Hg. A serum electrolyte panel shows sodium 141 mmol/L, potassium 4.4 mmol/L, chloride 100 mmol/L, CO_2 25 mmol/L, glucose 181 mg/dL, and creatinine 1.0 mg/dL. Which of the following would you most expect to be present in this patient?

 a. A prolactinoma

 b. Lung metastatic carcinoma

 c. An adrenal adenoma

 d. Excess licorice consumption

 e. Graves disease

6–3. A 55-year-old man has experienced episodic headaches for the past 3 months. On physical examination, his blood pressure is 185/110 mm Hg, with no other remarkable findings. Laboratory studies show sodium 145 mmol/L, potassium 4.3 mmol/L, chloride 103 mmol/L, glucose 91 mg/dL, and creatinine 1.3 mg/dL. An abdominal CT scan shows a 7-cm left adrenal mass. During surgery, as the surgeon is removing the left adrenal gland, the anesthesiologist notes a marked rise in blood pressure. Which of the following laboratory test findings would have been most likely have been present in this patient prior to surgery?

    a. Serum cortisol 90 nmol/L

    b. Urinary vanillylmandelic acid 25 μmol/d

    c. Serum ACTH 30 pmol/L

    d. Urinary free catecholamine 1090 nmol/d

    e. Aldosterone 300 pmol/L

6–4. A 44-year-old man has had headaches for 4 months. On physical examination, he is found to have a blood pressure of 170/110 mm Hg. Laboratory studies show a serum sodium of 147 mmol/L, potassium 2.3 mmol/L, chloride 103 mmol/L, glucose 82 mg/dL, and creatinine 1.2 mg/dL. His plasma renin activity is 0.1 ng/mL/h (normal values are 1.9 to 3.7 ng/mL/h), and his serum aldosterone 65 ng/mL. Which of the following abnormalities is the most likely cause for these findings?

    a. Pheochromocytoma

    b. Iatrogenic Cushing syndrome

    c. Pituitary adenoma

    d. Adrenal adenoma

    e. 21-Hydroxylase deficiency

SUGGESTED READINGS

Boscaro M, Barzon L, Fallo F, Sonino N. Cushing's syndrome. *Lancet.* 2001;357:783.

Eaton DC, Malik B, Saxena NC, Al-Khalili OK, Yue G. Mechanisms of aldosterone's action on epithelial Na⁺ transport. *J Membr Biol.* 2001;184:313.

Ehrhart-Bornstein M, Hinson JP, Bornstein SR, Scherbaum WA, Vinson GP. Intraadrenal interactions in the regulation of adrenocortical steroidogenesis. *Endocr Rev.* 1998;19:101.

Eisenhofer G, Kopin IJ, Goldstein DS. Catecholamine metabolism contemporary review with implications for physiology and medicine. *Pharmacol Rev.* 2004; 56:331.

Ganguly A. Current concepts: primary aldosteronism. *N Engl J Med.* 1998;339:1828.

McEwen BS. Protective and damaging effects of stress mediators. *N Engl J Med.* 1998;338:171.

Nelson HS. Drug therapy: β-adrenergic bronchodilators. *N Engl J Med.* 1995;333:499.

Newell-Price J, Trainer P, Besser M, Grossman A. The diagnosis and differential diagnosis of Cushing's syndrome and pseudo-Cushing's states. *Endocr Rev.* 1998;19:647.

Ngarmukos C, Grekin RJ. Nontraditional aspects of aldosterone physiology. *Am J Physiol Endocrinol Metab.* 2001;281:E1122.

Orth DN. Medical progress: Cushing's syndrome. *N Engl J Med.* 1995;332:791.

Stocco DM. StAR protein and the regulation of steroid hormone biosynthesis. *Annu Rev Physiol.* 2001;63:193.

Endocrine Pancreas

7

OBJECTIVES

▶ Identify the principal hormones secreted from the endocrine pancreas, their cells of origin, and their chemical nature.

▶ Understand the nutrient, neural, and hormonal mechanisms that regulate pancreatic hormone release.

▶ List the principal target organs for insulin and glucagon action and their major physiologic effects.

▶ Identify the time course for the onset and duration of the biologic actions of insulin and glucagon.

▶ Identify the disease states caused by oversecretion, undersecretion, or decreased sensitivity to insulin, and describe the principal manifestations of each.

The pancreas is a mixed exocrine and endocrine gland that plays a central role in digestion and in the metabolism, utilization, and storage of energy substrates. This chapter focuses on the endocrine function of the pancreas through the release of insulin and glucagon and the mechanisms by which these hormones regulate events essential to maintaining glucose homeostasis. Maintenance of glucose homeostasis is similar to the maintenance of calcium balance discussed in Chapter 5, in which several tissues and hormones interact in the regulatory process. In the case of glucose, the process involves a regulated balance among hepatic glucose release (from glycogen breakdown and gluconeogenesis), dietary glucose absorption, and glucose uptake and disposal by skeletal muscle and adipose tissue. The pancreatic hormones insulin and glucagon play central roles in regulating each of these processes, and their overall effects are in part modified by other hormones such as growth hormone, cortisol, and epinephrine. In addition to secreting insulin and glucagon, the endocrine pancreas also secretes somatostatin, amylin, and pancreatic polypeptide.

FUNCTIONAL ANATOMY

The pancreas is a retroperitoneal gland divided into a head, body, and tail that is located near the duodenum. Most of the pancreatic mass is composed of exocrine cells that are clustered in lobules (acini) divided by connective tissue and connected to a duct that drains into the pancreatic duct and into the duodenum. The product of the pancreatic exocrine cells is an alkaline fluid rich with digestive enzymes, which is secreted into the small intestine to aid in the digestive process. Embedded within the acini are richly vascularized, small clusters of endocrine cells called the **islets of Langerhans**, in which 2 endocrine cell types (β and α) predominate. The β-cells constitute most of the total mass of endocrine cells, and their principal secretory product is **insulin.** The α-cells account for approximately 20% of the endocrine cells and are responsible for **glucagon** secretion. A small number of δ-cells secrete **somatostatin**, and an even smaller number of cells secrete **pancreatic polypeptide**. The localization of these cell types within the islets has a particular pattern, with the β-cells located centrally, surrounded by α- and δ-cells.

The arterial blood supply to the pancreas is derived from the splenic artery and the superior and inferior pancreaticoduodenal arteries. Although islets represent only 1%–2% of the mass of the pancreas, they receive approximately 10%–15% of the pancreatic blood flow. The rich vascularization by fenestrated capillaries allows ready access to the circulation for the hormones secreted by the islet cells. Venous blood from the pancreas drains into the hepatic portal vein. Therefore, the liver, a principal target organ for the physiologic effects of pancreatic hormones, is exposed to the highest concentrations of pancreatic hormones. Following first-pass hepatic metabolism, the pancreatic endocrine hormones are distributed to the systemic circulation.

Parasympathetic, sympathetic, and sensory nerves richly innervate the pancreatic islets, and the respective neurotransmitters and neuropeptides released from their nerve terminals exert important regulatory effects on pancreatic endocrine hormone release. Acetylcholine, vasoactive intestinal polypeptide, pituitary adenylate cyclase-activating polypeptide, and gastrin-releasing peptide are released from the parasympathetic nerve terminals. Norepinephrine, galanin, and neuropeptide Y are released from sympathetic nerve terminals. Vagal nerve activation stimulates the secretion of insulin, glucagon, somatostatin, and pancreatic polypeptide. Sympathetic nerve stimulation inhibits basal and glucose-stimulated insulin secretion and somatostatin release and stimulates glucagon and pancreatic polypeptide secretion.

PANCREATIC HORMONES

Insulin

INSULIN SYNTHESIS, RELEASE, AND DEGRADATION

The process involved in the synthesis and release of insulin, a polypeptide hormone, by the β-cells of the pancreas is similar to that of other peptide hormones, as discussed in Chapter 1 (Figure 1–2). Preproinsulin undergoes cleavage of its signal peptide during insertion into the endoplasmic reticulum, generating proinsulin (Figure 7–1). Proinsulin consists of an amino-terminal β-chain, a carboxy-terminal α-chain, and a connecting peptide; known as the **C-peptide**, that links the α- and β-chains. Linking of the 2 chains allows proper folding of the molecule

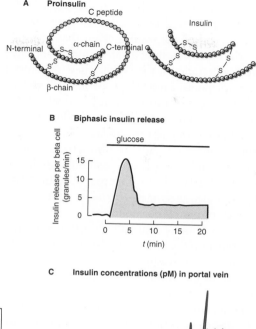

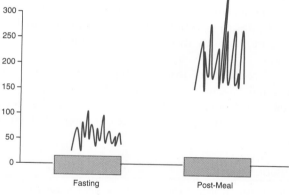

Figure 7–1. **A.** Insulin is a peptide hormone synthesized from preproinsulin. Preproinsulin undergoes posttranslational modification in the endoplasmic reticulum (ER) to form proinsulin. The active form of insulin is produced by modification of proinsulin by cleavage of the C-peptide structure linking the alpha and beta chains. Both insulin and the cleaved C-peptide are packaged in secretory granules and are coreleased in response to glucose stimulation. **B.** Insulin release occurs in a biphasic mode; from readily releasable secretory granules and from granules that must undergo a series of preparatory reactions including mobilization to the plasma membrane. **C.** In response to a meal, the increase in insulin release results from a higher frequency and amplitude of pulsatile release. Shown are portal insulin concentrations during basal state (left) and after a meal.

and the formation of disulfide bonds between the 2 chains. In the endoplasmic reticulum, proinsulin is processed by specific endopeptidases, which cleave the C-peptide exposing the end of the insulin chain that interacts with the insulin receptor, generating the mature form of insulin. Insulin and the free C-peptide are packaged into secretory granules in the Golgi. These secretory granules accumulate in the cytoplasm in 2 pools; a readily releasable (5%) and a reserve pool of the granules (more than 95%). On stimulation, the β-cell releases insulin in a biphasic pattern; initially from the readily releasable pool followed by the reserve pool of granules. Only a small proportion of the cellular stores of insulin are released even under maximal stimulatory conditions. Insulin circulates in its free form, has a half-life of 3–8 minutes, and is degraded predominantly by the liver, with more than 50% of insulin degraded during its first pass. Additional degradation of insulin occurs in the kidneys as well as at target tissues by insulin proteases following endocytosis of the receptor-bound hormone.

Exocytosis of secretory granule content results in the release of equal amounts of insulin and C-peptide into the portal circulation. The importance of C-peptide is that unlike insulin, it is not readily degraded in the liver. Thus, the relatively long half-life of the peptide (35 minutes) allows its release to be used as an index of the secretory capacity of the endocrine pancreas. C-peptide, may have some biologic action as recent evidence indicates that replacement of C-peptide improves renal function and nerve dysfunction in patients with type 1 diabetes. The receptor and signaling mechanisms involved in mediating these responses are still under investigation.

The amino acid sequence of insulin is highly conserved among species. In the past, porcine and bovine insulin were used to treat patients with diabetes. Currently, human recombinant insulin is available and has replaced animal-derived insulin, avoiding problems such as the development of antibodies to non-human insulin.

REGULATION OF INSULIN RELEASE

The pancreatic β-cell functions as a neuroendocrine integrator that responds to changes in plasma levels of energy substrates (glucose and amino acids), hormones (insulin, glucagon-like peptide I, somatostatin, and epinephrine), and neurotransmitters (norepinephrine and acetylcholine) by increasing or decreasing insulin release (Figure 7–2). Glucose is the principal stimulus for insulin release from the pancreatic β-cells. In addition, glucose exerts a permissive effect for the other modulators of insulin secretion.

The glucose-induced stimulation of insulin release is the result of glucose metabolism by the β-cell (see Figure 7–2). Glucose enters the β-cell through a membrane-bound glucose transporter 2 (GLUT 2) and undergoes immediate phosphorylation by glucokinase in the initial step of glycolysis, leading eventually to the generation of adenosine triphosphate (ATP) by the Krebs cycle. The resulting increase in intracellular ATP to adenosine diphosphate ratio inhibits (closes) the ATP-sensitive K^+ channels (K_{ATP}) in the β-cell, reducing the efflux of K^+. Decreased K^+ efflux results in membrane depolarization; activation

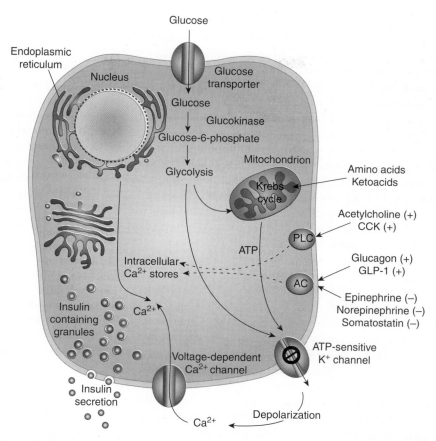

Figure 7–2. Regulation of insulin release. Glucose is the principal stimulus for insulin release from the pancreatic β-cell. Glucose enters the β-cell cell by a specific glucose transporter protein (GLUT 2) undergoes glycolysis leading to generation of ATP. The increased ATP/ADP ratio leads to inhibition and closure of the ATP-sensitive K⁺ channels (the target of sulfonylurea drugs), resulting in plasma membrane depolarization and opening of the voltage-dependent Ca²⁺ channels. The increased Ca²⁺ influx coupled with mobilization of Ca²⁺ from intracellular stores leading to the fusion of insulin-containing secretory granules with the plasma membrane and the release of insulin (and C-peptide) into the circulation. Addition factors can also stimulate insulin release from the β-cell, including hormones (glucagon-like peptide 1) and neurotransmitters (acetylcholine). Glucose synergizes with these mediators and enhances the secretory response of the β-cell to these factors. AC, adenylate cyclase; ADP, adenosine diphosphate; ATP, adenosine triphosphate; CCK, cholecystokinin; GLP 1, glucagon-like peptide-1; PLC, phospholipase C. (Modified, with permission, from Fajans SS, Bell GI, Polonsky KS. Mechanisms of disease: molecular mechanisms and clinical pathophysiology of maturity-onset diabetes of the young. *N Engl J Med*. 2001;345:971. Copyright © Massachusetts Medical Society. All rights reserved.)

(opening) of voltage-dependent Ca^{2+} channels, and increased Ca^{2+} influx. The increase in intracellular Ca^{2+} concentrations triggers the exocytosis of insulin secretory granules and the release of insulin into the extracellular space and into the circulation. It is important to note that the regulation of K^+ channels by ATP is mediated by the sulfonylurea receptor. This is the basis for the therapeutic use of sulfonylurea drugs in the treatment of diabetes.

The β-cell Ca^{2+} concentrations can also be elevated by amino acids through their metabolism and ATP generation, or by direct depolarization of the plasma membrane. Other factors (shown in Figure 7–2) that amplify the glucose-induced release of insulin from the β-cell include acetylcholine; cholecystokinin; gastrointestinal peptide, also known as glucose-dependent insulinotropic polypeptide; and glucagon-like peptide 1 (GLP 1). These substances all bind to cell surface receptors and trigger downstream signaling mechanisms controlling insulin release. Acetylcholine and cholecystokinin promote phosphoinositide breakdown, with a consequent mobilization of Ca^{2+} from intracellular stores, Ca^{2+} influx across the cell membrane, and activation of protein kinase C. GLP 1 increases levels of cyclic 3′,5′-adenosine monophosphate (cAMP) and activates cAMP-dependent protein kinase A. The generation of cAMP, inositol 1,4,5-trisphosphate, diacylglycerol, and arachidonic acid and the activation of protein kinase C amplify the Ca^{2+} signal by decreasing Ca^{2+} uptake by cellular stores and promoting both the phosphorylation and activation of proteins that trigger the exocytosis of insulin. Catecholamines and somatostatin inhibit insulin secretion through G protein–coupled receptor mechanisms, inhibition of adenylate cyclase, and modification of Ca^{2+} and K^+ channel gating.

The short-term regulation of insulin release is mediated through modification of proinsulin mRNA translation. Over longer periods, glucose also increases proinsulin mRNA content by both stimulating proinsulin gene transcription and stabilizing the mRNA. As mentioned above, the release of insulin in response to glucose is biphasic, with an initial rapid release of preformed insulin followed by a more sustained release of newly synthesized insulin. This biphasic response to glucose is a major characteristic of glucose-stimulated insulin secretion. The first phase occurs over a period of minutes, the second over an hour or more. Several hypotheses have been proposed to explain the biphasic nature of insulin secretion; including the involvement of 2 separate pools of insulin granules.

The release of insulin throughout the day is pulsatile and rhythmic in nature (see Figure 7–1). The pulsatile release of insulin is important for achieving maximal physiologic effects. In particular, it appears to be critical in the suppression of liver glucose production and in insulin-mediated glucose disposal by adipose tissue. Insulin release increases after a meal in response to the increases in plasma levels of glucose and amino acids. Secretion is the result of a combination of an increase in the total amount of insulin released in each secretory burst and an increased pulse frequency of a similar magnitude (see Figure 7–1). The synchronized increase in insulin release is thought to be the result of recruitment of β-cells to release insulin. Although it is not clear how the β-cells communicate with each other to synchronize the release of insulin, some of the proposed mechanisms include gap junctions allowing the passage of ions and small molecules; and propagation of membrane depolarization, aiding the synchronization between the cells. In addition, intra-pancreatic neural, hormonal, and substrate factors have been shown to play an important role in the pulsatile pattern of insulin release.

PHYSIOLOGIC EFFECTS OF INSULIN

Insulin produces a wide variety of effects that range from immediate (within seconds), such as the modulation of ion (K^+) and glucose transport into the cell; early (within minutes), such as the regulation of metabolic enzyme activity; moderate (within minutes to hours), such as the modulation of enzyme synthesis; to delayed (within hours to days), such as the effects on growth and cellular differentiation. Overall, the actions of insulin at target organs are anabolic and promote the synthesis of carbohydrate, fat, and protein, and these effects are mediated through binding to the insulin receptor (Table 7–1).

INSULIN RECEPTOR

The insulin receptor is part of the insulin-receptor family, which includes the insulin-like growth-factor receptor (Figure 7–3). The insulin receptor is a hetero-tetrameric glycoprotein membrane receptor composed of 2 α- and 2 β-subunits, linked by disulfide bonds. The extracellular α-chain is the site for insulin binding. The intracellular segment of the β-chain has intrinsic tyrosine kinase activity, which on insulin binding, undergoes autophosphorylation on tyrosine residues. The activated receptor phosphorylates tyrosine residues of several proteins known as **insulin receptor substrates** 1 through 4 (IRS-1–4); facilitating the interaction

Table 7–1. Insulin effects on carbohydrate, fat, and protein metabolism

Metabolic effects	Insulin stimulates	Insulin inhibits
Carbohydrate metabolism	Glucose transport in adipose tissue and muscle Rate of glycolysis in muscle and adipose tissue Glycogen synthesis in adipose tissue, muscle, and liver	Glycogen breakdown in muscle and liver Rate of glycogenolysis and gluconeogenesis in the liver
Lipid metabolism	Fatty acid and triacylglycerol synthesis in tissues Uptake of triglycerides from the blood into adipose tissue and muscle Rate of cholesterol synthesis in the liver	Lipolysis in adipose tissue, lowering the plasma fatty acid level Fatty acid oxidation in muscle and liver Ketogenesis
Protein metabolism	Amino acid transport into tissues Protein synthesis in muscle, adipose tissue, liver, and other tissues	Protein degradation in muscle Urea formation

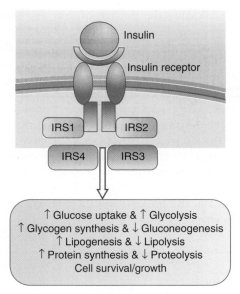

Figure 7–3. Insulin receptor signaling. Insulin binding to the receptor activates the intrinsic kinase activity of the intracellular domain of the receptor. This results in downstream activation of cellular events mediated through the phosphorylation of insulin receptor substrates (IRS). Downstream signaling pathways involved in insulin-mediated effects including the phosphatidylinositol 3-kinase (PI3K) and the mitogen-activated protein kinase (MAPK) cascades. Activation of phosphoinositide-3 kinase is a major pathway in the mediation of insulin-stimulated glucose transport and metabolism. Among the immediate effects of insulin is the active recruitment of glucose transporter 4 (GLUT 4), stored in intracellular vesicles to the cell surface. Exercise can also stimulate glucose transport by pathways that are independent of phosphoinositide-3 kinase and thought to involve 5′-adenosine monophosphate (AMP)-activated kinase.

of the insulin receptor with intracellular substrates. The result is the coupling of insulin receptor activation to signaling pathways, mainly the phosphatidylinositol 3-kinase (PI3K) and the mitogen-activated protein kinase (MAPK) pathways (see Figure 7–3).

The PI3K pathway involves phosphorylation of inositol phospholipids and the generation of phosphatidylinositol 3,4,5-trisphosphate and phosphatidylinositol 3,4-bisphosphate. These products, in turn, attract serine kinases to the plasma membrane, including the phosphoinositide-dependent kinase and different isoforms of protein kinase B, which, when activated, catalyze some of the cellular effects of insulin. The PI3K pathway is involved predominantly in mediating the metabolic effects of the hormone, including glucose transport, glycolysis, and glycogen synthesis, and plays a crucial role in the regulation of protein synthesis by insulin. Moreover, this pathway is involved in cell growth and transmits a strong antiapoptotic signal, promoting cell survival. The other main signaling pathway that is activated by insulin binding to its receptor is the MAPK pathway. Although signaling cascades in this pathway do not appear to play a significant role in the metabolic effects of insulin, they are involved in mediating the proliferative and differentiation effects elicited by insulin.

Signal transduction by the insulin receptor is not limited to its activation at the cell surface. The activated ligand-receptor complex is internalized into endosomes. Endocytosis of activated receptors is thought to enhance the insulin receptor tyrosine kinase activity on substrates that are distant from those readily accessible at the plasma membrane. Following acidification of the endosomal lumen, insulin dissociates from its receptor, ending the insulin receptor-mediated phosphorylation events, and promoting the degradation of insulin by proteases such as the acidic insulinase. The insulin receptor can then be recycled into the cell surface, where it becomes available for insulin binding again.

The number of available insulin receptors is modulated by exercise, diet, insulin, and other hormones. Chronic exposure to high insulin levels, obesity, and excess growth hormone all lead to a downregulation of insulin receptors. In contrast, exercise and fasting upregulate the number of receptors, improving insulin responsiveness.

INSULIN EFFECTS AT TARGET ORGANS

Early effects—Although the expression of insulin receptors is widespread, the specific effects of insulin on skeletal muscle glucose utilization dominate insulin action. Insulin mediates approximately 40% of glucose disposal by the body, the great majority (80%–90%) of which occurs in skeletal muscle. The movement of glucose into the cell is mediated by glucose transporters, with their own unique tissue distribution, summarized in Table 7–2.

Insulin-stimulated glucose transport is mediated through **GLUT 4**, most of which is sequestered intracellularly in the absence of insulin or other stimuli such as exercise. Insulin binding to its receptor results in increased GLUT 4 translocation through targeted exocytosis and decreased rate of its endocytosis. This is the underlying mechanism by which insulin stimulates glucose transport into fat and muscle cells.

Intermediate effects—The intermediate effects of insulin are mediated by modulation of protein phosphorylation of enzymes involved in metabolic processes in muscle, fat, and liver (Figure 7–4). In fat, insulin inhibits lipolysis and ketogenesis by triggering the dephosphorylation of hormone-sensitive lipase and stimulates lipogenesis by activating acetylcoenzyme A (acetyl-CoA) carboxylase. Dephosphorylation of hormone-sensitive lipase inhibits the breakdown of triglycerides to fatty acids and glycerol, the rate-limiting step in the release of free fatty acids mediated by lipolysis. This process thereby reduces the amount of substrate that is available for ketogenesis. Insulin antagonizes catecholamine-induced lipolysis through the phosphorylation and activation of phosphodiesterase, leading to a decrease in intracellular cAMP levels and a concomitant decrease in protein kinase A activity.

Table 7–2. Main features of glucose transporters (GLUTs)

Transporter	Expression	Function
GLUT 1	Ubiquitous, with particularly high levels in human erythrocytes and in the endothelial cells lining the blood vessels of the brain. Expressed in skeletal muscle and fat.	Glucose uptake by skeletal muscle and fat under basal conditions
GLUT 2	Low-affinity glucose transporter present in pancreatic β-cells, liver, intestine, and kidney	Functions in the glucose sensor system and ensures that glucose uptake by pancreatic β-cells and hepatocytes occurs only when circulating glucose levels are high
GLUT 3	Primarily in neurons	Together, GLUT 1 and GLUT 3 are crucial in allowing glucose to cross the blood-brain barrier and enter neurons
GLUT 4	Predominantly in striated muscle and adipose tissue. In contrast to the other GLUT isoforms, which are primarily localized on the cell membrane, GLUT 4 transporter proteins are sequestered in specialized storage vesicles that remain within the cell's interior under basal conditions.	The major insulin-responsive transporter
GLUT 5	Spermatozoa and small intestine	Predominantly a fructose transporter

In the liver, insulin stimulates the gene expression of enzymes involved in glucose utilization (eg, glucokinase, pyruvate kinase) and lipogenic enzymes and inhibits the gene expression of enzymes involved in glucose production (eg, phosphoenolpyruvate carboxykinase and glucose-6-phosphatase) (see Figure 7–4). Insulin stimulates glycogen synthesis by increasing phosphatase activity, leading to the dephosphorylation of glycogen phosphorylase and glycogen synthase. In addition, insulin-mediated dephosphorylation of inhibitory sites on hepatic acetyl-CoA carboxylase increases the production of malonylcoenzyme A (malonyl-CoA) and simultaneously reduces the rate at which fatty acids can enter hepatic mitochondria for oxidation and ketone body production.

In muscle, insulin stimulates glucose uptake and favors protein synthesis though phosphorylation of a serine/threonine protein kinase known as *mammalian target of rapamycin* (mTOR). In addition, insulin favors lipid storage in muscle as well as in adipose tissue. As discussed later, insulin deficiency leads to

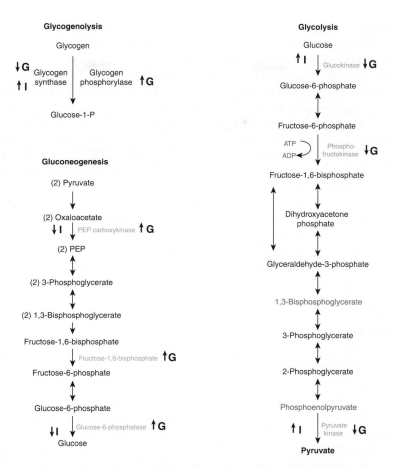

Figure 7–4. Glucagon and insulin effects on hepatic glucose metabolism. Binding of glucagon and insulin to their respective receptors stimulates a cascade of protein phosphorylation steps that activate (or inhibit) key enzymes involved in the regulation of glycogenolysis, gluconeogenesis, and glycolysis. The principal target enzymes for insulin- and glucagon-mediated effects are presented. The overall result is an increase in hepatic glucose output. ADP, adenosine diphosphate; ATP, adenosine triphosphate; G, glucagon; I, insulin; PEP, phosphoenolpyruvate.

glucose accumulation in blood, a decrease in lipid storage, and protein loss, resulting in negative nitrogen balance and muscle wasting.

Long-term effects—Sustained insulin stimulation enhances the synthesis of lipogenic enzymes and the repression of gluconeogenic enzymes. The growth-promoting and mitogenic effects of insulin are long-term responses mediated through the **MAPK pathway**. Both MAPK and particularly, the chronic activation of extracellular receptor kinase by insulin-receptor binding, lead to excessive cell growth. Although this pathway of insulin action is not as well elucidated as the effects that are mediated through the activation of IRS-PI3K, evidence suggests its involvement in the pathophysiologic consequences of chronic insulin elevations as those that occur in insulin resistant individuals.

Insulin levels are high (reflecting insulin resistance) during the development and early stages of type 2 diabetes. Chronic hyperinsulinemia has been linked to increased risk of cancers including endometrium, postmenopausal breast, colon, and kidney. Conditions that cause elevated insulin levels include high waist circumference, excess visceral fat, high waist-to-hip ratio, high body mass index, sedentary lifestyle, and high energy intake. In addition, the proliferative effects of chronic hyperinsulinemia influence vascular smooth muscle cells, which are responsible for the maintenance of vascular tone. These cells play an important role in the pathogenesis of several diseases, including hypertension, atherosclerosis, cardiovascular disease, and dyslipidemia, all of which are closely associated with insulin resistance and hyperinsulinemia. The molecular basis of insulin's effect on vascular smooth muscle cell growth and its association with hypertension are currently unclear.

Glucagon

GLUCAGON SYNTHESIS

Glucagon, is a 29–amino acid polypeptide hormone secreted by the α-cells of the islets of Langerhans, that plays an important role in the regulation of glucose homeostasis by producing antagonistic effects on insulin action. The primary sequence of glucagon is almost perfectly conserved among vertebrates, and it is structurally related to the secretin family of peptide hormones. Glucagon is synthesized as proglucagon and then proteolytically processed to yield glucagon. The prohormone proglucagon is expressed in the pancreas, and also in other tissues, such as enteroendocrine cells in the intestinal tract and in the brain. However, the processing of the prohormone differs among tissues. The 2 main products of proglucagon processing are glucagon in the α-cells of the pancreas and GLP 1 in the intestinal cells. GLP 1 is produced in response to a high concentration of glucose in the intestinal lumen. GLP 1 is known as an **incretin**, a mediator that amplifies insulin release from the β-cell in response to a glucose load. Glucagon has a short half-life (5–10 minutes) and is degraded mostly in the liver.

REGULATION OF GLUCAGON RELEASE

The mechanisms involved in the regulation and stimulus-secretion coupling of glucagon release are not as well understood as those for insulin. Glucagon release is inhibited by hyperglycemia (high blood-glucose levels) and stimulated by hypoglycemia (low blood-glucose levels). A meal rich in carbohydrates suppresses glucagon release and stimulates insulin release from the β-cells through intestinal release of GLP 1. Somatostatin also inhibits glucagon release. High amino acid levels following an amino acid–rich meal stimulate glucagon release. Epinephrine stimulates release of glucagon through a β_2-adrenergic mechanism (whereas it suppresses insulin release from β-cells through an α_2-adrenergic mechanism). Vagal (parasympathetic) stimulation increases glucagon release.

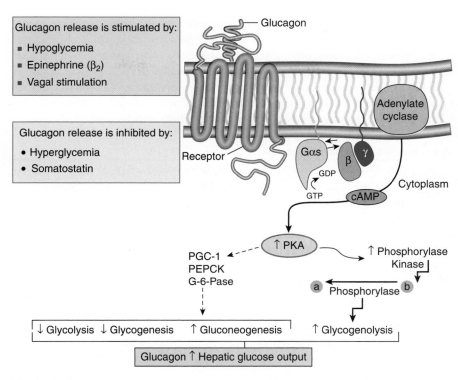

Figure 7–5. Glucagon receptor-mediated cellular effects. Glucagon binds to G protein–coupled receptor (GPCR) on target cells leading to activation of adenylate cyclase, elevation in cAMP and increased protein kinase A activity resulting in phosphorylation of enzymes responsible for control of glucose metabolism. The ultimate result is an increase in hepatic glucose production through increased gluconeogenesis and glycogenolysis. cAMP, cyclic 3′,5′-adenosine monophosphate; GDP, guanosine 5′-diphosphate; G-6-Pase, glucose-6-phosphatase; GTP, guanosine 5′-triphophate; PEPCK, phosphoenolpyruvate carboxykinase; PGC-1, peroxisome proliferator-activated receptor-coactivator-1; PKA, protein kinase A.

PHYSIOLOGIC EFFECTS OF GLUCAGON

The principal target tissue for glucagon is the liver. Glucagon's main physiologic effect is to increase plasma glucose concentrations by stimulating de novo hepatic glucose production through gluconeogenesis and glycogen breakdown; overall, these actions counteract the effects of insulin (Figure 7–5).

GLUCAGON RECEPTOR

Glucagon mediates its effects by binding to the glucagon $G\alpha_s$ protein–coupled receptor. The glucagon and GLP 1 peptide receptors belong to a family of G protein–coupled receptors that include those for secretin, calcitonin, vasoactive intestinal polypeptide, parathyroid hormone, and growth hormone-releasing factor. The glucagon receptor is expressed in liver, pancreatic β-cells, kidney, adipose tissue, heart, and vascular tissues, as well as in some regions of the brain, stomach, and adrenal glands. Glucagon binding activates adenylate cyclase and results in intracellular accumulation of cAMP, mobilization of intracellular Ca^{2+}, protein kinase A activation, and phosphorylation of effector proteins. The glucagon-receptor complex undergoes endocytosis into intracellular vesicles, where glucagon is degraded. The role of glucagon receptors in tissues other than the liver is still unclear.

GLUCAGON EFFECTS AT TARGET ORGANS

Glucagon stimulates hepatic glucose output by stimulating glycogen breakdown and gluconeogenesis and decreasing glycolysis (see Figure 7–5). The key enzymatic steps regulated by glucagon that mediate the stimulation of hepatic glucose output are summarized in Table 7–3. Glucagon has effects on adipose tissue that are relevant primarily during periods of stress or food deprivation, particularly when insulin release is suppressed.

In the adipocyte, glucagon stimulates protein kinase A–mediated phosphorylation (activation) of hormone-sensitive lipase, the enzyme that breaks down triglycerides (stored fat) into diacylglycerol and free fatty acids, releasing them into the circulation. Glycerol released into the circulation can be utilized in the liver for gluconeogenesis or for reesterification. Free fatty acids are used as fuel by most tissues, predominantly skeletal muscle and liver. In the liver, free fatty acids are used for reesterification, or they undergo β-oxidation

Table 7–3. Effects of glucagon on hepatic glucose metabolism

Effect on target enzyme	Metabolic response
Increased expression of glucose-6-phosphatase	Frees glucose to enter the circulation
Suppression of glucokinase	Decreases glucose entry into the glycolytic cascade
Phosphorylation (activation) of glycogen phosphorylase	Stimulates glycogenolysis
Inhibition of glycogen synthase	Inhibits glycogen synthesis
Stimulation of phosphoenolpyruvate carboxykinase expression	Stimulates gluconeogenesis
Inactivation of phosphofructokinase-2 (PFK-2) and activation of fructose-6-phosphatase. PFK-2 is the kinase activity and fructose-2,6-bisphosphatase (F-2,6-BPase) is the phosphatase activity of the bifunctional regulatory enzyme, phosphofructokinase-2/fructose-2,6-bisphosphatase (PFK-2/F-2,6-BPase).	Inhibits glycolysis Stimulates gluconeogenesis
Suppression of activity of the pyruvate kinase	Decreases glycolysis

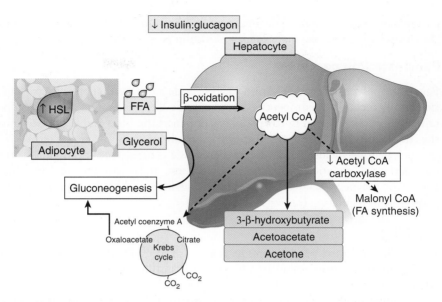

Figure 7–6. Process of ketogenesis in insulin deficiency. Insulin deficiency and high levels of counterregulatory hormones glucagon, epinephrine, and cortisol combine to increase the activity of hormone sensitive lipase and the release of free fatty acids, and decrease the activity of acetyl CoA carboxylase, thereby impairing the reesterification of FFA promoting fatty acid conversion to ketone bodies. The excess supply of fatty acyl CoA and deficiency in oxaloacetate leads to increased oxidation to ketone bodies with the resulting release of ketone bodies into the blood. CoA, coenzyme A; FFA, free fatty acid; HSL, hormone-sensitive lipase.

and conversion into ketone bodies (Figure 7–6). Thus, ketogenesis is regulated by the balance between the effects of glucagon and insulin at their target organs. The importance of this balance is evident during insulin deficiency and glucagon excess, as seen in uncontrolled diabetes (discussed later).

Somatostatin

Somatostatin is a 14–amino acid peptide hormone produced by the δ-cells of the pancreas. Its release is stimulated by high-fat, high-carbohydrate, and particularly protein-rich meals, and is inhibited by insulin. Somatostatin has a generalized inhibitory effect on virtually all gastrointestinal and pancreatic exocrine and endocrine functions. The regulation of its release is not well studied because of the difficulty in analyzing the small number of islet cells that produce this hormone. Further, the importance of endogenous paracrine inhibition of insulin and glucagon release is not well established. Because δ-cells are located in the periphery of the β-cells and because blood flows from the center of the islets of Langerhans toward the periphery, pancreatic somatostatin may have a limited contribution toward physiologic control of insulin and glucagon release. However, exogenous administration of somatostatin does suppress the release of both insulin and glucose and is used in the clinical setting for the management of insulin or glucagon producing tumors.

Pancreatic Polypeptide

Pancreatic polypeptide is a 36–amino acid peptide hormone that belongs to a peptide family including neuropeptide Y and peptide YY. It is produced in the endocrine type F cells located in the periphery of pancreatic islets and is released into the circulation after a meal, exercise, and vagal stimulation. The effects of pancreatic polypeptide include inhibition of pancreatic exocrine secretion, gallbladder contraction, modulation of gastric acid secretion, and gastrointestinal motility. Pancreatic polypeptide crosses the blood-brain barrier and has been postulated to play a role in regulating feeding behavior.

Amylin

Amylin, or islet amyloid polypeptide, is a 37–amino acid peptide hormone that belongs to the calcitonin family (calcitonin, calcitonin gene-related peptide, and adrenomedullin). Amylin is synthesized as a small precursor, undergoes post-translational modification (amidation), is stored in β-granules, and is released along with insulin and C-peptide. Plasma amylin concentrations increase after a meal or glucose infusion. Amylin appears to work with insulin to regulate plasma glucose concentrations in the bloodstream, suppressing the postprandial secretion of glucagon and slowing gastric emptying. In muscle, amylin opposes glycogen synthesis and activates glycogenolysis and glycolysis, thereby increasing lactate production. Circulating amylin is increased in obesity, hypertension, and gestational diabetes; it is low or absent in type 1 diabetes mellitus. Amylin is the main component of pancreatic islet amyloid, found in the vast majority of patients with non-insulin-dependent (type 2) diabetes mellitus, and is thought to contribute to destruction of the pancreatic β-cell. Amylin binds to a variant of the calcitonin G protein–coupled receptor. The modified calcitonin receptor has higher affinity for amylin, an effect mediated by transmembrane proteins known as receptor activity modifying proteins.

DISEASES ASSOCIATED WITH PANCREATIC HORMONES

Hormone-Producing Tumors

Excess pancreatic hormone production and release are usually caused by hormone-producing tumors, with insulinoma being the most frequent. Insulinomas produce excessive amounts of insulin, and patients present with episodes of hypoglycemia, confusion, aggressiveness, palpitations, sweating, convulsions, and even unconsciousness. These symptoms are mostly observed before breakfast and following physical exercise. The compensatory or counterregulatory response of the body includes the release of catecholamines, glucagon, cortisol, and growth hormone.

Glucagonomas are unusual tumors that may produce symptoms of diabetes. Excessive glucagon production by the tumor may also result in an overall catabolic effect on fat and muscle, leading to severe weight loss and anorexia. Somatostatinoma is a rare tumor that may cause moderate diabetes.

Diabetes Mellitus

The most common disease resulting from impaired pancreatic hormone release is diabetes mellitus. The 2 forms of diabetes, type 1 and type 2, are characterized by impaired insulin release. Type 1 diabetes, also known as insulin-dependent diabetes mellitus, is the result of β-cell destruction. It accounts for less than 5% of cases, and it occurs more frequently in younger people, hence its other name, *juvenile-onset diabetes*. Type 1 diabetes is characterized by the development of ketoacidosis in the absence of insulin therapy. Type 2 diabetes results from a loss of normal regulation of insulin secretion and accounts for more than 90% of diabetes cases. It is usually associated with obesity in adults and is characterized by mild hyperglycemia. It rarely leads to ketoacidosis. Type 2 diabetes is often part of "syndrome X" or "insulin-resistance syndrome," a metabolic syndrome characterized by hypertension, atherosclerosis, and central obesity.

The pathophysiology of the disease involves impaired entry of glucose into the cells and accumulation of glucose in the blood. This process results in increased plasma osmolarity and urinary loss of glucose, accompanied by excess loss of water and sodium (**polyuria**). The resulting dehydration triggers compensatory mechanisms such as thirst (**polydipsia**). The inability of the cells to utilize glucose resembles a state of cellular starvation, stimulating hunger (**polyphagia**) and triggering the activation of compensatory responses to increase the release and availability of fuel substrates through activation of lipolysis and proteolysis. Lack of insulin results in increased circulating levels of free fatty acids and gluconeogenic amino acids. These exceed the liver's capacity for their metabolic utilization, leading to the buildup of ketone bodies in the blood (diabetic ketoacidosis) and their urinary excretion.

Type 2 Diabetes

Type 2 diabetes is the result of decreased responsiveness of peripheral tissues to insulin action and inadequate responsiveness of the β-cells to glucose, which is ultimately followed by a net reduction in β-cell mass. Patients with type 2 diabetes secrete normal amounts of insulin during fasting, but in response to a glucose load (or a meal), they secrete considerably less insulin (70%) than nondiabetic patients. In addition to a reduction in insulin release, the pattern of insulin release is also altered following a meal, with pulses that are significantly smaller, sluggish, and erratic, particularly after dinner. This abnormality results in significantly higher levels of fasting glucose in these patients.

Regardless of the etiology (eg, abnormalities in glucose transport; abnormal insulin synthesis, processing, storage, or secretion), the earliest physiologic indication of β-cell dysfunction is a delay in the acute insulin response to glucose. The defect in the initial response to a glucose load leads to an excessive rise in plasma glucose, which in turn produces a compensatory and exaggerated second-phase hyperinsulinemic response. This initial period of sustained hyperinsulinemia downregulates the insulin receptors, decreasing the sensitivity of tissues to insulin action and producing a state of insulin resistance. The main pathologic defects in diabetes are excessive hepatic glucose production (reflected in elevated fasting glucose levels), defective β-cell secretory function, and peripheral insulin resistance.

Insulin Resistance

Insulin resistance is the inability of peripheral target tissues to respond properly to normal circulating concentrations of insulin. To maintain euglycemia, the pancreas compensates by secreting increased amounts of insulin. In patients with type 2 diabetes, insulin resistance may precede the onset of the disease by several years. Compensating for insulin resistance by an increase in insulin release is effective only temporarily. As insulin resistance increases, impaired glucose tolerance develops. Ultimately, failure or exhaustion of the pancreatic β-cell results in decreased insulin secretion. The combination of insulin resistance and impaired β-cell function characterizes clinical type 2 diabetes. Exercise has been demonstrated to increase glucose transport in skeletal muscle and to decrease insulin resistance in patients with type 2 diabetes. The increase in glucose transport resulting from exercise is not mediated through the insulin receptor, but involves increased cytosolic Ca^{2+} and the enzyme adenosine monophosphate (AMP)-activated protein kinase. AMP-activated protein kinase is activated during exercise and has been called a master metabolic switch because it phosphorylates key target proteins that control flux through metabolic pathways.

Clinical Evaluation of Diabetes

The diagnosis of diabetes is based on fasting glucose of at least 126 mg/dL; random glucose levels higher than 200 mg/dL in association with symptoms of diabetes (polyuria, polydipsia, and polyphagia); or persistent elevations in plasma glucose levels following an oral glucose load (greater than 200 mg/dL 2 hours after glucose ingestion). Glycated hemoglobin, resulting from glycosylation of hemoglobin is proportionate to blood glucose concentrations. Because the half-life of erythrocytes is approximately 60 days, the level of glycated hemoglobin reflects the prevailing mean blood glucose concentration over the preceding 6–8 weeks; providing a measure of chronic glycemia. The measurement of glycated hemoglobin is used to monitor glycemic control in patients with known diabetes. Normal values are 5% and targeted values in diabetic patients in treatment is <7%.

Treatment of the Diabetic Patient

The goal of therapy is tight glycemic control, which has been shown to delay the development of microvascular complications associated with diabetes. Because glucose homeostasis relies on regulated balance among hepatic glucose release, dietary glucose absorption, and skeletal muscle and adipose tissue glucose uptake and disposal; all 3 of these components have been targeted for pharmacologic treatment of diabetic patients. Some of the approaches used, in addition to conventional insulin, warrant mention because they affect the physiologic mechanisms of pancreatic hormone release and target organ effects on the control of glucose.

Sulfonylureas—Sulfonylureas increase insulin release by closing K^+-ATP channels in the pancreatic β-cell membrane. This action is mediated by binding of the drug to the sulfonylurea receptor subunit of the channel. Because type 1 diabetes is characterized by β-cell destruction, this approach is ineffective in those patients.

Biguanides—Biguanides, such as metformin, reduce hepatic glucose output (primarily through inhibition of gluconeogenesis and, to a lesser extent, glycogenolysis) and increase insulin-stimulated glucose uptake in skeletal muscle and adipocytes. In insulin-sensitive tissues (such as skeletal muscle), metformin facilitates glucose transport by increasing insulin receptor tyrosine kinase activity and enhancing glucose transporter trafficking to the cell membrane.

Alpha-glucosidase inhibitors—Alpha-glucosidase inhibitors delay the intestinal absorption of carbohydrates through inhibition of the brush-border enzymes that hydrolyze polysaccharides to glucose.

Thiazolidinediones—Thiazolidinediones reduce insulin resistance in skeletal muscle by activation of the gamma isoform of the peroxisome proliferator-activated receptor in the nucleus, thereby affecting the transcription of several genes involved in glucose and lipid metabolism and energy balance. Among the genes that are affected are those that code for lipoprotein lipase, fatty acid transporter protein, adipocyte fatty acid-binding protein, fatty acetyl-CoA synthase, malic enzyme, glucokinase, and the GLUT4.

Glucagon-like peptide—GLP 1 amplifies glucose-induced insulin release. GLP 1 increases insulin biosynthesis and insulin gene expression and has tropic and antiapoptotic effects on the pancreatic β-cells. GLP 1 suppresses glucagon release, hepatic glucose production, gastric emptying, and food intake.

COMPLICATIONS OF DIABETES

Complications of diabetes can be categorized as acute and chronic. Acute complications include hypoglycemia; diabetic ketoacidosis; and hyperglycemic, hyperosmolar nonketotic coma. Chronic complications of diabetes involve the vascular system (micro- and macrovascular damage), peripheral nerves, skin, and the lens. End-stage renal disease, autonomic neuropathy, and blindness, are more frequent in type 1 diabetes. Macrovascular disease leading to myocardial infarction and stroke are more likely in type 2 diabetic patients.

Hypoglycemia

A common complication of tight glycemic control is hypoglycemia resulting from excess insulin dose, fasting, or strenuous exercise. This results in an immediate activation of a systemic counterregulatory response involving sympathetic nervous system activation, glucagon release, followed by release of growth hormone and cortisol. Clinical manifestations range from tachycardia, palpitations, sweating, and tremors as glucose levels decrease to approximately 54 mg/dL, to irritability, confusion, blurred vision, tiredness, headache, and difficulty speaking when levels approach 50 mg/dL. Further decreases in glucose can lead to loss of consciousness or seizures.

Diabetic Ketoacidosis

Diabetic ketoacidosis is characterized by hyperglycemia, increased ketone bodies, and metabolic acidosis, resulting directly from decreased insulin availability and simultaneous elevations of the counterregulatory hormones glucagon, catecholamines, cortisol, and growth hormone. Diabetic ketoacidosis can be precipitated by infections, traumatic injury, and discontinuation of, or inadequate, insulin use.

In diabetic ketoacidosis, gluconeogenesis in the liver proceeds unopposed by the physiologic presence of insulin. The excess blood glucose increases osmolarity, which, if severe, can result in diabetic coma (see Figure 7–6). The lack of insulin and the high levels of counterregulatory hormones glucagon, epinephrine, and cortisol combine to increase the activity of hormone-sensitive lipase, increase the release of free fatty acids, and decrease the activity of acetyl-CoA carboxylase, thereby impairing the reesterification of free fatty acids and promoting fatty acid conversion into ketone bodies (see Figure 7–6). In the liver fatty acids undergo β-oxidation to acetyl-CoA. Acetyl-CoA condenses with oxaloacetate to form citrate in the entry step to the Krebs cycle (citric acid cycle or tricarboxylic cycle). However, a low-insulin-to-glucagon ratio favors gluconeogenesis; thus oxaloacetate is preferentially used for gluconeogenesis, decreasing its availability for condensation with acetyl-CoA. As a result, acetyl-CoA is diverted from entering the Krebs cycle and is used preferentially for ketone body formation or ketogenesis, the process by which fatty acids are transformed into acetoacetate and 3-hydroxybutyrate in hepatocyte mitochondria. The steps involved in ketogenesis are β-oxidation of fatty acids to acetyl-CoA, formation of acetoacetyl-CoA, and conversion of acetoacetyl-CoA to 3-hydroxy-3-methylglutaryl-CoA and then to acetoacetate, which is then reduced to 3-β-hydroxybutyrate. The enzymes involved in ketogenesis are summarized in Table 7–4. Acetoacetate can be spontaneously decarboxylated to acetone, a highly fat-soluble compound that is excreted slowly by the lungs and is responsible for the fruity odor of the breath of individuals with diabetic ketoacidosis.

During diabetic ketoacidosis, high amounts of ketone bodies are released into the blood, and a high ratio (3:1 or higher) of 3-β-hydroxybutyrate to acetoacetate is generated because of the highly reduced state of hepatic mitochondria. These ketone bodies can freely diffuse across cell membranes and serve as an energy source for extrahepatic tissues including the brain, skeletal muscle, and kidneys. Ketone bodies are filtered and reabsorbed in the kidney. At physiologic pH, ketone bodies, with the exception of acetone, dissociate completely. The resulting liberation of H^+ from ketone body metabolism exceeds the blood's buffering capacity, leading to metabolic acidosis with an increased anion gap. If severe, this condition can lead to coma.

Hyperglycemic Hyperosmolar Coma

Hyperglycemic coma is characterized by severe hyperglycemia, hyperosmolality, and dehydration in the absence of significant ketosis. It typically occurs in middle-aged or elderly patients with mild or occult diabetes. Lethargy and confusion

Table 7–4. Three principal enzymes involved in ketogenesis

Enzyme	Tissue	Function
Hormone-sensitive lipase	Adipocytes	Breaks down triglycerides, releasing fatty acids into the circulation
Acetyl-CoA carboxylase	Liver	Catalyzes the conversion of acetyl-CoA to malonyl-CoA, the primary substrate of fatty acid biosynthesis
HMG-CoA synthase	Liver	Involved in the conversion of acetyl-CoA to acetoacetate

CoA, coenzyme A; HMG, 3-hydroxy-3-methylglutaryl.

develop as serum osmolarity exceeds 300 mOsm/L, and coma can occur if osmolarity exceeds 330 mOsm/L. Underlying medical conditions such as renal insufficiency and congestive heart failure are common, and the presence of either worsens the prognosis. Precipitating events include infections such as pneumonia, cerebrovascular accident, or myocardial infarction, among others.

KEY CONCEPTS

1. *The pancreatic β-cell functions as a glucose sensor in the process of insulin release.*

2. *Insulin release is under nutrient, neural, and hormonal regulation.*

3. *The IRS-PI3K pathway mediates most of insulin's metabolic effects, and the MAPK pathway is mostly involved in mediating the proliferative responses.*

4. *The principal metabolic effects of insulin are to increase glucose utilization in skeletal muscle, suppress hepatic glucose production, and inhibit lipolysis.*

5. *Glucagon antagonizes insulin's effects by stimulating hepatic glucose release.*

6. *GLP 1 is an incretin that amplifies glucose-induced insulin release.*

7. *A disruption in the balance of insulin and glucagon leads to ketogenesis and hyperosmolar coma.*

STUDY QUESTIONS

7–1. In a patient with severe hypoglycemia (38 mg/dL), the differential diagnosis between self-administered insulin overdose and a tumor that produces excess insulin can be made by determining plasma levels of:

   a. Insulin

   b. Somatostatin

   c. C-peptide

   d. Gastrin

7–2. A 60-year-old man is found comatose by his relatives. Paramedics notice on physical examination that he has decreased skin turgor and dry mucous membranes. On arrival at the hospital, laboratory studies show blood glucose of 698 mg/dL, but no ketones in blood. Urine analysis is negative for ketone bodies and protein, but positive for glucose (4+). Which of the following is the most likely diagnosis?

   a. Islet cell tumor secreting glucagon

   b. Type 1 diabetes mellitus

   c. Cushing syndrome

   d. Ingestion of a large quantity of sugar

   e. Type 2 diabetes mellitus

7–3. A 57-year-old-female patient is brought to the emergency room with history of frequent urination, weight loss, and decreased oral intake. At presentation, the patient is lethargic, dehydrated, hypotensive, and tachycardic. Her caretaker reports that she was recovering from a recent bout of pneumonia. She had been diagnosed with type 2 diabetes 5 years prior to this incident. Which of the following laboratory findings are likely?

   a. Plasma glucose of 40 mg/dL

   b. Plasma osmolarity >350 mOsm/L

   c. Low blood pH

   d. High plasma ketones

7–4. A 21-year-old male diabetic patient is brought to the emergency room for abdominal pain, nausea, and vomiting of 16 hours duration. On examination, you notice that his insulin pump has stopped functioning. Which of the following are likely to be associated with his presentation?

   a. High plasma insulin levels

   b. Increased glucagon concentrations

   c. Increased serum ketones

   d. Increased blood pH

   e. Decreased hepatic glycogen breakdown

SUGGESTED READINGS

Bergsten P. Pathophysiology of impaired pulsatile insulin release. *Diabetes Metab Res Rev.* 2000;16:179.

Cefalu WT. Evaluation of alternative strategies for optimizing glycemia: progress to date. *Am J Med.* 2002;113(suppl 6A):23S.

Gerich JE. Matching treatment to pathophysiology in type 2 diabetes. *Clin Ther.* 2001;23:646.

Hauner H. The mode of action of thiazolidinediones. *Diabetes Metab Res Rev.* 2002;18(suppl 2):S10.

Kirpichnikov D, McFarlane SI, Sowers JR. Metformin: an update. *Ann Intern Med.* 2002;137:25.

Laffel L. Ketone bodies: a review of physiology, pathophysiology and application of monitoring to diabetes. *Diabetes Metab Res Rev.* 1999;15:412.

Lang J. Molecular mechanisms and regulation of insulin exocytosis as a paradigm of endocrine secretion. *Eur J Biochem.* 1999;259:3.

LeRoith D. Beta-cell dysfunction and insulin resistance in type 2 diabetes: role of metabolic and genetic abnormalities. *Am J Med.* 2002;113(suppl 6A):3S.

Porksen N, Grøfte T, Greisen J, et al. Human insulin release processes measured by intraportal sampling. *Am J Physiol Endocrinol Metab.* 2002;282:E695.

Richter EA, Derave W, Wojtaszewski JFP. Glucose, exercise and insulin: emerging concepts. *J Physiol.* 2001;535(pt 2):313.

Ryder JW, Chibalin AV, Zierath JR. Intracellular mechanisms underlying increases in glucose uptake in response to insulin or exercise in skeletal muscle. *Acta Physiol Scand.* 2001;171:249.

Saltiel AR, Pessin JE. Insulin signaling pathways in time and space. *Trends Cell Biol.* 2002;12:65.

Straub SG, Sharp GWG. Glucose-stimulated signaling pathways in biphasic insulin secretion. *Diabetes Metab Res Rev.* 2002;18:451.

Male Reproductive System

OBJECTIVES

▶ Describe the physiologic functions of the principal components of the male reproductive system.

▶ Describe the endocrine regulation of testicular function by gonadotropin-releasing hormone, follicle-stimulating hormone, luteinizing hormone, testosterone, and inhibin.

▶ Identify the cell of origin for testosterone, its biosynthesis, mechanism of transport within the blood, metabolism, and clearance. List other physiologically produced androgens.

▶ List the target organs or cell types, the cellular mechanisms of action, and the physiologic effects of testosterone.

▶ Describe spermatogenesis and the role of different cell types in this process.

▶ Understand the neural, vascular, and endocrine factors involved in the erection and ejaculation response.

▶ Compare and contrast the actions of testosterone, dihydrotestosterone, estradiol, and müllerian inhibitory factor in the process of sexual differentiation.

▶ Identify the causes and consequences of androgen oversecretion and undersecretion in prepubertal and postpubescent adult males.

In utero sexual differentiation, maturation, spermatogenesis, and ultimately reproduction are all functions of the male reproductive system that are under endocrine regulation. The 2 principal functions of the testicles, the adult male sex organs, are the production of sperm and the synthesis of testosterone. These processes ensure fertility and maintain male sexual characteristics, or virility. Testicular function is under central nervous system control in a classic neuroendocrine feedback loop with the gonadotropins follicle-stimulating hormone (FSH) and luteinizing hormone (LH) as the key hormonal signals. These gonadotropins, as discussed in Chapter 2, are under the influence of hypothalamic gonadotropin-releasing hormone (GnRH) stimulation. Additional paracrine, neural, and endocrine factors contribute to the complex regulation of the hypothalamic-pituitary-gonadal axis. This chapter discusses the basic principles of endocrine regulation of the male reproductive system.

FUNCTIONAL ANATOMY

The male reproductive organs include the testes (the central male sex organs), the vas deferens, the ejaculatory ducts, the penis, and the accessory glands, which include the prostate and bulbourethral glands (Figure 8–1). The testes consist of numerous lobules made of convoluted tubes (tubuli seminiferi) supported by loose connective tissue. The seminiferous tubules represent approximately 80%–85% of the testicular mass or volume. The tubules consist of a basement layer lined with epithelial (**Sertoli)** cells forming the walls of the seminiferous tubules. These tubules are lined with primitive germ cells (spermatogonia). The **Leydig cells** are embedded in the connective tissue are the endocrine cells responsible for the production of the most important circulating androgen, **testosterone**.

Sertoli cells form tight junctions creating a "blood-testis" barrier that functionally divide the seminiferous tubules into 2 compartments or environments for the development of spermatozoa. The basal compartment below the tight junctions has contact with the circulation and is the space in which spermatogonia develop to primary spermatocytes. The tight junctions open at specific times and allow progression of spermatocytes to the adluminal compartment, where meiosis is completed. The principal functions of Sertoli cells are as follows:

- Provide support for germ cells, forming an environment in which they develop and mature.

- Provide the signals that initiate spermatogenesis and sustain spermatid development.

- Regulate pituitary gland function and, in turn, control of spermatogenesis.

Together, the Sertoli and Leydig cells are the 2 principal cell types responsible for testicular function.

The tubuli seminiferi are united to form larger ducts called *tubuli recti*. These larger tubules form a close anastomosing network of tubes called the *rete testis*, terminating in the ductuli efferentes (see Figure 8–1). This tubular network carries the seminal fluid containing sperm from the testis to the epididymis; from here, spermatozoa enter the vas deferens and then the ejaculatory ducts. The ejaculatory ducts move semen (sperm containing fluid) into the urethra. The tubular network or excretory system and the accessory organs contribute to the final composition of sperm-containing semen through absorptive and secretory processes (summarized in Table 8–1). Sperm constitutes approximately 10% of the volume of the ejaculated semen, which is composed of testicular and epididymal fluid together with the secretory products of male accessory glands. Most of the volume of the ejaculate is formed by the seminal vesicles with the remainder consisting of epididymal fluids and secretions from the prostrate gland and bulbourethral glands.

The penis is composed of 2 functional compartments: the paired **corpora cavernosa** and the **corpus spongiosum**. The corpora cavernosa form the greater part of the substance of the penis and consist of bundles of smooth muscle fibers intertwined in a collagenous extracellular matrix. Interspersed within this parenchyma

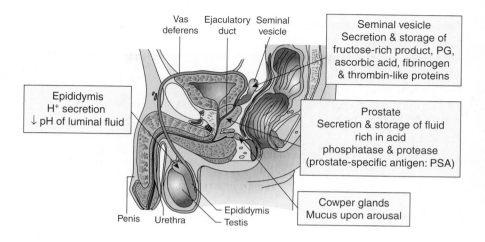

Vas deferens | Ejaculatory duct | Seminal vesicle

Seminal vesicle
Secretion & storage of fructose-rich product, PG, ascorbic acid, fibrinogen & thrombin-like proteins

Epididymis
H⁺ secretion
↓ pH of luminal fluid

Prostate
Secretion & storage of fluid rich in acid phosphatase & protease (prostate-specific antigen: PSA)

Cowper glands
Mucus upon arousal

Penis | Urethra | Epididymis | Testis

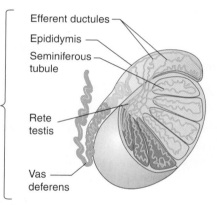

Sertoli (epithelial) cells

- Form blood-testes barrier
- Support spermatogonia
- Signal spermatogenesis
- Produce inhibin B

Leydig cells

- In connective tissue
- Produce testosterone

Efferent ductules
Epididymis
Seminiferous tubule
Rete testis
Vas deferens

Figure 8–1. Functional anatomy of the male reproductive system. The male reproductive organs include the testes, the vas deferens, the ejaculatory ducts, the penis, and the accessory glands, which include the prostate and bulbourethral glands. The testes consist of numerous lobules made of tubuli seminiferi supported by loose connective tissue. The tubuli seminiferi are united to form larger ducts called the tubuli recti. These larger tubules form a close anastomosing network of tubes called the *rete testis*, terminating in the ductuli efferentes. The tubular network carries the seminal fluid from the testis to the epididymis, from where spermatozoa enter the vas deferens and then enter the urethra through the ejaculatory ducts. The penis is composed of 2 functional compartments: the paired corpora cavernosa and the corpus spongiosum. The corpora cavernosa form the greater part of the substance of the penis and consist of bundles of smooth muscle fibers intertwined to form trabeculae, and containing numerous arteries and nerves. PG, prostaglandins. (Reproduced with permission from Widmaier EP, Raff H, Strang KT, eds. *Vander's Human Physiology: The Mechanisms of Body Function.* 11th ed. New York, NY: McGraw-Hill; 2007: figures 17–5 and 17–6.)

Table 8–1. Contribution of the excretory system and accessory organs to sperm production

Organ	Function
Excretory system	
Efferent ductules, vas deferens, ejaculatory duct, urethra	Movement of spermatozoa Fluid reabsorption
Epididymis	H⁺ secretion and acidification of luminal fluid Incapacitation of spermatozoa; glycoconjugation Reservoir for mature spermatozoa Phagocytosis of aging spermatozoa
Accessory glands	
Seminal vesicle	Secretion and storage of fructose-rich product (preferred energy substrate for sperm), prostaglandins, ascorbic acid, fibrinogen-like and thrombin-like proteins
Prostate	Secretion and storage of fluid rich in acid phosphatase and protease (prostate-specific antigen)
Cowper glands	Secretion of mucus into the urethra upon arousal

is a complex network of endothelial cell–lined sinuses, or lacunae, arteries, and nerve terminals. The penis is innervated by somatic and autonomic (both sympathetic and parasympathetic) nerve fibers. The somatic innervation supplies the penis with sensory fibers and supplies the perineal skeletal muscles with motor fibers. Autonomic nerves mediate vascular dilation leading to penile erection, stimulate prostatic secretions, and control smooth muscle contraction of the vas deferens during ejaculation.

The arterial blood supply to the male reproductive organs is predominantly derived from the superficial and deep external pudendal branches of the femoral artery, the superficial perineal branch of the internal pudendal artery, and the cremasteric branch from the inferior epigastric artery. Venous drainage follows the course of the corresponding arteries. Lymphatics drain into the inguinal lymph glands.

GONADOTROPIN REGULATION OF GONADAL FUNCTION

The primary functions of the testes are to produce spermatozoa and to produce the hormones involved in the regulation of reproductive function and virilization. These functions are regulated by the pituitary gonadotropins FSH and LH. LH and FSH circulate unbound in the plasma and have a half-life of 30 minutes (LH) and 1–3 hours (FSH). LH has higher amplitude fluctuations in plasma than FSH; FSH levels are more stable and show less variability.

The gonadotropins produce their physiologic responses by binding to cell membrane $G\alpha_s$ protein–coupled receptors located in the Leydig and Sertoli cells, leading to activation of adenylate cyclase and increased formation of cyclic 3′,5′-adenosine monophosphate (cAMP) (Figure 8–2; see Figure 1–5). The increase in intracellular cAMP results in the activation of protein kinase A and subsequent kinase-mediated protein phosphorylation, which mediates the cellular effects of the gonadotropins. This process is similar to that used for adrenocorticotropic hormone–mediated stimulation of adrenal steroid hormone production (discussed below).

LH is the principal regulator of testosterone production by the Leydig cells. FSH plays an important role in the development of the immature testis, particularly by controlling Sertoli cell proliferation and seminiferous tube growth.

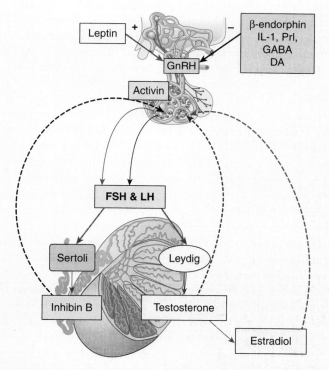

Figure 8–2. Negative feedback regulation of gonadotropin synthesis and release. Gonadotropin release from the anterior pituitary gland is controlled by the hypothalamic gonadotropin-releasing hormone (GnRH) pulse generator. Factors that stimulate GnRH release include norepinephrine (NE), neuropeptide Y (NPY), and leptin. Factors that inhibit GnRH release include β-endorphin, interleukin 1 (IL-1), γ-aminobutyric acid (GABA), and dopamine (DA) neurons. The activity of the pulse generator and the release of luteinizing hormone (LH) and follicle-stimulating hormone (FSH) are regulated by the gonadal hormones testosterone and inhibin B and by locally produced factors such as activin. Activin interacts with inhibin B, thus increasing FSH β-subunit synthesis. The negative feedback regulation exerted by testosterone is mediated by local conversion to 17β-estradiol.

Because the tubules account for approximately 80% of the volume of the testis, FSH is of major importance in determining testicular size, normally 4.1–5.2 cm in length and 2.5–3.3 cm in width in the adult male. FSH is important in the initiation of spermatogenesis during puberty. It is necessary for the production of androgen-binding protein by Sertoli cells and for the development of the blood-testis barrier.

Control of Gonadotropin Synthesis and Release

The overall regulation of FSH and LH secretion from the anterior pituitary was discussed in Chapter 3. The synthesis and release of the gonadotropins are regulated by neuroendocrine signals from the central nervous system, particularly the hypothalamus through the pulsatile release of GnRH, as well as by circulating hormones or their metabolites, as illustrated in Figure 8–2.

Pulsatile release of GnRH is determined by a pulse generator. The neuronal structures and chemical interactions that result in pulsatile GnRH release have not been fully elucidated. However, several central and peripheral signals modulate the activity of GnRH-releasing neurons. Some of these signals are stimulatory to GnRH release, such as norepinephrine and neuropeptide Y; others are inhibitory, such as β-endorphin and interleukin 1; others are both stimulatory and inhibitory, such as the estrogen 17β-estradiol. GnRH binds to a G protein–coupled receptor (G_q and G_{11}) in the anterior pituitary gonadotrophs, activating phospholipase C and leading to the stimulation of inositol trisphosphate, diacylglycerol and protein kinase C. Activation of inositol trisphosphate leads to an increase in intracellular Ca^{2+} concentrations. GnRH also indirectly stimulates cAMP, contributing to control of LH and FSH release. The ratio between LH and FSH production is determined by the frequency of GnRH pulses. Synthesis of FSH β-subunit is highest in response to low-frequency pulses of GnRH and is suppressed at higher-frequency pulses of GnRH. Higher frequency and amplitude of GnRH stimulation increase LH β-subunit synthesis.

LH stimulates testosterone production by the Leydig cell. Testosterone released into the circulation inhibits LH release in a negative feedback loop. At the level of the hypothalamus, testosterone inhibits GnRH release, and at the anterior pituitary, it decreases the gonadotropin-specific β-subunit synthesized (see Figure 8–2). Testosterone reduces LH levels and the LH pulse amplitude. It is important to mention that most of the inhibitory effect of testosterone on LH release is mediated by 17β-estradiol, a locally produced metabolite of testosterone aromatization (Figure 8–3). The negative feedback inhibition of FSH release occurs at the level of the pituitary and is mediated mainly by inhibin B, a Sertoli cell–derived peptide (discussed later).

Inhibin-Activin

In addition to the traditional feedback inhibition of gonadotropin hormone release described above (see Figure 8–2), locally produced factors (inhibin and activin) are also involved in regulation of gonadotropin release. **Inhibins** are

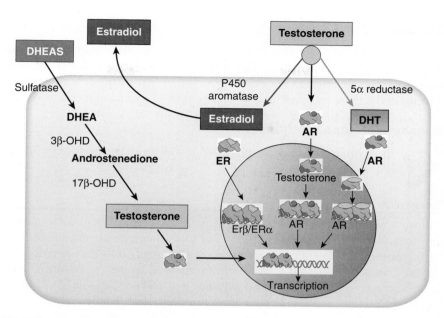

Figure 8–3. Receptor-mediated effects of testosterone at target tissues. Testosterone (a steroid hormone) enters the cell by passive diffusion and binds to the androgen (AR) receptor. Testosterone can be converted to dihydrotestosterone (DHT) by 5α-reductase and bind to the AR or it can be converted to 17β-estradiol by aromatase and either be released to act on a neighboring cell's estrogen receptors (ER) (paracrine mechanism), it can enter the circulation (endocrine effects), or it can bind to either the ER α or β. Intracellular testosterone can arise from androstenedione (Δ⁴A), dehydroepiandrosterone (DHEA), or dehydroepiandrosterone sulfate (DHEAS). The desulfated DHEA is converted to androstenedione by 3β-hydroxysteroid dehydrogenase (3β-OHD), and androstenedione transformed into testosterone by 17β-hydroxysteroid dehydrogenase (17β-OHD). Testosterone, DHT, and estradiol all bind to cytosolic steroid receptors. The cytosolic AR and ER is complexed to regulatory proteins (heat-shock proteins). Hormone binding results in the dissociation of the heat-shock protein complex, dimerization of the receptor, nuclear translocation, and DNA binding to regulatory elements. The final result is the activation of gene transcription.

peptide hormones that belong to the transforming growth factor beta (TGF-β) superfamily of growth factors. Inhibin B is produced by Sertoli cells in response to FSH stimulation (discussed later), and it produces feedback inhibition of FSH β-subunit production (and thus, FSH release). An additional factor involved in the regulation of FSH release is activin. **Activin** is expressed in several tissues including the pituitary. Its role is to antagonize inhibin B action, resulting in stimulation of FSH release. Thus, in addition to the negative feedback inhibition produced by gonadal androgens, the interaction between inhibin and activin contributes to the regulation of gonadotropin release.

GONADAL FUNCTION

The 2 principal physiologic functions of the testes—the production of hormones involved in sexual differentiation, maturation, and virilization and spermatogenesis—are closely related to each other. This chapter first discusses hormone production in the testes and then describes the process of spermatogenesis.

Gonadal Hormone Synthesis

 The 3 principal hormones produced by the testis are testosterone, estradiol, and inhibin.

TESTOSTERONE

Testosterone, produced by the Leydig cells, is the principal and most important testicular and circulating androgen. LH stimulates testosterone biosynthesis by increasing mobilization and transport of cholesterol into the steroidogenic pathway, an action that takes place within minutes; as well as by stimulating gene expression and activity of the steroidogenic enzymes (steroidogenic acute regulatory protein and P450scc), a slower process that requires several hours (Figure 8–4). As discussed in Chapter 6, steroidogenic acute regulatory protein (also found in the adrenal cortex cells) has a key role in the transfer of cholesterol from the outer to the inner mitochondrial membrane, the first step in steroid hormone biosynthesis, for the conversion of cholesterol to pregnenolone. Pregnenolone diffuses out of the mitochondria to the smooth endoplasmic reticulum, where it is further metabolized by the action of 3β-hydroxysteroid dehydrogenase to progesterone. Progesterone in turn is converted by a 2-step process to androstenedione by the action of 17α-hydroxylase. The conversion of androstenedione to testosterone is catalyzed by 17β-hydroxysteroid dehydrogenase. Note that up until this last enzymatic reaction, the enzymatic steps involved in testosterone synthesis are similar to those involved in androstenedione synthesis by the adrenal glands (see Figure 6–3). It is the activity of 17β-hydroxysteroid dehydrogenase and the enzymatic conversion of androstenedione to testosterone that are specific to the gonads.

INHIBIN

Inhibin is produced and released from the Sertoli cells in response to FSH stimulation and exerts both paracrine and endocrine responses. Inhibin belongs to the family of glycoprotein hormones and growth factors including TGF-β, müllerian-inhibiting substance (MIS), and activin. Inhibins are heterodimer glycoproteins consisting of an α- and a β-subunit ($β_A$ or $β_B$). Of the 2 forms of inhibin (α-$β_A$ and α-$β_B$), inhibin B is the physiologically important form in males. Its main function is to suppress the secretion of FSH from the pituitary in a classic negative feedback endocrine mechanism through binding to a membrane-spanning serine/threonine kinase receptor. Inhibin B secretion appears to be dependent on Sertoli cell proliferation, maintenance, and spermatogenesis, all of these functions regulated by FSH. Inhibin B levels correlate with total sperm count and testicular volume and can be used as an index of spermatogenesis.

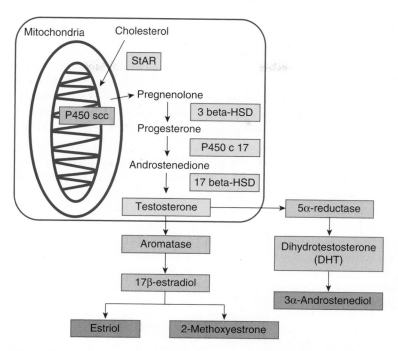

Figure 8–4. Key steps in testosterone biosynthesis and metabolism. Diagrammatic representation of the typical biochemical pathway and key enzymes involved in Leydig cell steroidogenesis that facilitate the biosynthesis of testosterone from the precursor cholesterol. Testosterone finally diffuses out of the Leydig cell and reaches the interstitial space and the peripheral circulation. In target cells, testosterone can be converted to the most potent androgen, dihydrotestosterone (DHT), by 5α-reductase or to 17β-estradiol by aromatase. Testosterone, dehydroepiandrosterone (DHEA), androstenedione, and 17β-estradiol are degraded in the liver to 17-ketosteroids or polar metabolites that are excreted in the urine. COMT, catechol-*O*-methyltransferase; HSD, hydroxysteroid dehydrogenase; scc, side chain cleavage; StAR, steroidogenic acute regulatory protein.

Activins, members of the same family of peptides as the inhibins, are homodimers or heterodimers of the β-subunit of the inhibins. They are synthesized in many adult tissues and cell types, and their receptors have been identified in those same tissues, a pattern more consistent with autocrine or paracrine mechanisms of action. At the pituitary, locally produced activin opposes inhibin's actions and favors the synthesis of β-FSH (see Figure 8–2).

ESTRADIOL

Testosterone conversion to 17β-estradiol is mediated by the enzyme **aromatase**, expressed in Leydig cells as well as in extragonadal tissues, particularly adipose tissue and placenta (see Figure 8–4). The contribution of 17β-estradiol produced by the Leydig cells to the total circulating estrogens in males is approximately 20%.

Gonadal Hormone Metabolism

Testosterone Metabolism

Most of the testosterone released into the circulation is bound to plasma proteins, primarily sex hormone-binding globulin (SHBG) and albumin (44% and 54%, respectively); both proteins made in the liver. In the testes, testosterone is bound to androgen-binding protein (ABP), a protein synthesized by Sertoli cells and released into the lumen of the seminiferous tubules. ABP has great similarity to SHBG. SHBG is expressed in several tissues, including brain, placenta, and testes and appears to function as part of a newly identified steroid-signaling system that is independent of the cytosolic androgen receptor. Unlike the effects mediated through binding to the intracellular steroid receptor produced by testosterone, SHBG interacts with a membrane form of the receptor and triggers cAMP signaling pathways. The physiologic relevance of the effects mediated through this pathway has not been elucidated.

At its target cells, testosterone can either have a direct androgen receptor–mediated effect or it can be metabolized to either 17β-estradiol through the action of aromatase or to **5α-dihydrotestosterone** (**DHT**) through the action of **5α-reductase** (see Figure 8–4).

Testosterone to Estradiol Conversion

The majority of estradiol in males is produced in adipose tissue through the aromatization of testosterone and, to a smaller extent, of adrenal-derived androstenedione. Aromatase expression is directly related to the degree of adiposity; it is dependent on cytokine stimulation and requires the presence of glucocorticoids. Although some of the 17β-estradiol produced in peripheral tissues is released into the circulation, not all estrogens produced from testosterone are involved in mediating endocrine responses. Some are involved in intracrine regulation of physiologic responses through estrogen receptor stimulation (see Figure 8–3). An example is the negative feedback regulation of GnRH in the hypothalamus and of gonadotropins in the anterior pituitary by testosterone. Another important example is the effect of testosterone on bones, where epiphysial closure is mediated through osteoblast and chondroblast aromatase conversion of testosterone to estradiol. In addition, the production of estrogens in the brain plays an important role in the masculinization of the brain during development and the maintenance of sexual behavior in the adult.

In the liver, testosterone is converted to androstenedione, which is then reduced and conjugated (glucuronidation) to form 17-ketosteroids (see Figure 8–4). A similar degradation pathway is used in the metabolism of dehydroepiandrosterone (DHEA) and androstenedione. After 17β-estradiol is produced by the testes or by the peripheral metabolism of testosterone, it is initially converted to estrone, which is converted into either catecholestrogens or 16α-hydroxyestrone. Catecholestrogens are degraded by catechol-O-methyltransferase (involved in catecholamine degradation; discussed in Chapter 6), while 16α-hydroxyestrone is converted to estriol before being conjugated in the liver and excreted by the kidney. Thus, the excretion of testosterone and its metabolites in the urine is approximately 50% in the form of 17-ketosteroids and 50% in the form of polar metabolites such as -diols, -triols, and conjugated forms.

TESTOSTERONE TO 5α-DIHYDROTESTOSTERONE CONVERSION

The conversion of testosterone to DHT in peripheral tissues, particularly in the skin, produces the most potent natural androgen (see Figure 8–4). Two isoenzymes (type 1 and type 2) of 5α-reductase are involved in the conversion of testosterone to DHT. The type 2 isoenzyme generates 3 times as much DHT as the type 1 isoenzyme and plays a critical role during sexual differentiation. During puberty, the contribution of the type 2 isoenzyme decreases and the type 1 reductase plays a more important role in adult males. A small amount of DHT can enter the circulation (approximately 10% of the total testosterone in blood) and can therefore exert effects at target cells that do not express 5α-reductase activity (see Figure 8–3). DHT is inactivated to the weak androgen 3α-androstenediol by the action of 3α-hydroxysteroid dehydrogenase. The enzymatic conversion of testosterone to DHT is irreversible. Because DHT is involved in some pathologic processes, the enzymatic conversion of testosterone to DHT has been used effectively as a target for pharmacologic interventions. Androgens stimulate the growth of prostate cancer and are also involved in benign prostatic hypertrophy. Finasteride, a 5α-reductase inhibitor, is currently used for the treatment of benign prostatic hyperplasia and prostate cancer.

ANDROGEN RECEPTOR-MEDIATED PHYSIOLOGIC EFFECTS

Both testosterone and DHT bind to identical androgen receptors on their target cells (see Figure 8–3). The androgen receptor is a member of the nuclear receptor superfamily and, like all other nuclear receptors; it consists of 3 functional domains involved in transcriptional regulation, DNA binding, and ligand binding. The ligand-free inactive cytosolic receptor is an inactive oligomer complexed to heat-shock proteins. On hormone binding, the oligomeric complex dissociates, undergoes a conformational change, and translocates into the nucleus. In the nucleus, it binds as a homodimer to DNA androgen response elements in the promotor region of target genes and functions as a nuclear transcription factor influencing the transcription of target genes and mediating androgen action.

The physiologic effects that are mediated by testosterone and DHT are related. DHT is the most potent activator of the androgen receptor, and the DHT-activated androgen receptor has a longer half-life, prolonging androgen action and amplifying the androgen signal. However, distinct physiologic responses can be attributed to each hormone (Table 8–2), in part determined by the localized conversion of testosterone to DHT. Testosterone controls sexual differentiation (development of the wolffian ducts), libido (the biologic need for sexual activity and sexual function), pubertal growth of the larynx, anabolic effects in muscle, and stimulation of spermatogenesis. In contrast, DHT plays a major role in embryonic and pubertal external virilization (eg, development of male external genitalia, urethra, and

Table 8–2. Specific actions of testosterone, dihydrotestosterone, and estradiol

Testosterone	DHT (5α-reductase activity)	17β-estradiol (aromatase activity)
Embryonic development of wolffian duct–derived structures	Embryonic development of the prostate	Epiphyseal closure
Postpubertal secretory activity	Descent of the testes	Prevention of osteoporosis
Pubertal growth of larynx and deepening of voice	Phallic growth	Feedback regulation of GnRH secretion
Anabolic effects on muscle and erythropoiesis	Male-pattern balding	
Inhibition of breast development	Development of pubic and underarm hair	
Stimulation of spermatogenesis Libido	Activity of sebaceous glands	

DHT, dihydrotestosterone; GnRH, gonadotropin-releasing hormone.

prostate, and growth of facial and body hair) and contributes to male-pattern balding in individuals with a genetic predisposition for baldness (Figures 8–5 and 8–6). Most of the effects of DHT are intracrine; they are mediated at target cells expressing 5α-reductase. However, as already mentioned a small amount enters the circulation (10% of testosterone levels) and may have some endocrine effects on cells that do not express 5α-reductase.

PHYSIOLOGIC EFFECTS OF ANDROGENS AT TARGET ORGANS

In addition to the regulation of LH release from the anterior pituitary, testosterone affects sexual development, maturation, and function, and contributes to the maintenance of fertility and secondary sexual characteristics in the adult male (see Figures 8–5 and 8–6). In addition, testosterone exerts overall anabolic effects in muscle and bone.

Sexual Development and Differentiation

Sexual differentiation in humans is genetically and hormonally controlled. Genes on the Y chromosome signal primordial cells in the embryonic gonad ridge to differentiate into Sertoli cells and stimulate newly migrated germ cells to differentiate as spermatogonia, developing into a testis (see Figure 8–5). The cells of the embryonic testis secrete hormones that lead to the development of male secondary sexual characteristics. The Sertoli cells secrete **müllerian inhibitory factor** or substance (MIF or MIS), causing regression of the **müllerian ducts.** The Leydig cells secrete testosterone, causing differentiation and growth of the **wolffian duct** structures. DHT causes growth of the prostate and penis and fusion of the labioscrotal folds (see Figure 8–6).

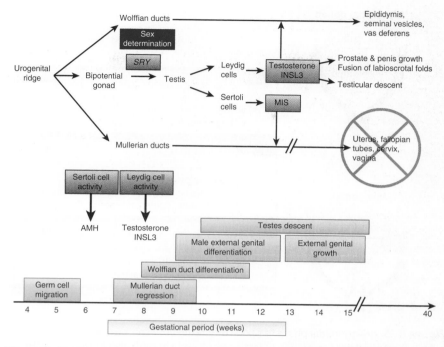

Figure 8–5. The bipotential gonad is differentiated into testes by the sex-determining region gene on the Y chromosome (*Sry*). This period of sex determination is followed by gonad differentiation of the different cell types of the testis. The Sertoli cells of the testis secrete müllerian-inhibiting substance (MIS or antimüllerian hormone [AMH]). The Leydig cells produce testosterone and insulin-like peptide 3 (INSL3). AMH (MIS) produces regression of the müllerian ducts. Testosterone stimulates the growth and differentiation of the wolffian ducts, growth of the penis and prostate. INSL3 participates in testicular descent; the final step in male sexual development. 5α-Dihydrotestosterone (DHT) produced from testosterone also participates in testis descent and development of the prostate.

The processes and factors involved in fetal development and sexual differentiation involve genetic, embryologic, histologic, and anatomic details not covered in this monograph. This section aims to summarize the key events in sexual differentiation as they pertain to endocrine regulation and function and to highlight the role of androgens in the determination of male sexual development.

SEX DETERMINATION

Mammalian sex determination leading to the development of male or female phenotype involves 3 sequential processes:

• Determination of the **genetic sex** of the embryo when an X- or a Y-bearing sperm fertilizes the oocyte

• Determination of the fate of the bipotential or nondifferentiated gonad and thus of **gonadal sex**

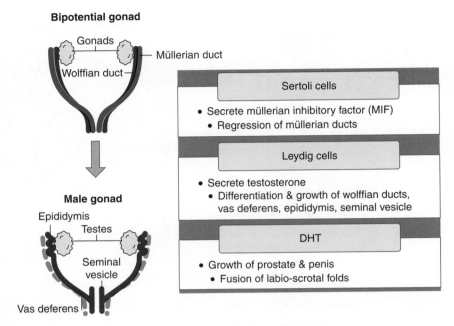

Figure 8–6. Postgonadal phase of sexual differentiation. This process is exclusively hormone dependent. Production of testosterone and antimüllerian hormone (AMH) ensures male development. Müllerian inhibitory factor (MIF) mediates apoptosis and regression of the müllerian ducts. The remaining wolffian ducts forms the vas deferens, epididymis, and seminal vesicle. This process is dependent primarily on testosterone secreted by Leydig cells. The differentiation of external male genitalia is regulated particularly through the actions of 5α-dihydrotestosterone (DHT), synthesized predominantly by type 2 testosterone reductase. Following androgen-dependent virilization of the urogenital system, the testes migrate from their site of origin next to the kidney into the scrotum, a process mediated by testosterone and insulin-like growth factor 3.

- Differentiation of male or female internal and external genitalia, or determination of **phenotypic sex.**

The determination of genetic sex is mediated through the chromosomal set, which in the normal male is 46,XY. The subsequent sexual differentiation is determined by genetic factors. Several sex-specific genes have been found to regulate gonadal differentiation and subsequent male or female reproductive tract development. One of the first genes involved in sexual differentiation is a gene on the Y chromosome called *SRY* (sex-regulating region of the Y). The product of the SRY gene is a protein that stimulates the neutral gonadal tissues to differentiate into testes, thereby determining gonadal sex. SRY is necessary and sufficient to initiate the male development cascade. If the SRY gene is mutant or missing on the Y chromosome, the embryo develops into a female.

SEXUAL DIFFERENTIATION

The process of differentiation of the human male gonads begins in the sixth week of gestation (see Figure 8–5). The first morphologically identifiable event is the development of precursor Sertoli cells, which aggregate to form the seminiferous cords, which are then infiltrated by primordial germ cells. By the end of the ninth week, the mesenchyme that separates the seminiferous cords gives rise to the interstitial cells, which differentiate as steroid-secreting Leydig cells. It is thought that the placenta-derived hormone, human chorionic gonadotropin (hCG), might be responsible for the initial development of Leydig cells because the onset of testosterone production precedes LH secretion. Hence, gonadotropic control of fetal testicular steroidogenesis is mediated initially by placenta-derived hCG and later by LH. The resulting increase in fetal testosterone production stimulates Leydig cell proliferation, increases the expression of steroidogenic enzymes (particularly 3β-hydroxysteroid dehydrogenase and 17α-hydroxylase), and increases the expression of the androgen receptor in the target tissues.

The postgonadal phase of sexual differentiation or external genitalia differentiation is almost exclusively hormone dependent (see Figures 8–5 and 8–6). Once the gonads have differentiated into testes, the secretion of testicular hormones is sufficient to promote masculinization of the embryo. The production of testosterone and antimüllerian hormone (AMH) during a critical time in early gestation ensures male development. Initially, both the male (mesonephric or wolffian) and female (paramesonephric or müllerian) internal genital ducts are present. In females, the mesonephric ducts regress, and the paramesonephric ducts develop into the uterine tubes, uterus, and upper vagina. In males, starting at the eighth week of gestation, AMH mediates the regression of the paramesonephric or müllerian ducts. AMH is a member of the TGF-β family that is expressed in the Sertoli cell from the beginning of testicular differentiation up to puberty. AMH binds to the type 2 AMH serine/threonine kinase receptors expressed in the surrounding mesenchyme of the müllerian ducts leading to apoptosis and regression of the müllerian ducts. The mesonephric duct system (wolffian ducts) remains and forms the vas deferens, epididymis, and seminal vesicle. This process is dependent primarily on testosterone. In the female, in the absence of androgens, the wolffian ducts regress and the müllerian ducts are spared from apoptosis, developing into the uterus, fallopian tubes, and vagina. Estrogens do not appear to be essential for normal sexual differentiation of either sex, as shown by normal genital development in males with a mutant estrogen receptor gene or with aromatase deficiency. The differentiation of external male genitalia is regulated particularly through the actions of DHT. During the developmental period, as already mentioned, the expression of the type 2 testosterone reductase is higher than that for the type 1 reductase. The capacity for converting testosterone to DHT is greater for the former isoenzyme.

Following müllerian duct regression and androgen-dependent virilization of the urogenital system, the testes migrate from their site of origin next to the kidney into the scrotum. This is the final critical event in male sexual differentiation. The 2-step process of transabdominal migration followed by descent into the extraabdominal scrotal sac finalizes sexual differentiation in the male and is completed during the late gestational period. The descent of the testis results from the regression of the cranial suspensory ligament, which connects them to the abdominal wall through the gubernaculum. Regression of the cranial suspensory ligament, transabdominal migration, and the final descent of the testis into the scrotum are mediated by testosterone and **insulin-like growth factor 3**. This hormone, also known as Leydig insulin-like hormone or relaxin-like factor, is a member of the insulin and insulin-like growth factor peptide hormone family. In humans, failure of complete testicular descent into the scrotum (cryptorchidism) is one of the most common congenital abnormalities, involving approximately 3% of male births. Cryptorchidism is important because spermatogenesis requires lower temperatures (as in the scrotum) than those found intraabdominally. If untreated, cryptorchidism can lead to infertility, and it has been associated with an increased risk of testicular tumors.

SEXUAL MATURATION AND FUNCTION

Puberty—Puberty is the physiologic transition between childhood and adulthood and involves the development of secondary sexual characteristics and the pubertal growth spurt. The process takes place over a period of approximately 4 years. Puberty is triggered by increased pulsatile secretion of GnRH by the hypothalamus, leading to increases in serum gonadotropins and, thus, to increases in gonadal secretion of sex steroids. The hypothalamic-pituitary-gonadal system is active during the neonatal period but enters a dormant state in the juvenile, prepubertal period. During the initial phase of puberty, plasma levels of LH increase primarily during sleep. These sleep-associated surges are later present throughout the day and mediate or result in an increase in circulating testosterone levels.

Puberty is preceded by adrenarche, a period characterized by increased adrenal production of DHEA and androstenedione at around 6–8 years of age that is not associated with increased production of adrenocorticotropic hormone or cortisol. The peak concentrations of DHEA and androstenedione are reached during late puberty and early adulthood. During this stage, there is some conversion of adrenal-derived androgens to testosterone, resulting in a small increase in circulating testosterone levels. The signal that triggers upregulation of the synthesis of DHEA and androstenedione is not known.

The increase in pulsatile release of GnRH is essential for the onset of puberty. However, the mechanism controlling the pubertal increase in GnRH release is still unclear. Leptin, a hormone secreted from adipose tissue (see Chapter 10), has been shown to have a permissive role in the timing of the activation of the GnRH pulse generator. The increase in the amplitude of GnRH pulses triggers a cascade of events including increases in the amplitude of FSH and LH pulses, followed by marked increases in gonadal sex hormone production. Accompanying the increase in gonadal steroid production during puberty is an increase in the amplitude of growth hormone secretory bursts. Together, growth hormone and gonadal steroids are responsible for producing normal pubertal growth. During the adolescent growth spurt, growth velocity increases from the prepubertal rate of 4–6 cm per year to as much as 10–15 cm per year. The physiologic changes associated with puberty are summarized as follows:

- Leydig cell maturation and initiation of spermatogenesis
- Testis enlargement; reddening and wrinkling of scrotal skin
- Pubic hair growth from the base of the penis
- Penis enlargement
- Prostate, seminal vesicle, and epididymis growth
- Facial (mustache and beard) and extremities hair growth, regression of scalp line
- Larynx enlargement, thickening of the vocal cords and deepening of the voice
- Enhanced linear growth
- Increased muscle mass and hematocrit
- Increased libido and sexual potency

Maturity and senescence—Sexual maturity is achieved at approximately age 16–18 years. During this stage, sperm production is optimal, plasma gonadotropins are normal, and most sexual anatomic changes have been completed. Beginning at age 40, there is a gradual decline in circulating testosterone levels, followed at age 50 by a reduction in sperm production. Testosterone levels in healthy, aging men decline on the order of 100 ng/dL per decade, accompanied by increases in SHBG resulting in an overall decrease in free and bioavailable testosterone levels. In addition, aging is associated with decreased testosterone to estradiol ratio, decreased LH pulse frequency, loss of the diurnal rhythm of testosterone secretion, and diminished accumulation of 5α-reduced steroids in reproductive tissues. These hormonal changes are well established by the age of 50 years. This period of androgen deficiency is called *andropause* and is characterized by diminished sexual desire and erectile capacity; fatigue and depression; decreased intellectual activity, lean body mass, body hair, and bone mineral density; and increased visceral fat and obesity. These age-related physiologic changes are caused by decreased testosterone, DHEA androstenedione, and growth hormone production.

Fertility and Secondary Sexual Characteristics

SPERMATOGENESIS

Spermatogenesis is the process of continuous germ cell differentiation to produce spermatozoa (Figure 8–7). Spermatogenesis is initiated at the time of puberty, is compartmentalized within the blood-testis barrier, and is mainly under FSH regulation. Spermatogenesis involves 4 basic processes:

Proliferation of spermatogonia (stem cells) giving rise to spermatocytes (diploid cells)—Spermatogonia line the seminiferous tubule near the basement membrane. They originate at puberty by proliferation of the gonocytes and are derived from primordial germ cells. One or 2 divisions of spermatogonia occur

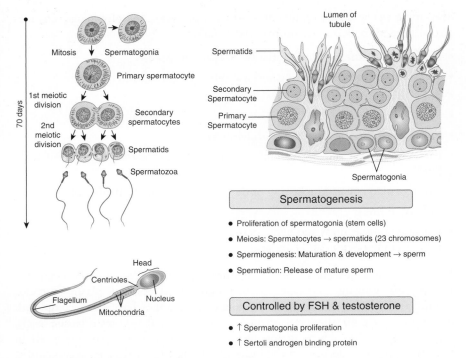

Figure 8–7. Schematic representation of key events in spermatogenesis. The process of spermatogenesis involves proliferation (mitosis) of spermatogonia, producing primary spermatocytes (diploid cells; 46 chromosomes). Spermatocytes undergo 2 meiotic divisions to yield spermatids, or haploid cells (23 chromosomes). Spermatids undergo a process of maturation (spermiogenesis) and development into spermatozoa. During this last phase, spermatozoa acquire the key elements for their function (see Table 8–3). This continuous process takes approximately 70 days. At any given time, cells from all steps of spermatogenesis can be identified in the testes.

to maintain their population in a stem cell pool (see Figure 8–7). Of the cells resulting from these mitotic divisions, some spermatogonia stay in the "resting" pool, whereas the remaining spermatogonia proliferate several times and undergo 1–5 stages of division and differentiation. After the last division, the resulting cells are termed *primary spermatocytes*. The "resting" or stem cell spermatogonia remain dormant for a time and then join a new proliferation cycle of spermatogonia. These cycles of spermatogonial divisions occur before the previous generation of cells has completed spermatogenesis, so that multiple stages of the process are occurring simultaneously in the seminiferous tubules. This overlap ensures a residual population of spermatogonia that maintain the ability of the testis to continuously produce sperm.

Meiosis of spermatocytes to yield spermatids (haploid cells; 23 chromosomes)—The primary spermatocytes undergo 2 divisions; the first

Table 8–3. Key events in spermiogenesis and their functional importance in sperm function

Key event	Functional importance
Nuclear chromatin condensation	Haploid chromatin carries either X or Y chromosome
Acrosome development	The acrosome is a large secretory vesicle that overlies the nucleus in the apical region of the sperm head and contains enzymes needed for mucus penetration and fertilization
Repositioning of spermatids; development and growth of flagellum	Microtubular structure provides motility, allowing sperm movement (3 mm/min) through the genital tract
Formation of mitochondrial sheath around flagellum	Provides energy (fructose-derived ATP) for flagellar movement

ATP, adenosine triphosphate.

meiotic division produces 2 secondary spermatocytes. Division of the secondary spermatocytes completes meiosis and produces the spermatids.

Spermiogenesis, or maturation and development of spermatids into spermatozoa (sperm)—This phase is characterized by nuclear and cytoplasmic changes that provide spermatozoa with key elements for their function. The main events during this phase involve spermatid condensation of nuclear material, formation of the acrosome, repositioning of the spermatid to allow formation and elongation of tail structures, mitochondrial spiral formation, and removal of extraneous cytoplasm, resulting in spermatozoa. Each of the features acquired during this step plays an important role in sperm function, as summarized in Table 8–3.

Spermiation—This is the final process of release of mature sperm from the Sertoli cells into the tubule lumen.

Throughout spermatogenesis, the germ cells move from the basal to the adluminal region of the seminiferous tubule into the compartment protected by the blood-testis barrier. The mitotic phase occurs in the basal compartment, whereas the meiotic and postmeiotic phases occur in the luminal compartment. The overall results of spermatogenesis are the following: cell proliferation and maintenance of a reserve germ cell population, reduction in chromosome number and genetic variation through meiosis, and production of spermatozoa.

REGULATION OF SPERMATOGENESIS

Spermatogenesis is dependent on gonadotropin stimulation and testosterone production. FSH stimulates proliferation and secretory activity of the Sertoli cells, whereas LH stimulates the production of testosterone. Testosterone in turn stimulates spermatogenesis through receptor-mediated events in the Sertoli cells. The LH-induced rise in intratesticular testosterone plays an essential role in the initiation and maintenance of spermatogenesis by the Sertoli cells. Testosterone produced by the Leydig cells are transported to the developing germ cells bound to ABP produced by the Sertoli cell in response to FSH stimulation and released into the adluminal compartment. The synthesis of ABP requires that the Sertoli cell be under androgen influence, underscoring the importance of testosterone in Sertoli cell function and the reliance on paracrine mechanisms of hormone action.

Anabolic and Metabolic Effects of Androgens

In bone, the main physiologic effect of testosterone is to reduce bone resorption by increasing osteoblast lifespan and proliferation. Testosterone enhances bone formation, increases periosteal apposition of bone, increases protein synthesis, and decreases protein breakdown, having an overall anabolic effect in bone and skeletal muscle. Much of testosterone's action on bone results from its aromatization to 17β-estradiol and the estrogen receptor. Testosterone-derived estrogen is a critical sex hormone in the pubertal growth spurt, skeletal maturation, accrual of peak bone mass, and maintenance of bone mass in the adult. It stimulates chondrogenesis in the epiphysial growth plate, increasing pubertal linear growth. At puberty, estrogen promotes skeletal maturation and the gradual, progressive closure of the epiphysial growth plate and the termination of chondrogenesis. In the adult, estrogen is important in maintaining the constancy of bone mass through its effects on remodeling and bone turnover.

Testosterone inhibits lipid uptake and lipoprotein lipase activity in adipocytes, stimulates lipolysis by increasing the number of lipolytic β-adrenergic receptors, and inhibits differentiation of adipocyte precursor cells. Androgens stimulate resting metabolic rate and lipid oxidation and enhances glucose disposal by increasing the expression of glucose transporters on the plasma membrane of adipocytes.

NEUROENDOCRINE AND VASCULAR CONTROL OF ERECTION AND EJACULATION

The physiologic process of human reproduction involves the fertilization of a mature ovum through the deposition of sperm-containing semen in the vagina of the female. This event involves penile erection and ejaculation of the sperm-containing semen at the time of copulation. Penile erection results from smooth muscle relaxation mediated by a spinal reflex involving central nervous processing and integration of tactile, olfactory, auditory, and mental stimuli. Corporeal vasodilatation and corporeal smooth muscle relaxation allow increased blood flow into the corpus cavernosum. The concordant contraction of the perineal skeletal muscles leads to a temporary increase in corpus cavernosum blood pressure above mean systolic arterial pressure, helping to increase penile firmness.

Corporeal vasodilatation is mediated by the parasympathetic nervous system. Parasympathetic fibers directly innervating the corporeal smooth muscle and sinusoidal endothelial cells release acetylcholine, stimulating the production of constitutive endothelial nitric oxide. Nitric oxide produced locally in the smooth muscle cell, or reaching it by diffusion from the adjacent endothelial cells, is the major mediator of smooth muscle relaxation through activation of guanylate cyclase and increased production of cyclic guanosine monophosphate (cGMP). The inactivation of cGMP phosphodiesterase, the enzyme that degrades cGMP with the drug sildenafil, preserves smooth muscle relaxation, and prolongs the erection period. This is used commercially to treat erectile dysfunction.

The ejaculation phase of the sexual response consists of 2 sequential processes: emission and ejaculation. Emission is the deposition of seminal fluid into the posterior urethra and is mediated by simultaneous contractions of the ampulla of the vas deferens, the seminal vesicles, and the smooth muscles of the prostate. The second process is ejaculation, which results in expulsion of the seminal fluid from the posterior urethra through the penile meatus. This process is controlled by sympathetic innervation of the genital organs and occurs as a result of a spinal cord reflex arc. Detumescence of the penis following ejaculation and maintenance of the flaccid penis in the absence of sexual arousal, are produced by sympathetic corporeal vasoconstriction and corporeal smooth muscle contraction by noradrenergic, neuropeptide Y, and endothelin-1 fibers.

DISEASES OF TESTOSTERONE EXCESS OR DEFICIENCY

Hypergonadism—Excess androgen activity in childhood leads to precocious puberty, defined as the appearance of male secondary sex characteristics before age 9 years (see Table 8–2). Hypothalamic tumors, activating mutations of the LH receptor, congenital adrenal hyperplasia, and androgen-producing tumors are all causes of premature virilization. Two types of precocious puberty can be identified: gonadotropin dependent and independent.

Hypogonadism—Decreased testosterone production, or hypogonadism, can be caused by disorders at the hypothalamic/pituitary level (hypogonadotropic or secondary hypogonadism) or by testicular dysfunction (hypergonadotropic or primary hypogonadism). Hypogonadotropic hypogonadism can be caused by abnormalities in hypothalamic GnRH secretion or action, associated with impaired gonadotropin secretion by the anterior pituitary. This condition may result from genetic defects including Kallmann syndrome; adrenal hypoplasia; mutations of the GnRH receptor, LH, or FSH β-subunits; pituitary tumors (including prolactinoma); trauma; or surgery.

Abnormal testicular function in the presence of elevated gonadotropin levels (hypergonadotropic or primary hypogonadism) is caused by testicular damage or impaired testicular development, which can be either congenital or acquired following chemotherapy or radiation. Causes include cryptorchidism, gonadal dysgenesis, varicocele, enzyme defects in testosterone biosynthesis, or LH receptor defects. Klinefelter syndrome is the most common sex chromosome disorder, in which affected males carry an additional X chromosome. This genetic abnormality results in male hypogonadism, androgen deficiency, and impaired spermatogenesis. Klinefelter syndrome is the most common genetic cause of human male infertility. Hyperprolactinemia from any cause results in both reproductive and sexual dysfunction because of prolactin inhibition of GnRH release, resulting in hypogonadotropic hypogonadism.

Clinical Presentation

Excess testosterone in the prepubescent male is associated with the appearance of all the changes of puberty at a very early age. These changes include enlargement of the penis and testicles; appearance of pubic, underarm, and facial hair; spontaneous erections; production of sperm; development of acne; and deepening of the voice.

Androgen deficiency leads to severe symptoms, which differ according to the time of onset. Androgen deficiency during early childhood results in short stature, lack of deepening of the voice, female distribution of secondary hair, anemia, underdeveloped muscles, and genitalia with delayed or absent onset of spermatogenesis and sexual function. Androgen deficiency in the adult after normal virilization has been completed leads to a decrease in bone mineral density (bone mass), decreased bone marrow activity resulting in anemia, alterations in body composition associated with muscle weakness and atrophy, changes in mood and cognitive function, and regression of sexual function and

Table 8–4. Normal values of semen parameters according to World Health Organization (1992)

Standard tests	
Volume	>2 mL
pH	7.2–8.0
Sperm concentration	$>20 \times 10^6$ spermatozoa/mL
Total sperm count	$>40 \times 10^6$ spermatozoa/ejaculate
Motility	>50% with forward progression (categories a and b) or >25% with rapid progression (category a) within 60 min of ejaculation
Morphology	>30% with normal forms
Vitality	>75% or more live, *ie*, excluding dye
White blood cells	$<1 \times 10^6$/mL
Immunobead test	<20% spermatozoa with adherent particles
Mixed agglutination reaction test	<10% spermatozoa with adherent particles
Optional tests	
α-Glucosidase (neutral)	>20 mU per ejaculate
Zinc (total)	>2.4 μmol per ejaculate
Citric acid (total)	>52 μmol per ejaculate
Acid phosphatase (total)	>200 U per ejaculate
Fructose (total)	>13 μmol per ejaculate

spermatogenesis. In the adult male, androgen deficiency decreases nocturnal erections and libido.

Evaluation of Hypogonadism

Sparse facial, axillary, and pubic hair and small penis and testicles characterize the clinical presentation of the prepubescent male patient with hypogonadism. Low plasma levels of testosterone should be interpreted in conjunction with LH levels to distinguish between hypo- and hypergonadotropic forms of hypogonadism. Similar to the functional tests described for other endocrine organs, a challenge test with intravenously injected GnRH to determine the gonadotropin and testosterone response 25 and 40 minutes later is used to assess the gonadotropin reserve capacity of the pituitary. When the response is absent, a prolonged period (7 days) of GnRH can be used to further stimulate the anterior pituitary gonadotrophs. In adults, fertility assessment by semen evaluation is also indicated. Semen analysis is interpreted according to normal values shown in Table 8–4.

KEY CONCEPTS

Testicular function is under LH and FSH regulation. LH and FSH production and release are under hypothalamic GnRH stimulation and feedback inhibition by gonadal hormones.

Leydig cells synthesize testosterone. Sertoli cells support spermatogenesis and form the blood-testis barrier.

The main functions of the testes are testosterone production and spermatogenesis.

The main hormones produced by the testis are testosterone, estradiol, and inhibin.

Testosterone can be metabolized to DHT, a more potent androgen, or to 17β-estradiol, an estrogen.

Androgens exert their physiologic effects through modulation of gene transcription.

Three essential testis-derived hormones regulate male sexual development: androgens, AMH, and insulin-like growth factor 3.

STUDY QUESTIONS

8–1.   A 20-year-old male patient presents to the doctor's office complaining about continuous growth, lack of facial hair development, and smaller penis and testicles
than his college friends. Laboratory values include total testosterone 1 ng/mL and
LH 1.5 mU/mL. Thyroid-stimulating hormone and prolactin levels are normal. He
has no history of medications, drug use, or disease. GnRH stimulation test over a
7-day period produces elevations in circulating levels of LH. Continued growth in
this case is caused by:

a. Increased estrogen production

b. Decreased inhibin release

c. Decreased testosterone production

d. Decreased sensitivity to LH stimulation

8–2.   In the patient described above, it was observed that in addition to being much
taller than young adults his age, his arms were very long. The excessive height and
arm length resulting from delayed epiphyseal growth plate closure is caused by:

a. Increased DHT formation

b. Decreased adrenal DHEA production

c. Decreased estradiol production

d. Increased estriol production

8–3.   A college football player purchases online natural hormone analogs to increase his
muscle mass. After a year of hormone analog injections his muscle mass increases
significantly, he develops acne, and notices that his sclera has a yellowish tint.
Consultation with the team's physician leads to a complete physical examination
that reveals small testicular size. Being a newlywed, he wants to determine his fertility status, and test results show sperm count of 10×10^6 spermatozoa/ejaculate.
Which of the following is the underlying mechanism for these manifestations?

a. Decreasing circulating levels of DHT

b. Suppression of FSH release from the pituitary

c. Increased testicular testosterone concentrations

d. Increasing aromatase activity

8–4.   A 15-year-old male underweight high school student is brought to the family physician because of what appears to be a delay in the onset of puberty. The most
likely mechanism underlying this defect is:

a. Decreased aromatase activity

b. Increased DHT production

c. Decreased leptin production

d. Cryptorchidism

SUGGESTED READINGS

Habert R, Lejeune H, Saenz JM. Origin, differentiation and regulation of fetal and adult Leydig cells. *Mol Cell Endocrinol.* 2001;179:47.

Hughes IA. Minireview: sex differentiation. *Endocrinology.* 2001;142:3281.

Kandeel FR, Koussa VK, Swerdloff RS. Male sexual function and its disorders: physiology, pathophysiology, clinical investigation, and treatment. *Endocr Rev.* 2001;22:342.

MacLaughlin DT, Teixeira J, Donahoe PK. Perspective: reproductive tract development—new discoveries and future directions. *Endocrinology.* 2001;142:2167.

Nef S, Parada LF. Hormones in male sexual development. *Genes Dev.* 2000;14:3075.

Simoni M, Gromoll J, Nieschlag E. The follicle-stimulating hormone receptor: biochemistry, molecular biology, physiology, and pathophysiology. *Endocr Rev.* 1977;18:739.

Welt C, Sidis Y, Keutmann H, Schneyer A. Activins, inhibins, and follistatins: from endocrinology to signaling. A paradigm for the new millennium. *Exp Biol Med.* 2002;227:724.

Female Reproductive System

OBJECTIVES

▶ Describe oogenesis, its relationship to follicular maturation, and the roles of pituitary and ovarian factors in their regulation.

▶ Describe gonadotropin control of ovarian function.

▶ List the target organs and principal physiologic actions of estrogen and progesterone and how they interact with each other.

▶ Describe the cellular mechanisms of action for estrogen and progesterone.

▶ Describe the endometrial (proliferative and secretory phases) and ovarian events that occur throughout the menstrual cycle and correlate them with the changes in blood levels of pituitary and ovarian hormones.

▶ Identify the pathways of sperm and egg transport required for fertilization and for movement of the embryo to the uterus.

▶ Describe the principal endocrine functions of the placenta, particularly in rescue of the corpus luteum and maintenance of pregnancy, and the fetal adrenal-placental interactions involved in estrogen production.

▶ Understand the roles of oxytocin, relaxin, and prostaglandins in the initiation and maintenance of parturition.

▶ Explain the hormonal regulation of mammary gland development during puberty, pregnancy, and lactation, and explain the mechanisms that control milk production and secretion.

▶ Explain the physiologic basis for the effects of steroid hormone contraceptive methods.

▶ Describe the age-related changes in the female reproductive system, including the mechanisms responsible for these changes, throughout life from fetal development to senescence.

The principal functions of the female reproductive system are to produce the ova for sperm fertilization and to provide the appropriate conditions for embryo implantation, fetal growth and development, and birth. Endocrine regulation of the reproductive system is directed by the hypothalamic-pituitary-ovarian axis. Ovarian-derived hormones regulate the hypothalamic-pituitary-gonadal axis in a classical negative feedback pattern. Throughout the ovarian cycle, a selected follicle is stimulated to undergo growth and development, culminating in ovulation. The remnants of the follicle undergo reorganization into the **corpus luteum**, a

temporary endocrine organ that plays a central role in preparation and maintenance of the initial stages of pregnancy. Parallel changes occur in endometrial
morphology and function throughout the ovarian cycle in preparation for implantation of a fertilized ovum. Ovarian and placental hormones maintain pregnancy
and prepare the breast for lactation. This chapter describes the basic principles of
the neuroendocrine regulation of this hypothalamic-pituitary-ovarian axis.

FUNCTIONAL ANATOMY

The female reproductive organs include the ovaries, the uterus and fallopian tubes,
and the breasts or mammary glands (Figure 9–1). Their growth, development, and
function are under hormonal regulation. The ovaries store and release the ovum
and produce the 2 principal female sex hormones, estrogen and progesterone.
Functionally, the ovaries consist of an outer cortex layer containing different-size
follicles and an inner medulla consisting of vascular connective tissue and hilar
cells. The primordial follicle contains a primary oocyte surrounded by epithelial
(pregranulosa) cells separated from the ovarian stroma by a basement membrane.
During follicular development, the epithelial cells differentiate into **granulosa**
cells, and a layer of cells from the ovarian stroma is transformed into **theca** cells.
The larger, more mature follicles are filled with a transparent albuminous fluid
and consist of an external fibrovascular coat, connected with the surrounding
stroma of the ovary by a network of blood vessels; and an internal coat, consisting of several layers of nucleated cells (granulosa cells) anchored in the zona
pellucida, a glycoprotein-rich eosinophilic material surrounding the oocyte. The
zona pellucida forms the corona radiata, which close to the time of ovulation is
separated from the granulosa cells and expelled with the oocyte. Formation of
the follicles begins before birth, and their development and maturation continue
uninterrupted from puberty until the end of a woman's reproductive life, as discussed later.

The female genital tract is derived from the müllerian ducts (see Chapter 8;
Figure 8–6) and consists of the uterus, fallopian tubes, and vagina (see Figure 9–1).
The fallopian tubes extend from each of the superior angles of the uterus and consist of the isthmus, the ampulla, and the infundibulum, which opens into the
abdominal cavity and is surrounded by ovarian fimbriae and attached to the ovary
(see Figure 9–1). The epithelial lining of the fallopian tubes has secretory and ciliated cells that contribute to sperm movement, aiding in fertilization and facilitating the movement of the zygote (fertilized ovum) to the uterus for implantation
and fetal development. These functions are also aided by the rhythmic contraction
of the smooth muscle walls.

The uterus is composed of 3 layers: serous, muscular, and mucous. The muscular coat accounts for the bulk of the uterus and consists of bundles of smooth
muscle fibers, organized in layers and intermixed with loose connective tissue,
blood vessels, lymphatic vessels, and nerves. The mucous membrane, or endometrium, is lined by columnar ciliated secretory epithelium that undergoes cycles
of proliferation, differentiation, and breakdown every 28 days in preparation for

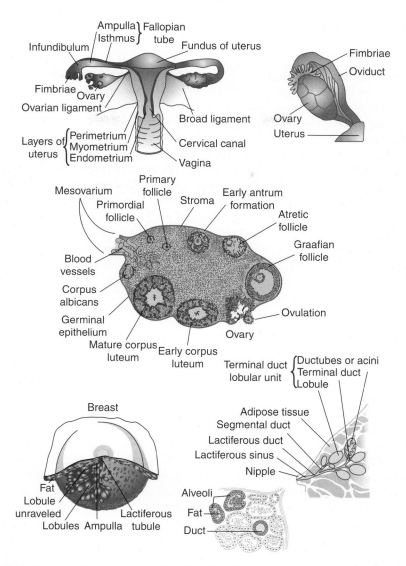

Figure 9–1. Functional anatomy of the female reproductive tract. The female reproductive organs include the ovaries, the uterus and fallopian tubes, and the breasts or mammary glands. The ovaries consist of an outer cortex layer that contains different-sized follicles and their remains undergoing apoptosis, embedded in connective tissue. The fallopian tubes extend from each of the superior angles of the uterus and consist of the isthmus, the ampulla, and the infundibulum, which opens into the abdominal cavity and is surrounded by ovarian fimbriae and attached to the ovary. The cilia of the epithelial lining of the fallopian tubes contribute to sperm movement, aiding in fertilization, and facilitate movement of the zygote (fertilized ovum) to the uterus for implantation and fetal development. The breast is organized into lobes made of lobules, connected by connective tissue, blood vessels, and ducts. The lobules consist of a cluster of rounded alveoli, which open into excretory lactiferous ducts and unite to form larger ducts made of longitudinal and transverse elastic fibers. These ducts converge toward the areola, beneath which they form ampullar dilatations, which serve as reservoirs for the milk.

embryo implantation. The arterial blood supply to the female reproductive tract is provided by branches of the hypogastric and ovarian arteries from the abdominal aorta. The veins correspond with the arteries and end in the uterine plexuses. The nerves are derived from the hypogastric and ovarian plexuses and from the third and fourth sacral nerves.

The breast consists of glandular tissue organized in lobes connected by fibrous tissue, with fat deposits interspersed between the lobes (see Figure 9–1). The mammary lobes themselves are made of lobules connected by connective tissue, blood vessels, and ducts. The lobules consist of a cluster of rounded alveoli, which open into excretory lactiferous ducts and unite to form larger ducts made of longitudinal and transverse elastic fibers. These ducts converge toward the areola, beneath which they form ampullar dilatations, which serve as reservoirs for the milk. The arterial blood supply to the breast is derived from the thoracic branches of the axillary, the intercostal, and the internal mammary arteries. The veins drain into the axillary and internal mammary veins.

GONADOTROPIN REGULATION OF OVARIAN FUNCTION

Pulsatile release of gonadotropin-releasing hormone (GnRH) from the hypothalamus stimulates pulsatile pituitary release of luteinizing hormone (LH) and follicle-stimulating hormone (FSH). As already mentioned in Chapter 8, GnRH secretion is regulated by dopamine, serotonin, β-endorphin, and norepinephrine. Both FSH and LH bind to G protein–coupled receptors, causing activation of the Gα-stimulatory (Gα$_s$) subunit, which leads to cyclic 3′,5′-adenosine monophosphate (cAMP)-mediated stimulation of steroidogenic events (described in Chapters 6 and 8) culminating in ovarian production of **estradiol** and **progesterone**; the 2 principal hormones involved in the regulation of ovarian function and control of the reproductive cycle (Figure 9–2). The variations in pulsatile release of the gonadotropins result in a cyclic response of ovarian function. Each cycle lasts 28 days and can be divided into 2 phases (follicular and luteal) of 14 days each.

Follicular phase— During the follicular phase, FSH stimulates follicular recruitment and growth and estrogen synthesis. Before the selection of the follicle for ovulation, granulosa cells are responsive only to FSH. As follicular maturation progresses, the coupling between FSH receptor stimulation and the activation of adenylate cyclase becomes more and more efficient, leading to a steady increase in cAMP production. The accumulation of FSH-induced cAMP results in upregulation of LH receptors, allowing LH to act as a surrogate for FSH in **granulosa cells**. Low gonadotropin levels (especially FSH) lead to granulosa cell death and follicular atresia.

Luteal phase—LH is responsible for ovulation and corpus **luteum** formation and for progesterone and estrogen production by the corpus luteum. Activation of the LH receptors in theca cells stimulates androstenedione production, providing the substrate for the enzymatic conversion to 17β-estradiol that is mediated by the enzyme aromatase in granulosa cells.

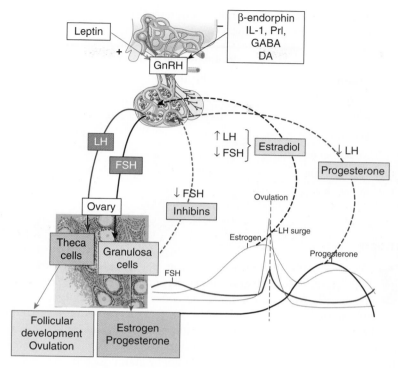

Figure 9–2. Hypothalamic-pituitary-ovarian axis. Gonadotropin synthesis and release and differential expression are under both positive and negative feedback control by ovarian steroid and peptide hormones. Ovarian hormones can decrease gonadotropin release both by modulating gonadotropin-releasing hormone (GnRH) pulse frequency from the hypothalamus and by affecting the ability of GnRH to stimulate gonadotropin secretion from the pituitary itself. Estradiol enhances luteinizing hormone (LH) and inhibits follicle-stimulating hormone (FSH) release, whereas inhibins A and B (gonadal glycoprotein hormones) reduce FSH secretion. After ovulation, ovarian progesterone production predominates. Progesterone increases hypothalamic opioid activity and slows GnRH pulse secretion, favoring FSH production and decreasing LH release. Inhibin B peaks early in the follicular phase, whereas inhibin A peaks in the midluteal phase. The increasing inhibin B levels in the midfollicular phase act at the pituitary gonadotroph to offset activin signaling and suppress FSH biosynthesis from early follicular phase levels. The decrease in inhibin A at the end of the luteal phase creates an environment in which FSH levels can again increase. GABA, γ-aminobutyric acid; DA, dopamine; IL-1, interleukin 1; NE, norepinephrine; NPY, neuropeptide Y; Prl, prolactin.

OVARIAN HORMONE SYNTHESIS

Ovarian production of steroid hormones (progesterone, estrogen, and testosterone) and peptide hormones (inhibins) varies throughout the ovarian cycle. The production and secretion rates of the principal ovarian steroid hormones are summarized in Table 9–1.

Table 9-1. Production and secretion rates of principal female sex steroid hormones

Hormone	Production/Secretion rate (mg/d)	
	Follicular	Luteal
Progesterone	2/1.7	25/24
Estradiol	0.09/0.08	0.25/0.24
Estrone	0.11/0.08	0.26/0.15
Androstenedione	3.2/2.8	NC
Testosterone	0.19/0.06	NC

NC, no change.

Estrogen

The production of estrogen involves coordinated enzymatic activities between the **theca** and **granulose cells** of the **ovarian follicle** (Figure 9–3). Theca cells express the enzymes necessary to convert cholesterol to androgens (mainly androstenedione) but lack the enzymes necessary to convert androgens to estradiol. Granulosa cells can convert androgens to estradiol, and they can produce progesterone, but they are unable to synthesize androgens. Thus, theca cell–produced androgens are aromatized to estradiol by granulosa cells (see Figure 9–3). More than 95% of circulating estradiol is directly secreted by the ovaries, with a smaller contribution from peripheral conversion of estrone to estradiol in premenopausal women.

Androgens

Female androgens are derived from the adrenal glands (dehydroepiandrosterone and androstenedione), from the ovaries (androstenedione and testosterone), and from peripheral conversion of androstenedione and dehydroepiandrosterone to testosterone. Ovarian androgen secretion parallels that of estrogen throughout the menstrual cycle, whereas adrenal androgen production does not fluctuate throughout the menstrual cycle. Most of the circulating testosterone in females is derived from the peripheral conversion of androstenedione by 17β-hydroxysteroid dehydrogenase. The conversion of testosterone to dihydrotestosterone in peripheral tissues is limited in females because of higher levels of sex hormone-binding globulin in females than in males, as well as by the peripheral conversion to estrogen by aromatase, protecting females from virilization by dihydrotestosterone.

Progesterone

The preovulatory LH surge results in luteinization of granulosa and theca cells, altering the steroidogenic pathway so that progesterone becomes the primary steroid hormone produced by each of these cell types after luteinization. The changes leading to the ability to produce progesterone include increased expression of the

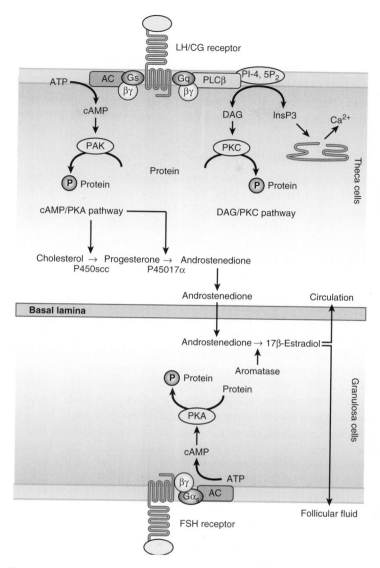

Figure 9–3. Theca and granulosa cells coordinate the production of estrogen. The secretion of estradiol by the dominant follicle requires cooperation between theca cells, which synthesize androstenedione and testosterone, and granulosa cells of mature follicles, which convert androgens to estradiol and estrone. Androgen synthesis in theca cells results from the activity of 3 enzymes: cholesterol side-chain cleavage (P450scc), 17α-hydroxylase-lyase (P450C17), and 3β-hydroxysteroid dehydrogenase (3β-HSD). Luteinizing hormone (LH) induces steroidogenic acute regulatory protein (StAR), which allows the entry of cholesterol into mitochondria. In granulosa cells, the enzyme 17β-hydroxysteroid dehydrogenase transforms androstenedione into testosterone in follicles from the primary stage. In mature follicles, follicle-stimulating hormone (FSH) stimulates the activity of aromatase, which transforms testosterone into 17β-estradiol. AC, adenylate cyclase; ATP, adenosine triphosphate; cAMP, cyclic adenosine monophosphate; DAG, diacylglycerol; InsP$_3$, inositol 1,4,5-trisphosphate; PI-4,5P$_2$, phosphatidylinositol 4,5-bisphosphate; PKA, protein kinase A; PKC, protein kinase C; PLCβ, phospholipase Cβ.

enzymes involved in the conversion of cholesterol to progesterone (cholesterol side-chain cleavage cytochrome P450 complex and 3β-hydroxysteroid dehydrogenase) and decreased expression of the enzymes that convert progesterone to estrogens (17α-hydroxylase cytochrome P450 and aromatase cytochrome P450).

Inhibins, Activins, and Follistatin

Inhibin production by granulosa cells of mature follicles is regulated by FSH and LH, and by local factors such as growth factors (epidermal, transforming, and insulin-like) and hormones (androstenedione, activin, and follistatin) in an autocrine and paracrine way. In clinical practice, inhibin B is a good marker of granulosa cell function under the control of FSH, whereas inhibin A is a marker of corpus luteum function under the control of LH. Inhibins contribute to the regulation of LH and FSH release through endocrine feedback regulation at the anterior pituitary.

Activin production by the granulosa cells changes during **folliculogenesis** and its effects are probably limited to paracrine action on granulosa cells. Activin promotes granulosa cell proliferation, upregulates FSH receptor expression on granulosa cells, and modulates steroidogenesis in both granulosa and theca cells. In the pituitary-ovarian axis, activin is a physiologic antagonist to inhibin and specifically stimulates pituitary FSH synthesis and secretion.

Activin-binding protein, follistatin, is a product of granulosa cells. Its basal expression increases with differentiation of granulosa cells. Its function is to neutralize the effect of activin on steroid production. The physiologic endocrine role of follistatin is not completely understood, but its effects are most likely autocrine or paracrine on ovarian steroidogenesis.

OVARIAN CYCLE

The ovarian cycle is divided into a follicular and a luteal phase (Figure 9–4).

The follicular phase begins on day 1 of the cycle, the first day of menses, and corresponds to the growth and development of a dominant follicle. Throughout the reproductive life span of the woman (from puberty to menopause), a single mature oocyte is produced each month. Most of the human oocytes (germ cells) present during uterine development are destined to undergo apoptosis, or programmed cell death. Only follicles that are responsive to FSH stimulation (approximately 350) will enter the final stage of development and progress to ovulation. At mid cycle (day 14), the rising levels of estrogen stimulate a surge in LH release, which stimulates ovulation 24–36 hours later.

The luteal phase begins after ovulation, with the reorganization of the remnants of the ovulatory follicle and the formation of the corpus luteum (see Figure 9–4). The corpus luteum is a transient endocrine organ that produces progesterone, and to a lesser extent estradiol and inhibin A. The corpus luteum is under LH regulation. The luteal phase ends when there is no fertilization and placental-mediated survival of the corpus luteum discussed below.

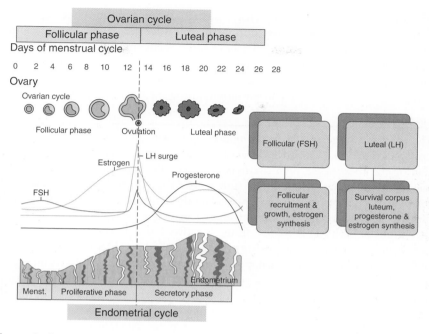

Figure 9-4. Hormonal events during the ovarian and endometrial cycles. Plasma concentrations of inhibins, estrogen, progesterone, luteinizing hormone, and follicle-stimulating hormone (FSH) during the human menstrual cycle correspond to proliferative and secretory changes in the endometrium and to follicular development and ovulation.

Ovarian Regulation of Gonadotropin Release

Gonadotropin release is under negative and positive feedback regulation by estradiol, progesterone, and inhibins A and B. Progesterone and 17β-estradiol act both in the hypothalamus and the pituitary, and inhibins act at the level of the pituitary (see Figure 9-2). The contributions of these ovarian hormones vary according to the stage of the ovarian cycle.

FOLLICULAR PHASE

During this phase, the dominant follicle produces high concentrations of 17β-estradiol and inhibin B. Although initially estradiol exerts negative feedback on FSH and LH release, as concentrations of estradiol increase, toward the end of the follicular phase, a switch from negative to positive feedback occurs. High estradiol levels in the hypothalamus and pituitary lead to low-amplitude, high-frequency pulses (every 90 minutes) of LH, resulting in a midcycle LH surge. The estradiol-mediated stimulation of the LH surge results from an increased responsiveness of gonadotropic cells to GnRH (following exposure to increasing estradiol levels), an increase in GnRH receptor number, and a GnRH surge, triggered by the effect on the hypothalamus of increasing estradiol concentrations (see Figures 9–2 and 9–4). Inhibin B levels rise during the follicular phase and decrease immediately before the LH peak, with a brief surge occurring 2 days after ovulation. Inhibin A levels increase in the late follicular phase to reach a peak concentration on the day of the LH and FSH surge. The concentration then falls briefly before rising to reach a maximum concentration during the midluteal phase.

LUTEAL PHASE

The midcycle surge in LH levels induces ovulation, resumption of meiosis, and promotes the formation and survival of the corpus luteum during the luteal phase. During the luteal phase, high circulating concentrations of progesterone (produced by the corpus luteum) suppress the frequency and the amplitude of LH release, resulting in an overall decrease in LH by blocking the surges of GnRH, downregulating pituitary GnRH receptor expression, and decreasing gene expression of the α- and β-subunits of both LH and FSH. Thus, negative feedback regulation by progesterone during the luteal phase prevents a second LH surge. The marked suppression of GnRH and LH pulse frequency achieved by high progesterone levels during the luteal phase allows enrichment of gonadotroph FSH levels. Inhibin B levels remain low during the luteal phase. Inhibin A is secreted by the granulosa cells during the luteal phase, and its concentration falls during luteal regression synchronously with estradiol and progesterone, remaining low during the early follicular phase.

Unless the corpus luteum is stimulated by human chorionic gonadotropin (hCG), a placental hormone (described later), it regresses. Regression or lysis of the corpus luteum and the associated decrease in progesterone levels leads to an increase in FSH release toward the beginning of the next ovarian cycle. During the luteal-follicular transition, following the midcycle rise in FSH secretion, the inhibin B concentration rises and peaks 4 days after the peak FSH concentration is reached.

Oogenesis and Formation of the Dominant Follicle

Unlike the fetal testis, the fetal ovary begins germ cell development (oogenesis) early in fetal life. During early intrauterine development (15 weeks), primordial germ cells (oogonia) proliferate and migrate to the genital ridge. On their arrival in the fetal ovary, some of the oogonia continue mitotic proliferation and some begin to undergo apoptosis (Figure 9–5). Some of these oogonia begin (but do not complete) meiosis and become oocytes. These cells have 2 X chromosomes. By 6 months postpartum, all oogonia have been converted to oocytes. At or near birth, the meiotic process is arrested at prophase of the first meiotic division. The oocytes remain arrested in the diplotene stage of the first meiotic prophase until they are recruited to grow and mature (by FSH) to produce an ovum or they undergo apoptosis. During the first days of postnatal life, the oocytes recruit somatic follicular cells, which are organized into a finite number of "resting" primordial follicles. Primordial follicles are composed of an outer layer of granulosa cells and a small oocyte, both enveloped in a basal lamina. The pool of primordial follicles in the female ovary reaches its maximum number at approximately 20 weeks of gestational age and then decreases in a logarithmic fashion throughout life until complete depletion occurs during menopause. When reproductive life is initiated, less than 10% of the primordial follicles are left.

Folliculogenesis, or formation of the dominant follicle, consists of 2 stages: the gonadotropin-independent (preantral) period and the gonadotropin-dependent (antral or graafian) period. Primordial follicular growth up to the antral stage (up to 0.2 mm) occurs during fetal life and infancy and is gonadotropin independent (see Figure 9–5). Primary follicles are formed when the flattened epithelial cells become cuboidal and undergo mitosis. The antral follicle growth phase is characterized by granulosa cell proliferation, expression of FSH and steroid hormone receptors, and association of the theca cells with the growing follicle and granulosa cells, leading to formation of the secondary follicles. Tertiary follicles are formed following further theca cell hypertrophy and development. Their antrum is filled with estrogen-rich fluid, and the theca interstitial cells start to express FSH and LH receptors. The mechanisms that trigger initiation of follicular growth are still not completely understood, but are thought to involve bidirectional communication between germ and somatic cells through gap junctions and paracrine factors, including cytokines and growth factors (insulin-like growth factor 1 [IGF-1], epidermal and fibroblast growth factors, and interleukin 1β). When follicles reach a size of 2–5 mm, approximately 50% enter the selection growth phase and are rescued from apoptosis. This final developmental phase of follicular growth begins approximately 85 days before ovulation in the luteal phase of the cycle preceding ovulation (see Figure 9–5).

During this gonadotropin-dependent growth phase, follicles grow exponentially, and FSH stimulates estrogen production from granulosa cells, follicular fluid formation, cell proliferation, and LH receptor expression in the dominant follicle. Selection of a dominant follicle is dictated by sensitivity to FSH action, which is locally modulated by antimüllerian hormone (AMH).

AMH or müllerian-inhibiting substance discussed in Chapter 8 as it pertains to sex differentiation in the male embryo, is a peptide growth factor and member of the large transforming growth factor beta family of growth and differentiation factors. AMH is expressed in the granulosa cells of the recruited primordial follicles, and continues to be expressed in the growing follicles that have undergone recruitment from the primordial follicle pool but that have not been selected for dominance. This pattern of expression suggests an important role in the regulation of both the number of growing follicles and their selection for ovulation. Because the number of growing follicles is correlated to the size of the primordial follicle pool size, a marker such as AMH that reflects all follicles that have made the transition from the primordial follicle pool to the growing pool has been proposed to be a good indirect marker of ovarian reserve. FSH and inhibin B levels have also been proposed to serve as predictors of the ovarian reserve.

The average time between primary follicle development and ovulation is 10–14 days (see Figure 9–5).

During follicular recruitment, the oocyte enters a growth phase that leads to the completion of the first meiotic division. The resumption of meiosis is mediated

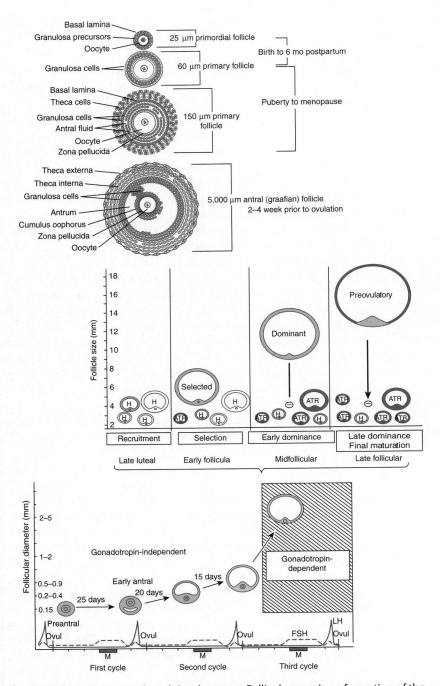

Figure 9–5. Follicle growth and development. Folliculogenesis, or formation of the dominant follicle, consists of 2 stages: the gonadotropin-independent (preantral) period and the gonadotropin-dependent (antral or graafian) period. Primordial follicular growth up to the antral stage occurs during fetal life and infancy and is gonadotropin independent. The final developmental phase of follicular growth, in which antral follicles are protected from apoptosis, begins approximately 85 days before ovulation. One dominant follicle is recruited in the luteal phase of the cycle preceding ovulation. Atr, atretic; FSH, follicle-stimulating hormone; LH, luteinizing hormone.

by the midcycle surge in LH. LH acts on mature follicles to terminate the program of gene expression associated with folliculogenesis. The transcription of genes that control granulosa cell proliferation (ie, IGF-1, FSH and estrogen receptors, cyclin D2) and those that encode steroidogenic enzymes is rapidly turned off by LH-mediated increases in intracellular cAMP. In addition, LH induces genes involved in ovulation (ie, progesterone receptor, cyclooxygenase-2) and luteinization (ie, cell cycle inhibitors, steroidogenic enzymes, transcription factors, and protein kinases). At this stage, mRNA synthesis virtually ceases and does not resume until 1–3 days after the egg has been fertilized, when the final phases of meiosis are completed. One preovulatory follicle is selected every cycle, approximately 350 times during the female reproductive life span.

OVULATION

 The surge of LH induces follicular rupture and ovulation, releasing the oocyte and corona radiata into the peritoneal cavity, close to the opening of the fallopian tubes (Figure 9–6). Follicle rupture is an inflammatory

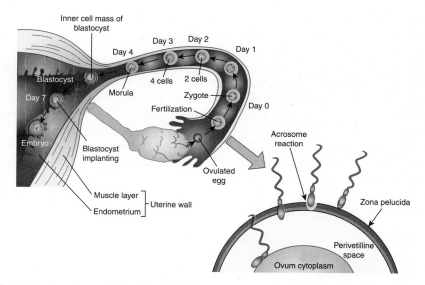

Figure 9–6. Fertilization and embryo migration. Sperm binds to the zona pellucida and undergoes the acrosome reaction, releasing its enzymatic contents, which are necessary for penetration of the zona pellucida. In addition, cortical granules in the ovum release their contents, preventing multiple sperm from fertilizing 1 ovum. Once the sperm penetrates the zona pellucida and begins entry into the perivitelline space, the sperm repositions itself from its original orientation with binding at the tip of the head to binding in an equatorial or sideways position, leading to fusion with the egg plasma membrane and formation of the zygote. This leads to completion of the meiotic division and initiation of mitotic divisions while the zygote is being propelled through the fallopian tubes through both ciliary movements by the epithelium and rhythmic contractions of the smooth muscle walls. The embryo enters the uterine cavity (where implantation occurs) as a blastocyst on day 4 following fertilization.

process that involves cyclooxygenase-2, plasminogen activator, and metalloproteinases. Ciliary movement on the mucous membrane of the fimbria aids movement of the ovum into the fallopian tubes. Throughout the preovulatory stage, the oocyte, granulosa cells, and theca cells acquire specific functional characteristics: The oocyte becomes competent to undergo meiosis; granulosa cells acquire the ability to produce estrogens and respond to LH via the LH receptor; and theca cells begin to synthesize increasing amounts of androgens that serve as substrates for the aromatase enzyme in the granulosa cells.

FORMATION OF THE CORPUS LUTEUM

Following ovulation, the reorganization of the follicle leads to formation of the corpus luteum, composed of small (theca) and large (granulosa) cells, fibroblasts, endothelial cells, and immune cells. Small amounts of bleeding into the antral cavity occurring during ovulation lead to the formation of the corpus hemorrhagicum and the invasion by macrophages and mesenchymal cells, leading to revascularization of the corpus luteum. The corpus luteum, a temporary endocrine gland, continues to produce and secrete progesterone and estradiol, playing a key role in regulating the length of the ovarian cycle, maintaining gestation in its early stages, and suppressing LH and FSH release through the inhibition of GnRH release.

If fertilization occurs, the corpus luteum continues to grow and function for the first 2–3 months of pregnancy. Regression of the corpus luteum is prevented by placental production of hCG during the initial gestational period. hCG stimulates the granulosa-lutein cells to produce progesterone, 17-hydroxyprogesterone, estrogen, inhibin A, and relaxin, a polypeptide hormone from the insulin/IGF hormone family. Relaxin regulates the synthesis and release of metalloproteinases, mediators of tissue (uterus, mammary gland, fetal membranes, birth canal) growth and remodeling, in preparation for birth and lactation. After the first trimester of pregnancy, the corpus luteum slowly regresses as the placenta assumes the role of hormone biosynthesis for the maintenance of pregnancy.

LUTEOLYSIS

Luteolysis is the process of lysis or regression of the corpus luteum if fertilization does not occur within 1–2 days of ovulation. Luteolysis marks the end of the female reproductive cycle and involves an initial decline in progesterone secretion (functional luteolysis), followed by changes in the cellular structure leading to gradual corpus luteum involution (structural or morphologic luteolysis) to form a small scar of connective tissue known as the **corpus albicans**.

ENDOMETRIAL CYCLE

The ovarian cycle is accompanied by cyclic growth and shedding of the endometrium controlled by estrogen and progesterone (see Figure 9–4). Three distinct phases can be identified in the endometrium throughout the menstrual cycle.

Proliferative Phase

The proliferative phase corresponds to the follicular phase of the ovary (see Figure 9–4). It is characterized by estrogen-induced endometrial epithelial cell proliferation and upregulation of estradiol and progesterone receptor expression. The preovulatory endometrial proliferation leads to relative hypertrophy of the uterine mucosa. This is the initial phase of endometrial maturation in preparation for implantation of the embryo.

Secretory Phase

This phase corresponds to the ovarian luteal phase and is characterized by pro-gesterone-induced differentiation of the endometrial epithelial cells into secretory cells. During the secretory phase, there is a short, well-defined period of uterine receptivity for embryo implantation (referred to as the "implantation window").

Menstrual Phase

The menstrual period is characterized by shedding of the endometrium, result-ing from proteolysis and ischemia in its superficial layer. Proteolytic enzymes accumulate in membrane-bound lysosomes during the first half of the postovu-latory period. The integrity of the lysosomal membrane is lost with the decline in estrogen and progesterone on day 25, resulting in lysis of the glandular and stromal cells and the vascular endothelium. Ischemia caused by vasoconstriction of endometrial vessels during the early part of the menstrual period results in rupture of the capillaries, leading to bleeding. In addition, a significant increase in prostaglandin F2α in the late secretory endometrium stimulates release of acid hydrolases from lysosomes and enhances myometrial contractions, aiding in the expulsion of degenerated endometrium.

Fertilization

Fertilization is the union of the 2 germ cells, the ovum and the sperm, restor-ing chromosome number and initiating the development of a new individual. The final steps of mammalian oogenesis (and of spermatogenesis) prepare eggs (and sperm) for fertilization. In preparation for ovulation, fully grown oocytes undergo "meiotic maturation," preparing them to interact with sperm. A very low proportion (approximately 0.002%) of the sperm deposited into the vagina migrates up the female reproductive tract to the ampullary-isthmic junction of the fallopian tubes (see Figure 9–6), the site of fertilization. During this trajec-tory, sperm undergo activation or "capacitation," a series of changes in the sperm plasma membrane that increase its affinity for the zona pellucida, enabling the sperm to bind to the ovum and to undergo the acrosome reaction. In the fallopian tubes, sperm bind to the zona pellucida, leading to fusion of the ovum and sperm plasma membranes to form a single "activated" cell, the zygote (see Figure 9–6). This simple process requires several events.

Sperm acrosome reaction and penetration of the ovum's zona pellucida—
Sperm binding to the zona pellucida primes the sperm cell to initiate the acrosome

reaction. The acrosome reaction involves fusion of the acrosome with the sperm plasma membrane and exocytosis of its enzymatic contents (proteases and glycosidases) required for sperm penetration. During or after the acrosome reaction, the fertilizing sperm penetrates through the zona pellucida and fuses with the ovum plasma membrane. In this process, the sperm initially binds with the tip of its head to the ovum, which is followed by release in binding of the tip of the sperm head and an equatorial (parallel) binding, allowing incorporation of the acrosomal membrane into the ovum cytoplasm and fusion of the 2 cells.

Cortical and zona reaction—Fusion of the sperm and the ovum triggers the second meiotic division of the ovum, leading to the formation of the mature oocyte and the second polar body. In addition, this fusion triggers mechanisms that prevent fertilization of the ovum by multiple sperm, such as exocytosis of cortical granules (cortical reaction) from the oocyte, resulting in proteolysis of zona pellucida glycoproteins, as well as cross-linking of proteins forming the perivitelline barrier. The fusion of the sperm and ovum reconstitutes a diploid cell, called the zygote.

During migration of the zygote through the fallopian tubes toward the site of implantation in the uterine cavity, mitosis yields a morula and then a blastocyst. The outer cells of the blastocyst; the **trophoblast** cells, participate in the implantation process and form the fetal components of the **placenta**.

Implantation

The human embryo (blastocyst) enters the uterus 3 days before implantation. As mentioned earlier, the "window of implantation" corresponds to the short period of endometrial receptivity for the embryo, between days 20 and 24 of the menstrual cycle. Morphologically, this optimal period for implantation is characterized by the presence of columnar epithelium with microvilli and an increase in stromal cell proliferation. Implantation involves cytokine induction of adhesion molecule expression in endometrial cells, followed by invasion requiring enzymatic digestion of the extracellular matrix with simultaneous control of hemostasis and angiogenesis within decidual tissues. These enzymatic processes are mediated by proteinases, metalloproteinases, collagenases, gelatinases, stromelysins, metallolastases, and urokinase. Both the growth of the trophoblast and invasion are required for successful embryo implantation and placental development.

PHYSIOLOGIC EFFECTS OF OVARIAN HORMONES

Estrogen

ESTROGEN SYNTHESIS, TRANSPORT, AND METABOLISM

The primary source of estradiol in women is the granulosa cell of the ovaries. However, as already mentioned, both granulosa and theca cells and both gonadotropins (FSH and LH) are required for the production of estrogen (see Figure 9–3). In premenopausal women, 17β-estradiol produced by the ovaries is the chief circulating estrogen. Serum estradiol concentrations are low in preadolescent girls and increase at menarche. In the adult woman, they fluctuate from approximately 100 pg/mL in the follicular phase to approximately 600 pg/mL at the time of ovulation. The highest rates of production and serum concentrations are seen in the preovulatory phase and the lowest during the premenstrual phase (see Figure 9–4). Estradiol levels increase significantly during pregnancy. After menopause, serum estradiol concentrations decrease to values similar to or lower than those in men of a similar age.

Most of the estradiol released into the blood circulates bound to sex hormone-binding globulin and to albumin, with only 2%–3% circulating in the free form. Estradiol (as well as androstenedione) is converted to estrone (a weak estrogen) in peripheral tissues (Figure 9–7). Estrone is converted to estriol, primarily in the liver. Estrogens are metabolized by sulfation or glucuronidation, and the conjugates are excreted into the urine. Estrogen can also be metabolized through hydroxylation and subsequent methylation to form catechol- and methoxy-estrogens.

ESTROGEN RECEPTOR-MEDIATED (GENOMIC) EFFECTS

The estrogen receptors are members of the superfamily of steroid hormone receptors that function as transcription factors, altering gene expression on activation (see Figure 9–7). Two subtypes of estrogen receptors have been identified. They differ in structure, are encoded by different genes, and differ in tissue distribution. Estrogen receptor alpha (α) is considered the classic estrogen receptor. It is found predominantly in endometrium, breast cancer cells, and ovarian stroma. Estrogen receptor beta (β) is found predominantly in granulosa cells and in several nonreproductive target tissues, including the kidney, intestinal mucosa, lung parenchyma, bone marrow, bone, brain, endothelial cells, and prostate gland.

Estrogen receptors are mostly nuclear, but are also found in the cytoplasm. The process of hormone-receptor binding and translocating to the nucleus is similar to that used by adrenal steroid hormones testosterone.

PHYSIOLOGIC ACTIONS OF ESTROGEN AT TARGET ORGANS

Reproductive System
Estrogen exerts multiple effects in reproductive organs (Figure 9–8).

Uterus—Estrogen promotes endometrial proliferation, sensitizes uterine smooth muscle to the effects of oxytocin by increasing the expression of oxytocin receptors and contractile proteins, and increases watery cervical mucus production.

Ovary—Estrogen exerts potent mitotic effects on granulosa cells.

Breast—Estrogen stimulates growth and differentiation of the ductal epithelium, induces mitotic activity of ductal cylindric cells, and stimulates the growth of connective tissue. The density of estrogen receptors in breast tissue is highest in the follicular phase of the menstrual cycle and falls after ovulation. Estrogen can also indirectly affect mammary gland development by elevating prolactin and progesterone levels and inducing progesterone receptors in mammary epithelium. The growth-promoting effects of estrogen have been implicated in breast and endometrial cancer.

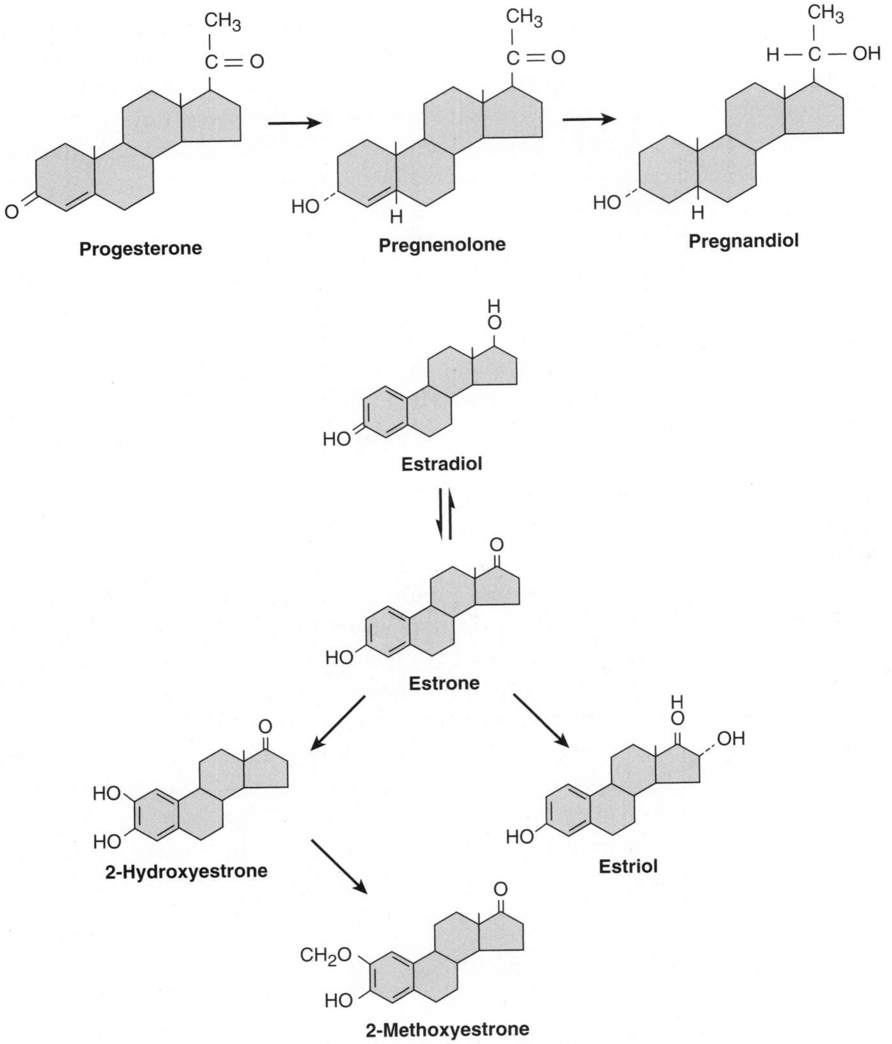

Figure 9–7. Metabolic fate of progesterone and estrogen. Progesterone and estrogen are degraded primarily in the liver. Estradiol and androstenedione are converted to estrone (a weak estrogen) in peripheral tissues. Estrone is converted to estriol, primarily in the liver. Estrogens are metabolized by sulfation or glucuronidation, and the conjugates are excreted into the urine. Estrogen can also be metabolized through hydroxylation and subsequent methylation to form catechol- and methoxyestrogens (not shown).

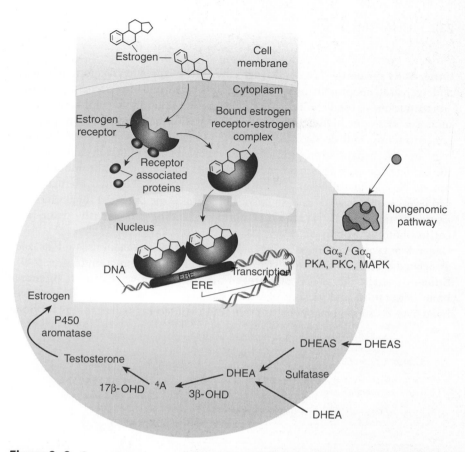

Figure 9–8. Genomic and nongenomic effects of estrogen. 17β-estradiol (E₂) diffuses into the cell and binds to either estrogen receptor (ER)α or ERβ, forming homo- or heterodimers. Binding involves dissociation of the receptor from chaperone proteins and translocation into the nucleus, where the hormone-receptor complex binds to estrogen responsive elements and modulates gene transcription (genomic effects). Recently, it has been shown that estrogen can produce rapid effects that do not require gene transcription. These nongenomic mechanisms involve activation of an estrogen receptor localized in the plasma membrane and linked to second-messenger systems, producing immediate responses as well as converging with the genomic pathway. The figure also illustrates intracrine extragonadal estrogen synthesis, prevalent during menopause. Estradiol is derived from testosterone, from androstenedione (Δ⁴A), and from dehydroepiandrosterone (DHEA) or dehydroepiandrosterone sulfate (DHEAS). The desulfated DHEA is converted to Δ⁴A by 3β-hydroxysteroid dehydrogenase (3β-OHD), and the Δ⁴A is transformed into testosterone by 17β-hydroxysteroid dehydrogenase (17β-OHD). Testosterone can then be converted into either estradiol or androstenedione, which in turn can be converted to estrone and then to estradiol by the type I isoenzyme. Some of the family of 17β-hydroxysteroid dehydrogenase isoenzymes (eg, type II isoenzyme) can convert estradiol to estrone, providing an additional mechanism for the regulation of estrogen synthesis and metabolism. ERE, estrogen response element; MAPK, mitogen-activated protein kinase; PKA, protein kinase A; PKC, protein kinase C. (Modified, with permission, from Gruber CJ, Tschugguel W, Schneeberger C, Huber JC. Mechanisms of disease: production and actions of estrogens. *N Engl J Med.* 2002;346:340. Copyright © Massachusetts Medical Society. All rights reserved.)

Other body systems—Liver—Estrogen affects the expression of apoprotein genes and increases lipoprotein receptor expression, resulting in a decrease in serum concentrations of total cholesterol and low-density lipoprotein (LDL) cholesterol, increases in serum high-density lipoprotein (HDL) cholesterol and triglyceride concentrations, and decreases in serum lipoprotein A concentrations. Estrogen regulates the hepatic expression of genes involved in coagulation and fibrinolysis. Estrogen decreases plasma concentrations of fibrinogen, antithrombin III and protein S, and plasminogen activator inhibitor type 1. Elevated plasma estrogen levels are associated with an overall increase in the potential for fibrinolysis. Estrogen stimulates the synthesis of hormone-binding proteins (thyroxine- and cortisol-binding globulins).

Central nervous system—Estrogen has neuroprotective actions, and its age-associated decline is associated with a decline in cognitive function (Figure 9–9). **Bone**—Overall, the effects of estrogen are antiresorptive. Estrogen promotes bone maturation and closure of epiphysial plates in long bones. It conserves bone mass by suppressing bone turnover and maintaining balanced rates of bone

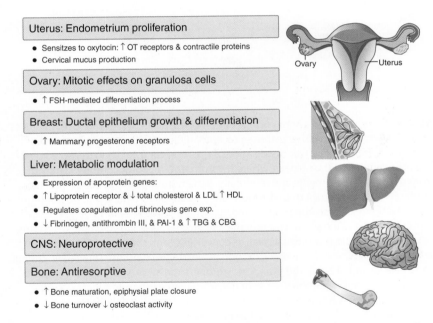

Uterus: Endometrium proliferation
- Sensitzes to oxytocin: ↑ OT receptors & contractile proteins
- Cervical mucus production

Ovary: Mitotic effects on granulosa cells
- ↑ FSH-mediated differentiation process

Breast: Ductal epithelium growth & differentiation
- ↑ Mammary progesterone receptors

Liver: Metabolic modulation
- Expression of apoprotein genes:
- ↑ Lipoprotein receptor & ↓ total cholesterol & LDL ↑ HDL
- Regulates coagulation and fibrinolysis gene exp.
- ↓ Fibrinogen, antithrombin III, & PAI-1 & ↑ TBG & CBG

CNS: Neuroprotective

Bone: Antiresorptive
- ↑ Bone maturation, epiphysial plate closure
- ↓ Bone turnover ↓ osteoclast activity

Ovary   Uterus

Figure 9–9. Systemic effects of estrogen. In addition to its reproductive organ effects, estrogen has neuroprotective effects and reduces perimenopausal mood fluctuations in women. Estrogen is cardioprotective and may protect against colon cancer, and it has vasodilatory effects. In the liver, estrogen stimulates the uptake of serum lipoproteins and the production of coagulation factors. Estrogen protects against bone loss. In the skin, it increases skin turgor and collagen production and reduces the depth of wrinkles. CBG, cortisol-binding globulin; FSH, follicle-stimulating hormone; HDL, high-density lipoprotein; LDL, low-density lipoprotein; OT, oxytocin; PAI-1, plasminogen activator inhibitor-1; TBG, testosterone-binding globulin.

formation and bone resorption. Estrogen affects the generation, life span, and functional activity of both osteoclasts and osteoblasts. It promotes synthesis of osteoprotegerin, decreases osteoclast formation and activity, and increases osteoclast apoptosis.

NONGENOMIC EFFECTS OF ESTROGEN

Some rapid effects of estrogen cannot be explained by a transcriptional mechanism (nongenomic) and are the result of direct estrogenic action on cell membranes mediated by cell membrane forms of estrogen receptor (see Figure 9–7). Although these receptors remain largely uncharacterized, they are thought to resemble their intracellular counterparts. Examples of some of the rapid nongenomic effects of estrogen include direct effects on the vasculature and activation of growth factor–related signaling pathways. Estrogen can cause short-term vasodilatation by both endothelium-dependent and endothelium-independent pathways. Estrogen produces short-term vasodilatation and reduces vascular smooth muscle tone through the increased formation and release of endothelial nitric oxide and prostacyclin and the opening of calcium channels mediated by cyclic guanosine monophosphate. Estrogen inhibits apoptosis of endothelial cells and promotes their angiogenic activity in vitro and may protect against atherosclerosis. At pharmacologic concentrations, estrogen inhibits the influx of extracellular calcium into vascular smooth muscle cells by an effect on L-type calcium channels.

 Estrogen promotes rapid activation of growth factor–related signaling pathways through mitogen-activated protein kinase signaling cascades in several tissues, including osteoblasts, endothelial cells, neurons, and human breast cancer cells.

Progesterone

Progesterone is the predominant ovarian hormone produced in the luteal phase. It is produced by both theca and granulosa cells of the corpus luteum in response to LH stimulation. The majority of progesterone secreted circulates bound to albumin. The principal targets of progesterone are the reproductive tract and the hypothalamic-pituitary axis. The degradation of progesterone is similar to that of androgens and estrogens and occurs primarily in the liver.

PROGESTERONE RECEPTOR-MEDIATED EFFECTS

Progesterone exerts most of its effects by directly regulating gene transcription through 2 specific progesterone receptor proteins, termed *A* and *B*, located in target tissues such as the breast, uterus, brain, central nervous, and cardiovascular systems. These progesterone receptor proteins arise from a single gene and act as ligand-inducible transcription factors, regulating the expression of genes by binding specific progesterone responsive elements on the DNA (as described for estrogen and adrenal steroid hormones). The expression of progesterone receptors is upregulated by estrogen and downregulated by progesterone in most target tissues. Thus, progesterone receptor expression in the uterus is increased during the first half of the menstrual cycle and decreased during the luteal phase.

In general, progesterone acts on the reproductive tract to prepare it for initiation and maintenance of pregnancy. The major physiologic roles of progesterone are mediated in the uterus and ovary, where it stimulates the release of mature oocytes, facilitates implantation, and maintains pregnancy through stimulation of uterine growth and differentiation and suppression of myometrial contractility. In the brain, progesterone modulates sexual behavior and regulates body temperature. Increased progesterone levels during the luteal phase increase both core and skin temperatures. This results in a biphasic pattern of body core temperature throughout the menstrual cycle, with a higher temperature in the luteal phase of the cycle.

Physiologic Actions of Progesterone at Target Organs

 Effects on the uterus during early pregnancy—Progesterone induces stromal differentiation; stimulates glandular secretions, and modulates cyclic proliferation during the menstrual cycle.

Progesterone induces uterine cell proliferation and differentiation in early pregnancy producing an environment that supports early embryonic development.

Promotion and maintenance of implantation—Progesterone plays a major role in preparing the endometrium for implantation of a fertilized ovum, stimulates the synthesis of enzymes responsible for lysis of the zona pellucida.

Effects on uterine contractility—Progesterone induces quiescence of the myometrium (Figure 9–10). Several mechanisms are involved including: increasing resting membrane potential and preventing electrical coupling between myometrial cells; decreasing extracellular calcium influx required for contraction by downregulating gene expression of subunits of voltage-dependent calcium channels; blocking the ability of estradiol to induce membrane expression of α-adrenergic receptors (α-adrenergic activation causes contractions); decreasing prostaglandin synthesis; increasing prostaglandin inactivation; and opposing the stimulatory effects of estrogen on endometrial prostaglandin F2α expression. Progesterone maintains the levels of relaxin, inhibiting spontaneous or prostaglandin-induced myometrial contraction, and contributes to the maintenance of implantation and early pregnancy by increasing the collagen framework and distensibility of the uterus.

At the end of pregnancy, the decrease in progesterone levels is associated with increased prostaglandin synthase activity and prostaglandin F2α production, enhancing uterine contractility. The antiprogestin mifepristone antagonizes all of the actions of progesterone on prostaglandin synthesis and catabolism and stimulates prostaglandin production, thereby producing its abortive effects.

Effects on lactation—In the mammary gland, progesterone stimulates lobular-alveolar development in preparation for milk secretion. Progesterone antagonizes prolactin's effects in mid- to late pregnancy, preventing milk protein synthesis before parturition. The sudden fall in circulating progesterone that occurs with parturition is associated with a concurrent increase in prolactin secretion and the onset of lactation.

Antiestrogen actions—Progesterone antagonizes estrogen induction of many of the known hormone-responsive genes. This effect is mediated by downregulation

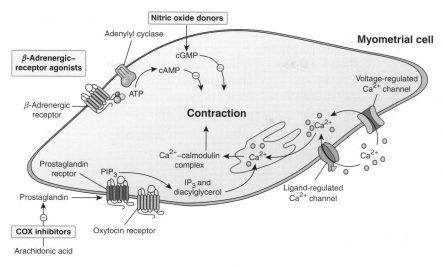

Figure 9–10. Factors that affect uterine contractility. Smooth muscle contraction is mediated through Ca⁺⁺-calmodulin activation of myosin light chain kinase, the enzyme that phosphorylates myosin light chain. Uterine contraction is stimulated by prostaglandin F (PGF) and oxytocin (OT). Uterine contraction is decreased by several agents including β-adrenergic agonists, NO, relaxin and PGI₂ The mechanism involves an increase in either cAMP or cyclic GMP. Indomethacin inhibits prostaglandin synthesis from arachidonic acid. β-adrenergic agonists, relaxin, and PGI₂ increase intracellular cAMP. cAMP, activates PKA, which then phosphorylates MLCK to reduce its ability to bind Ca-CAM or phosphorylates a membrane-binding site for Ca²⁺ that increases Ca⁺⁺ binding and reduces free intracellular Ca⁺⁺ concentrations. ATP, adenosine triphosphate; cAMP, cyclic adenosine monophosphate; cGMP, cyclic guanosine monophosphate; COX, cyclooxygenase; IP₃, inositol 1,4,5-trisphosphate; PIP₃, phosphatidylinositol trisphosphate; Ca-CAM, calcium-calmodulin.

of cytoplasmic and nuclear estrogen receptor protein concentrations, decreasing the active estrogen concentration (and antagonizing the action of estrogen receptor at the molecular level), particularly in the uterus.

The Placenta

STRUCTURE AND PHYSIOLOGIC FUNCTION

The placenta is derived from 2 major cell types, which are the source of the principal placental hormones. The outer cell mass of the blastocyst, the precursor to the trophoblast, is in contact with the endometrium and undergoes proliferation and tissue penetration during implantation. The trophoblast has 2 cell populations: an inner cytotrophoblast and an outer invasive syncytiotrophoblast. The maternal side of the placenta contains fetal chorionic villi that provide an extensive surface area for nutrient and gas exchange between the fetal and maternal circulation. The villi are covered with multinucleated syncytiotrophoblast and trophoblast stem cells, stromal cells, and blood vessels. The villous cytotrophoblast cells are entirely secluded from maternal elements, with the exception of any molecules that might be transported across the placenta by the syncytiotrophoblast. By contrast, the extravillous trophoblast cells are continuously exposed to maternal tissues. The middle layer of the placenta consists of densely packed cytotrophoblast cell columns and serves as structural support for the underlying villi.

The physiologic functions of the placenta can be classified as follows:

- Supportive, allowing embryo implantation into the uterus and transporting nutrients and oxygen necessary for fetal growth
- Immune, suppressing the local immune system to prevent immunologic rejection of the fetus by the mother
- Endocrine, including hormone synthesis, transport, and metabolism to promote fetal growth and survival

Inability of the placental unit to perform these functions leads to multiple complications of human pregnancy, including abortion, miscarriage, impaired fetal growth, and preeclampsia.

Endocrine Function of the Placenta

The placenta produces cytokines, hormones, and growth factors that are essential for regulation of the feto-maternal unit. In addition, the placenta expresses enzymes involved in hormone metabolism, playing an important role in protection of the fetus from maternal adrenal-derived androgens through aromatase activity and from glucocorticoids through the activity of 11β-hydroxysteroid dehydrogenase type II (see Chapter 6). The principal placental hormones are as follows.

Human chorionic gonadotropin (hCG)—hCG is a heterodimeric glycoprotein from the same hormone family as LH, FSH, and TSH. It is produced by the syncytiotrophoblast and released into the fetal and maternal circulation. It is known as the hormone of pregnancy and is the basis for the pregnancy test. hCG is detected in serum at day 6–8 after implantation, and its levels peak at 60–90 days of gestation, declining thereafter. hCG has structural and functional similarity to LH, and exerts its physiologic effects through binding to the LH receptors. The main function of hCG is to maintain the corpus luteum to ensure the production of progesterone until placental production takes over. In addition, hCG plays an important role in fetal development through the regulation of testosterone production by the fetal Leydig cells (see Chapter 8). Regulation of hCG release from the placenta is not completely understood, but evidence indicates that its paracrine regulation involves placenta-derived GnRH, activin, and inhibin. Maternal hCG levels are a useful index of functional status of the trophoblast (placental health).

Human placental lactogen and growth hormone—The human growth hormone (hGH) and human placental lactogen (hPL) gene family is important in the regulation of maternal and fetal metabolism and the growth and development of the fetus. hPL is produced by the syncytiotrophoblast and is secreted into both the maternal and fetal circulations after the sixth week of pregnancy. In the fetus, hPL modulates embryonic development; regulates intermediary metabolism; and stimulates the production of IGFs, insulin, adrenocortical hormones, and pulmonary surfactant. During pregnancy, hGH-V, a growth hormone (GH) variant expressed by the placenta, becomes the predominant GH in the mother. This hormone has structural and functional similarity to pituitary GH (it differs by 13 amino acids) and is not released into the fetus. Starting from the 15th to the 20th week of gestation up to term of pregnancy, placental GH gradually replaces maternal pituitary GH, which becomes undetectable. hGH-V stimulates IGF-1 production and modulates maternal intermediary metabolism, increasing the availability of glucose and amino acids to the fetus. Placental GH is not detectable in the fetal circulation, and thus it does not appear to have a direct effect on fetal growth. However, its physiologic role is thought to involve modulation of placental development through an autocrine or paracrine mechanism because of GH receptor expression by the placenta.

Progesterone—The major source of progesterone during the initial phase of pregnancy is the corpus luteum, which is under hCG regulation. Starting from about week 8 of gestation, the placenta (syncytiotrophoblast) becomes the principal source of progesterone, leading to increasing levels of maternal progesterone from 25 ng/mL during the luteal phase to 150 ng/mL during the last trimester of pregnancy. Because the placenta is unable to produce cholesterol from acetate, cholesterol for placental progesterone synthesis is derived from circulating LDL. LDL binds to the LDL receptor in trophoblast cells and undergoes endocytosis; cholesterol is released and processed through the steroidogenic hormone pathway (see Chapter 6). As discussed earlier, progesterone plays an important role in maintaining uterine quiescence during pregnancy, inhibiting prostaglandin synthesis and modulating the immune response to preserve pregnancy.

Estrogen—The main source of estrogen during the initial phase of pregnancy is the corpus luteum, being replaced later by placental production. The principal estrogen produced by the syncytiotrophoblast cells of the placenta is estriol. The production of estrogen by the placenta requires coordinated interaction between fetal and maternal adrenal gland steroid hormone production (feto-placental unit of steroid biosynthesis). The placenta lacks 17α-hydroxylase and 17, 20-desmolase and is thus unable to convert progesterone to estrogen or to produce androgens. This lack of placental androgen production protects the female fetus from masculinization; protection is also aided by the strong aromatase activity that inactivates maternal and fetal adrenal-derived androgens. Therefore, maternal and fetal adrenal-derived androgens (dehydroepiandrosterone sulfate [DHEAS]) are required for 17β-estradiol and estriol production. Estriol is synthesized through the aromatization of 16α-hydroxyandrostenedione derived from 16α-hydroxyepiandrosterone sulfate produced by the fetal liver and desulfated in the placenta (Figure 9–11); 16α-hydroxyepiandrosterone sulfate is derived from DHEAS produced in the fetal adrenal gland. The enzymes involved are placental sulfatase (DHEAS deconjugation), 3β-hydroxysteroid dehydrogenase (pregnenolone to progesterone conversion), and aromatase. Plasma and urinary levels of estriol increase significantly

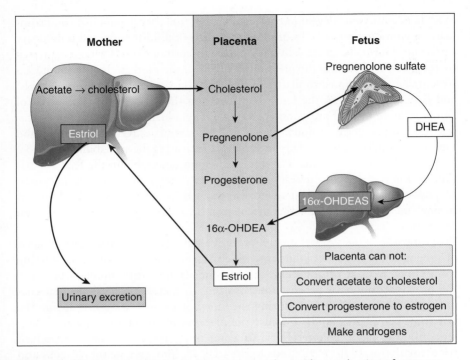

Figure 9–11. Feto-placental unit of hormone synthesis. The production of estrogen by the placenta requires the coordinated interaction between fetal and maternal adrenal gland steroid hormone production. The placenta lacks 17α-hydroxylase and is thus unable to convert progesterone to estrogen or to produce androgens. Fetal adrenal-derived androgens (dehydroepiandrosterone sulfate [DHEAS]) are required for 17β-estradiol and estrone production. Estriol is synthesized through the aromatization of 16α-hydroxyandrostenedione derived from 16α-hydroxyepiandrosterone sulfate (16α-OHDEAS) produced by the fetal liver and desulfated in the placenta; 16α–hydroxyepiandrosterone sulfate in turn is derived from DHEAS produced in the fetal adrenal gland. 16α-OHDEA, 16α-hydroxyepiandrosterone; DHEA, dehydroepiandrosterone; LDL, low-density lipoprotein.

throughout pregnancy. The principal physiologic effects of estrogen during pregnancy include stimulation of uterine growth, prostaglandin synthesis, thickening of the vaginal epithelium, sensitization to oxytocin effects, and growth and development of the mammary epithelium.

Corticotropin-releasing hormone—Corticotropin-releasing hormone (CRH) is produced by the syncytiotrophoblast and trophoblast cells of the placenta. Its structure and function are similar to those of hypothalamus-derived CRH. The CRH concentration increases exponentially throughout pregnancy and peaks during labor. Placental production of CRH has been linked to the length of gestation in humans. CRH is secreted into the maternal circulation in large amounts during the third trimester of pregnancy and may play an important role in the onset of labor. CRH exerts a number of functions within the intrauterine environment, such as induction of prostaglandin production and maintenance of placental blood flow.

Pregnancy and Lactation

HORMONAL CONTROL OF PARTURITION

Uterine contractility during pregnancy and parturition can be divided into at least 4 distinct phases.

Phase 0—During pregnancy, the uterus is maintained in a relatively quiescent state, mainly through the effects of progesterone. Additional factors involved in modulation of uterine activity during this period are prostacyclin, relaxin, parathyroid hormone-related peptide, and CRH. In general, their effects are the result of increased intracellular concentrations of cAMP or cyclic guanosine monophosphate and inhibition of intracellular calcium release, resulting in decreased myosin light chain kinase activity. The initiation of parturition results from the transition from the quiescent phase (phase 0) to a phase of activation (phase 1).

Phase 1—This phase of parturition is associated with activation of uterine function and is characterized by release from the inhibitory mechanisms maintaining uterine quiescence throughout pregnancy and activation of factors promoting uterine activity. These factors include uterine stretch and tension caused by the fully grown fetus, activation of the fetal hypothalamic-pituitary-adrenal axis, and increased prostaglandin synthesis. Mechanical stretch or hormonal priming leads to upregulation of gene expression of proteins that facilitate smooth muscle contraction, including connexins (key components of gap junctions), prostaglandin and oxytocin receptors, and ion channel proteins.

Phase 2—This phase of parturition is a period of active uterine contraction and is stimulated by prostaglandins, oxytocin, and CRH. Prostaglandins, particularly those produced in the intrauterine tissues, play a central role in the initiation and progression of labor. They induce myometrial contractility and help produce the changes associated with cervical softening at the onset of labor.

Phase 3—This postpartum phase involves uterine involution after delivery of the fetus and placenta and is mainly caused by the effects of oxytocin.

MAMMARY GLAND DEVELOPMENT

Mammary gland development represents a complex program of cell proliferation, cell differentiation, and morphogenesis. Most mammary gland development occurs during the postnatal period and involves branching and extension of ductal growth points and secretory lobules into a fatty stroma. Ductal development in the mammary gland supports the establishment of alveolar structures during pregnancy before the onset of lactogenesis and is regulated by the associated alterations in key hormones and growth factors during the various reproductive states (Figure 9–12).

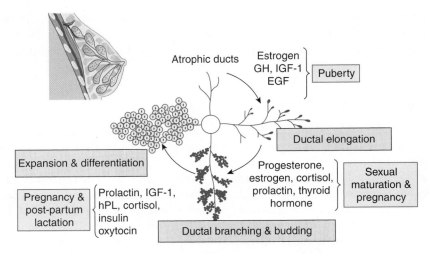

Figure 9–12. Hormonal regulation of breast development and lactogenesis. Mammary gland development is initiated at puberty through the action of estradiol and growth factors and is further regulated during pregnancy through the effects of prolactin and human placental lactogen (hPL). Throughout pregnancy, progesterone inhibits lactogenesis. This inhibitory effect is removed following parturition, when prolactin levels act unopposed to stimulate lactogenesis. Suckling, through neuroendocrine reflexes stimulates the release of oxytocin from the posterior pituitary, producing the milk "let-down" reflex. Ductal elongation is mediated by estrogen, growth hormone (GH), insulin-like growth factor 1 (IGF-1), and epidermal growth factor (EGF). Ductal branching and alveolar budding are regulated by progesterone, prolactin, and thyroid hormone. Progesterone stimulates ductal side branching and alveolar development. Prolactin acts directly on mammary epithelium to induce alveolar development. Both progesterone and prolactin synergize to stimulate proliferation of ductal epithelium

Ductal elongation is mediated by estrogen, GH, IGF-1, and epidermal growth factor. At the onset of puberty, estrogen production stimulates the developmental process from the immature breast consisting of a nipple, a few small ductal elements, and an underlying fat pad. The terminal end bud directs ductal growth, elongation, and branching into the fat pad.

Ductal branching and alveolar budding are influenced by progesterone, prolactin, and thyroid hormone. Progesterone stimulates ductal side branching and alveolar development. Prolactin acts directly on mammary epithelium to induce alveolar development. Both progesterone and prolactin synergize to stimulate proliferation of ductal epithelium. In the postpubertal female, during the luteal phase, progesterone stimulates the sprouting of alveolar structures from the sides of the ducts. During pregnancy, prolactin, progesterone, and hPL levels increase, and the terminal duct lobular units undergo expansion and differentiation of the secretory function.

The stage of mammary differentiation into a secretory function in preparation for lactogenesis is called *stage I lactogenesis*. During pregnancy, progesterone, estrogen, prolactin, hPL, and GH act synergistically to prepare the breast for lactation by promoting lobuloalveolar development. The elevated levels of progesterone prevent milk production during this period. With the progression of pregnancy, the circulating levels of prolactin continue to increase. During the third trimester, prolactin levels increase more than 10-fold. The increase in prolactin levels is the result of estrogen-induced increase in lactotrophs and prolactin synthesis in the anterior pituitary during gestation.

The second stage (stage II lactogenesis) is initiated after termination of pregnancy. The sudden decrease in circulating progesterone that accompanies parturition, in association with the concurrent increase in prolactin secretion mark the onset of lactation. The removal of the inhibition of synthesis of α-lactalbumin, and β-casein by the decrease in progesterone action allow prolactin, insulin, and glucocorticoids to stimulate the synthesis of the milk proteins. Continuous milk production is maintained by prolactin secretion from the anterior pituitary (see Chapter 3) throughout the period of lactation. Prolactin is the main regulator of milk protein synthesis; a process that requires the presence of glucocorticoids and insulin. Pharmacologic analogs of dopamine such as bromocriptine inhibit lactogenesis through the inhibition of prolactin release. Weaning, or cessation of the lactation period, is followed by involution of the terminal duct lobular units mediated by alveolar cell apoptosis and gland remodeling, returning the breast to its mature quiescent state.

HORMONAL CONTROL OF MILK SECRETION AND EJECTION

The onset of adequate milk production during the postpartum period requires developed mammary epithelium, persistent elevation in plasma prolactin (approximately 200 ng/mL), and a decrease in circulating levels of progesterone. Milk secretion from the mammary glands is triggered by stimulation of tactile receptors in the nipples by sucking (see Chapter 2). Oxytocin produces contraction of the myoepithelial cells of the lactiferous ducts, sinuses, and breast tissue alveoli. The immediate process (30 seconds to 1 minute) of milk flow in response to sucking is called the *milk let-down reflex*, and persists throughout the lactation period. Milk production increases during the first 36 hours postpartum from a volume of less than 100 mL/d to an average of 500 mL/d at approximately day 4 postpartum. The composition of breast milk changes considerably during this period as well.

AGE-RELATED CHANGES IN THE FEMALE REPRODUCTIVE SYSTEM

Puberty

Female puberty is initiated by low-amplitude nocturnal pulses of gonadotropin release, which increase serum estradiol concentrations. The increased synthesis and secretion of estrogen by the ovary cause the progressive skeletal maturation that eventually leads to epiphysial fusion and the termination of linear growth. The onset of puberty causes a rapid increase in bone mass that correlates with bone age. The initial stage of puberty (at age 8–13 years) in girls involves breast development, accompanied by ovarian and follicular growth. This is followed by androgen- plus estrogen-induced pubic and axillary hair growth and the onset of menses (approximately at age 13 years), indicating sufficient estrogen production to stimulate endometrial proliferation. The first cycles are usually anovulatory, becoming fully ovulatory after 2–3 years. In girls, leptin serum concentrations increase dramatically as pubertal development progresses, and this increase in leptin levels parallels the increase in body fat mass. As mentioned in Chapter 8, leptin is considered to play a permissive role in the initiation of puberty.

Menopause

Menopause is the permanent cessation of menstruation resulting from loss of ovarian follicular activity. Menopause is preceded by a perimenopausal period, starting when the first features of impending menopause begin (ie, irregular menstrual bleeding and cycle frequency) and lasting until at least 1 year after the final menstrual period. During the menopausal transition, gonadotropins, estradiol, and inhibin show a marked degree of variability in their circulating levels. Within 1–2 years after the final menstrual period or the onset of menopause, FSH levels are markedly elevated, LH levels are moderately high, and estradiol and inhibin levels are low or undetectable. The resultant ovarian changes include short follicular phases with early ovulation and luteal insufficiency characterized by lower levels of progesterone secreted for shorter periods of time compared with the luteal phase of younger women. Postmenopausally, adrenal androstenedione is the major source of estrogen, and serum testosterone levels decrease moderately.

Starting from age 36 years, ovarian follicular apoptosis accelerates, leading to a steady decline in ovarian estradiol production (Figure 9–13). This loss of ovarian function results in a 90% loss of circulating estradiol; serum estradiol concentrations are often lower than 20 pg/mL. However, extragonadal estrogen synthesis increases as a function of age and body weight, and most of the estradiol is formed by extragonadal conversion of testosterone. The predominant estrogen in menopausal women is the weak estrogen estrone, produced through aromatase conversion of androstenedione.

The decline in ovarian function associated with the perimenopausal period is also responsible for an early decline in the release of inhibin B (inhibitor of FSH secretion), leading to an increase in follicular phase FSH. The decrease in serum inhibin B is believed to reflect the age-related decrease in ovarian follicle reserve, which is the primary source of serum inhibin B. The later increase in serum LH during the menopausal transition is caused by the cessation of ovarian follicle development. Despite a 30% decrease in GnRH pulse frequency with aging, there is an increase in the overall amount of GnRH secreted. FSH levels gradually increase with age in women who continue to cycle regularly. The consequences of loss of ovarian function during reproductive life may be severe. Symptoms include hot flashes, night sweats, vaginal dryness and dyspareunia

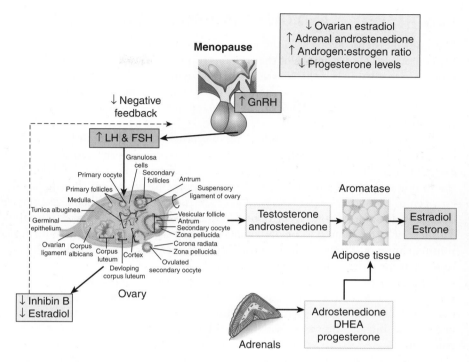

Figure 9–13. Changes in gonadotropin and ovarian hormone production associated with aging. Lower levels of inhibin B and estradiol result in impaired negative feedback regulation of gonadotropin release, increasing follicle-stimulating hormone (FSH) and luteinizing hormone (LH). Production of androstenedione and testosterone during early menopause continues, with some conversion to estradiol by aromatase activity in adipose tissue. Adrenal-derived androstenedione is converted to estrone, principally in adipose tissue. DHEA, dehydroepiandrosterone; GnRH, gonadotropin-releasing hormone.

(painful intercourse), loss of libido, loss of bone mass with subsequent osteoporosis, and abnormalities of cardiovascular function, including a substantial increase in the risk of ischemic heart disease. As already mentioned, estrogens (like androgens) have general metabolic roles that are not directly involved in reproductive processes. These include actions on vascular function, lipid and carbohydrate metabolism, bone, and brain. Within these sites, aromatase action can generate high levels of estradiol locally without significantly affecting circulating levels. Circulating C_{19} steroid precursors are essential substrates for extragonadal estrogen synthesis. The levels of these androgenic precursors decline markedly with advancing age in women. This is thought to contribute to the greater risk of bone mineral loss and fracture, and possibly the decline in cognitive function, in women as compared with men.

CONTRACEPTION AND THE FEMALE REPRODUCTIVE TRACT

The multiple steps involved in the regulation of ovarian hormone production, the consequent modifications of the endometrium, and the regulation of uterine motility are all under tight control, ensuring ovulation, fertilization, implantation, and maintenance of pregnancy. Multiple approaches have been implemented for contraception. Some of the principal interventions are summarized in Table 9–2.

Combined oral contraceptive pills contain synthetic estrogen (ethinyl estradiol or mestranol) together with one of several synthetic progestogens and produce a range of effects on the female reproductive tract. Their main mode of action is the inhibition of ovulation; both estrogen and progestogen inhibit the ability of estrogen to produce a preovulatory surge of LH. The degree of follicular activity occurring during oral contraceptive use depends on the type and dose of steroid. The dose of estrogen used in modern contraceptive preparations is likely to be the minimal amount (20 µg ethinyl estradiol) that will reliably suppress FSH enough to prevent the growth of an ovulatory follicle.

Natural methods, such as the rhythm method, are based on the identification of a period for intercourse with less likelihood of fertilization that relies on knowledge of the life span of an ovum (24 hours) and of sperm (3 days) and of the interval between ovulation and menstruation, which is generally constant (14 days). The time of ovulation is determined by charting basal core

Table 9–2. Principal contraceptive methods

Method	Mechanism involved
Steroid contraceptives	Combination estrogen-progestin: constant concentrations over a 21-day period followed by 7 days rest Phasic estrogen-progestin: varying concentrations throughout the 21-day period and 7 days of placebo Progestin only: constant progesterone dose daily
Intrauterine devices	Prevent blastocyst implantation by altering the endometrial lining Some release progesterone, modifying the endometrial lining
Barrier methods: condoms, foam, and diaphragms	Prevent fertilization by either interfering with the access of sperm to the uterine cavity or destroying sperm in the vaginal cavity
Sterilization	Surgically disrupts the continuity of the fallopian tubes, impairing access of the fertilized ovum to the uterine cavity and implantation
Abortive	Antiprogestin mifepristone produces an increase in prostaglandin F2α synthesis, leading to expulsion of the embryo
Rhythm	Relies on changes in mucus thickness and body temperature throughout the menstrual cycle, indicating a "safe" period for intercourse

temperature or using sensors for urinary LH levels throughout the cycle. The likelihood of conception is greatest during the follicular or preovulatory phase, during ovulation, and during the immediate postovulatory phase. Thus, for a typical 28- to 30-day cycle, the abstinence period would fall at about days 10–19 of the menstrual cycle.

DISEASES OF OVERPRODUCTION AND UNDERSECRETION OF OVARIAN HORMONES

Alterations in female reproductive endocrine function are of multiple etiologies and produce manifestations that range from precocious puberty to infertility, depending on the age at presentation. The most frequent are abnormalities in the menstrual cycle, consisting of either absent menstruation (amenorrhea) or excess bleeding (metrorrhagia), and infertility. Abnormalities of ovarian development and function are usually caused by gonadal dysgenesis and rarely by defects in the synthesis of ovarian steroids. In general, increased ovarian hormone production can be caused by increased gonadotropin release (hypergonadotropic hypergonadism) related to tumors, brain inflammatory diseases, and head injury, among other causes, or it can result from excess hormone production by ovarian tumors. Hypogonadotropic hypergonadism may be caused by congenital adrenal hyperplasia, activating mutations of the α-subunit of the G_s protein, and excess aromatase (the last enzymatic step in estrogen synthesis) activity. Decreased ovarian hormone production can be genetic (eg, FSH and LH receptor gene mutations, mutation of the β-subunit of FSH, enzymatic deficiencies) or acquired (eg, radiation) despite adequate gonadotropin release (hypergonadotropic hypogonadism). Decreased ovarian hormone production caused by impaired gonadotropin release (hypogonadotropic hypogonadism) is rare and may result from GnRH receptor gene mutations, lesions in the hypothalamic area, and other causes.

KEY CONCEPTS

1. *Gonadotropin release is under negative and positive feedback regulation by ovarian steroid and peptide hormones.*

2. *Estrogen synthesis requires LH and FSH regulation of coordinated metabolism by granulosa and theca cells of the ovarian follicle.*

3. *FSH stimulates estrogen synthesis and ovarian follicle growth and maturation.*

LH stimulates ovulation and corpus luteum progesterone and estrogen synthesis.

 The corpus luteum is a temporary endocrine organ that plays a central role during the initial stages of pregnancy.

 The ovarian cycle produces cyclic changes in steroid hormone production, which in parallel produce marked morphologic and functional changes in the endometrium, preparing it for embryo implantation.

 Estrogen has important systemic effects affecting the risk of cardiovascular disease, osteoporosis, and endometrial and breast cancer.

 Progesterone ensures uterine quiescence and prevents lactogenesis during pregnancy.

 Mammary gland morphologic development occurs during puberty and is functionally modified during pregnancy by prolactin and hPL, ensuring lactogenesis.

STUDY QUESTIONS

9–1. A 30-year-old female patient arrives at your office because of missed menstrual periods for 2 months. Her history indicates regular menstrual periods in the past. During physical examination, you suspect that she may be pregnant. Which laboratory values would be compatible with your diagnosis?

  a. Low plasma progesterone and high LH

  b. High prolactin, low LH, and low progesterone

  c. High urinary estradiol and low progesterone

  d. High urinary hCG and high plasma progesterone

9–2. A 5-month-pregnant woman is referred to your office with newly diagnosed hypertension. You are concerned that the fetus and placenta may be compromised. To assess fetal and placental health, which of the following hormone measurements would be most informative?

  a. Urinary estriol and serum hCG

  b. Serum progesterone and prolactin

  c. Serum LH and hPL

  d. Urinary estriol and serum progesterone

9–3.   A 32-year-old women complains of amenorrhea since delivery of a baby 15 months previously, despite the fact that she did not breastfeed her baby. The delivery was complicated by excessive hemorrhage that required transfusion of 2.5 liters of blood. She has also been fatigued and has gained an additional 10 pounds (4.5 kg) since the baby was born. Laboratory data is likely to show the following:

    a. High serum LH

    b. Normal serum estradiol

    c. Increased prolactin

    d. Decreased T_3

    e. Increased ACTH

9–4.   A 55-year-old woman stopped menstruating approximately 3 months ago. Worried that she may be pregnant, she decided to have a pregnancy test. The test came back negative. Which of the following series of tests results would confirm that the woman is postmenopausal?

    a. Decreased LH, decreased FSH, increased estrogen

    b. Decreased LH, increased FSH, decreased estrogen

    c. Increased LH, decreased FSH, decreased estrogen

    d. Increased LH, increased FSH, decreased estrogen

    e. Increased LH, increased FSH, increased estrogen

SUGGESTED READINGS

Chabbert Buffet N, Djakoure C, Maitre SC, Bouchard P. Regulation of the human menstrual cycle. *Front Neuroendocrinol*. 1998;19:151.

Challis JR, Sloboda DM, Alfaidy N, et al. Prostaglandins and mechanisms of preterm birth. *Reproduction*. 2002;124:1.

Graham JD, Clarke CL. Physiological action of progesterone in target tissues. *Endocr Rev*. 1997;18:502.

Kaipia A, Hsueh AJW. Regulation of ovarian follicle atresia. *Annu Rev Physiol*. 1997;59:349.

McEwen BS. Invited review: Estrogens effects on the brain: multiple sites and molecular mechanisms. *J Appl Physiol*. 2001;91:2785.

Mendelsohn ME, Karas RH. Mechanisms of disease: the protective effects of estrogen on the cardiovascular system. *N Engl J Med*. 1999;340:1801.

Neville MC, Morton J. Physiology and endocrine changes underlying human lactogenesis II. *J Nutr*. 2001;131:3005S.

Niswender GD, Juengel JL, Silva PJ, Rollyson MK, McIntush EW. Mechanisms controlling the function and life span of the corpus luteum. *Physiol Rev*. 2000;80:1.

Wassarman PM. Mammalian fertilization: molecular aspects of gamete adhesion, exocytosis, and fusion. *Cell*. 1999;96:175.

Endocrine Integration of Energy and Electrolyte Balance

10

OBJECTIVES

- ▶ Identify the normal range of plasma glucose concentrations and the hormonal regulation of its metabolism, storage, and mobilization.
- ▶ Identify the specific roles of insulin, glucagon, glucocorticoids, catecholamines, growth hormone, and thyroid hormone in the regulation of energy substrate utilization, storage, and mobilization.
- ▶ Describe the hormonal regulation of energy substrate metabolism during the fed and fasted states and understand the consequences of its dysregulation.
- ▶ Identify the mechanisms involved in the maintenance of long-term energy balance.
- ▶ Identify the normal range of dietary sodium intake, its body distribution, and routes of excretion. Explain the roles of antidiuretic hormone, aldosterone, angiotensin, and atrial natriuretic hormone in the regulation of sodium balance.
- ▶ Identify the normal range of dietary potassium intake, its body distribution, and routes of excretion. Explain the hormonal regulation of plasma potassium concentration, distribution, and balance in the acute and chronic settings.
- ▶ Identify the normal range of dietary calcium intake, its body distribution, and routes of excretion. Explain the hormonal regulation of plasma calcium concentration through bone resorption, renal excretion, and intestinal absorption.
- ▶ Identify the normal range of dietary phosphate intake, its body distribution, and routes of excretion. Explain the hormonal regulation of plasma phosphate concentration through exchange with bone, renal excretion, and dietary intake and absorption.

In the first chapter, several of the key functions of the endocrine system that maintain homeostasis were outlined. Subsequent chapters described the specific physiologic effects of individual hormones, the mechanisms that regulate their production and release, and the consequences of isolated excess or deficiency. The presentation of this material would not be complete without an attempt to integrate some of these actions into the overall regulation of specific functions. Although a complete description of the integrative control of physiologic function is beyond the scope of this book, this chapter integrates many of the concepts already presented. It describes how the different arms of the neuroendocrine system interact to regulate and maintain basic functions, which include energy substrate balance, blood volume and blood pressure, and preservation of bone mineral density (BMD). Finally, it presents an integrated discussion of the neuroendocrine mechanisms involved in mediating the stress response.

NEUROENDOCRINE REGULATION OF ENERGY STORAGE, MOBILIZATION, and UTILIZATION

Two distinct phases directly related to the ingestion of a meal alternate throughout the day in the regulation of energy metabolism. The **fed state** reflects overall **anabolic metabolism**, during which energy is stored in the form of energy-rich compounds (adenosine triphosphate [ATP], phosphocreatinine), glycogen, fat, and proteins. The **fasted or catabolic phase** is the period during which endogenous energy sources are utilized.

The anabolic and catabolic phases alternate to preserve adequate glucose supply to the brain as well as sufficient energy to maintain body functions, such as thermoregulation (maintaining a constant core temperature), food digestion, and physical activity. The 2 hormones at the core of maintaining this balance are insulin and glucagon (see Chapter 7); in particular, their ratio plays a critical role in the dynamic regulation of substrate metabolism (summarized in Table 10–1). However, several other established and newly discovered hormones participate in the regulation of energy metabolism to different extents, according to age, sex, nutritional state, and metabolic demands of the individual.

The autonomic nervous system interacts with the endocrine system in the modulation of glucose and fat metabolism. Hence, the system is in fact under neuroendocrine regulation. The autonomic nervous system exerts its effects both directly and indirectly. For example, activation of the sympathetic

Table 10–1. Regulation of metabolic processes by insulin/glucagon ratios

Anabolic ↑I:G	Metabolic process	Catabolic ↓I:G
↑	Glycogen synthesis (liver and muscle)	↓
↓	Glycogen breakdown	↑
↓	Gluconeogenesis	↑
↑	Triglyceride synthesis (hepatocytes and adipose tissue)	↓
↑	Muscle protein synthesis	↓
↑	Lipogenesis and triglyceride formation	↓
↓	Lipolysis	↑
↓	Free fatty acid oxidation	↑
↓	Ketone body formation	↑
↓	Muscle proteolysis	↑

G, glucagon; I, insulin.

nervous system through norepinephrine release directly stimulates skeletal muscle glycogenolysis and hepatic glucose output. The indirect effects of the autonomic nervous system are exemplified by sympathetic activation of the adrenal medulla (see Chapter 6), stimulating the release of epinephrine. Epinephrine stimulates the pancreatic release of glucagon and suppresses the release of insulin, resulting in an increase in the glucagon to insulin ratio and an overall increase in hepatic glucose production.

To simplify the discussion of the neuroendocrine regulation of substrate metabolism, a brief summary of overall substrate regulation and the principal hormones involved will be presented as they pertain to the fed (anabolic) and fasted (catabolic) states.

Neuroendocrine Regulation of Energy Metabolism During the Fed State

Glucose

Blood glucose regulation occurs through interactions among hormonal, neural, and hepatic autoregulatory mechanisms. As described in detail in Chapter 7, the pancreatic hormones insulin and glucagon play central roles in the tight control of blood glucose concentrations. Following a meal (postprandial state), in response to the increase in pancreatic insulin release, glucose uptake is increased in muscle, fat, and the hepatosplanchnic bed; hepatic glucose output is suppressed; and glycogen synthesis is increased.

Glucose disposal by insulin-sensitive tissues is regulated initially by an increase in glucose transport and enzyme phosphorylation leading to the activation of glycogen synthase, phosphofructokinase, and pyruvate dehydrogenase (see Figure 7–5). The majority of insulin-stimulated glucose taken up is stored as glycogen. Hormonally induced changes in intracellular fructose 2,6-bisphosphate concentrations play a key role in muscle glycolytic flux and both glycolytic and gluconeogenic flux in the liver.

Fat

Most of the body's energy reserve is stored in adipose tissue in the form of triglycerides. During periods of caloric excess or abundance, fat is stored in the form of triacylglycerol in the adipocytes. The principal hormone involved in lipogenesis is insulin, through activation of lipogenic and glycolytic enzymes. Opposing the effects of insulin are growth hormone (GH; discussed in Chapter 3) and leptin (described later), which inhibit lipogenesis (Figure 10–1). The balance between lipogenesis and lipolysis followed by fatty acid oxidation determines the overall accumulation of body fat.

Protein

The whole-body protein pool, as well as that of individual tissues, is determined by the balance between protein synthesis and degradation (see Figure 10–1). These in turn are principally regulated by interactions among hormonal, nutritional, neural, and inflammatory mediators. Hormonally, regulation of protein metabolism

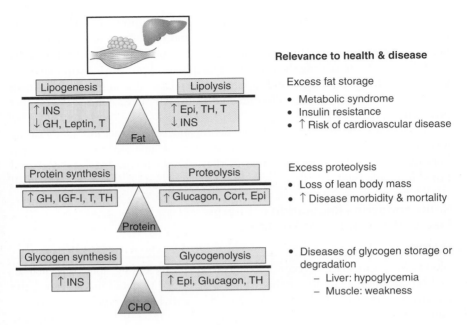

Figure 10–1. Hormonal factors controlling fat, protein, and carbohydrate (CHO) stores and balance. Adipose, protein, and carbohydrate (CHO in the form of glycogen) stores are the result of balanced synthesis and degradation under hormonal regulation by insulin (INS), growth hormone (GH), leptin, testosterone (T), epinephrine (Epi), thyroid hormone (TH), insulin-like growth factor 1 (IGF-1), and cortisol (Cort). Excess, deficiencies, or impaired regulation of adipose, protein, and carbohydrate stores have direct implications on health and disease as illustrated above.

is predominantly under the influence of insulin, GH, and insulin-like growth factor-1 (IGF-1). During the fed state, insulin acts primarily to inhibit proteolysis, and GH stimulates protein synthesis. IGF-1 has antiproteolytic effects during the postabsorptive state that progress to stimulation of protein synthesis in the fed state or when amino acids are provided. GH and testosterone are of particular importance during growth and development, as well as during adulthood and senescence. Thyroid hormones are also required for normal growth and development. Thyroid hormones stimulate bone growth indirectly by increasing secretion of GH and IGF-1 and directly by activating gene transcription.

Neuroendocrine Regulation of Energy Metabolism During the Fasted State

During the fasted postabsorptive state, catabolism of stored energy sources provides the energy required for bodily functions. The total amount of energy produced per unit of time by a given individual is referred to as the **metabolic rate**. The amount of energy expended by an awake, resting individual, measured 12–14 hours following the last meal, at normal (or thermoneutral) body temperature is called the **basal metabolic rate** (BMR). The BMR is the amount of energy required to maintain breathing, brain activity, enzymatic activity, and other functions without any physical movement of the individual. Any deviation from the basal condition, such as changes in body temperature (fever or hypothermia), the level of activity of the individual (exercise or sleeping), or time from the last meal (fed or fasted), will affect the metabolic rate. In addition, BMR can be directly affected by hormone action, particularly thyroid hormones, which increase body temperature and increase Na^+/K^+-adenosine triphosphatase (ATPase) activity, resulting in an increase in the BMR. In a healthy individual, BMR averages 2000 kcal/d. Hence, the recommended dietary allowance of calories is derived from the BMR, age, sex, and level of activity of any given individual. The BMR can be estimated clinically by measuring the amount of oxygen consumed with the use of indirect calorimetry.

GLUCOSE

In the resting postabsorptive state, release of glucose from the liver through glycogenolysis and gluconeogenesis is the key regulated process. During fasting, hepatic glucose production is increased and peripheral glucose utilization is inhibited. Initially, hepatic glucose output is derived from breakdown of hepatic glycogen stores (a maximum of 70–80 g in humans) through glycogenolysis. Following an overnight fast, glycogenolysis provides approximately 50% of the overall hepatic glucose output. As hepatic glycogen stores are depleted during a period of prolonged fasting (approximately 60 hours), the contribution of glycogenolysis to hepatic glucose output becomes negligible, with hepatic gluconeogenesis predominating. Glycogenolysis depends on the relative activities of glycogen synthase and phosphorylase, the latter being the more important (see Figure 7–5). Gluconeogenesis is regulated by the activities of fructose-1,6-diphosphatase, phosphoenolpyruvate carboxykinase, pyruvate kinase, and pyruvate dehydrogenase, and by the availability of the principal gluconeogenic precursors, lactate, glycerol, glutamine, and alanine.

A smaller, yet significant amount (approximately 25%) of systemic glucose production in the postabsorptive state is derived from renal gluconeogenesis. The proximal tubule cells produce glucose at a rate similar to that of glucose utilization by the renal medulla. Overall, the kidney is not a net producer of glucose. Thus, in the postabsorptive state, blood glucose homeostasis is the result of hormonal regulation of glycogenolysis, gluconeogenesis, and glucose uptake.

FAT

The amount of energy stored as triglycerides in adipose tissue is substantial. For example, an adult with 15 kg of body fat has enough energy to support the whole body energy requirements (8.37 MJ; 2000 kcal) for about 2 months. After an overnight fast, most of the resting energy requirement is provided by oxidation of fatty acids derived from adipose tissue. Lipolysis in adipose tissue is mostly dependent on the concentrations of hormones (epinephrine stimulates lipolysis, and insulin inhibits lipolysis). During a period of acute energy deprivation or prolonged starvation, lipolysis mobilizes triglycerides, providing nonesterified fatty acids as energy substrates for tissues such as muscle, heart, and liver; and substrates for glucose (glycerol) and lipoprotein (free fatty acids) synthesis to the liver. Unlike most other tissues, the brain cannot utilize fatty acids for energy when blood glucose levels become compromised. In this case, ketone bodies (discussed in Chapter 7) provide the brain with an alternative source of energy, amounting to nearly two-thirds of the brain's energy needs during periods of prolonged fasting and starvation.

The release of glycerol and free fatty acids from adipose tissue is under negative regulation by insulin and is stimulated primarily by catecholamines (see Chapter 7). During fasting, plasma insulin levels decrease and plasma GH and glucagon both increase. As the fasting period progresses, or more frequently during periods of acute glucose deficiency (insulin-induced hypoglycemia) or increased energy demand (as with strenuous exercise), catecholamines play an important role in the stimulation of lipolysis.

PROTEIN

Unlike excess fat and glucose, which are stored as fat and glycogen in adipose tissue, liver, and muscle, there is no storage pool for body protein. Therefore, under catabolic conditions, essential proteins are degraded. Glucagon, cortisol, and epinephrine together favor muscle protein breakdown and hepatic amino acid uptake, some of which can be utilized for gluconeogenesis (see Figure 10–1). The effects of glucagon are predominantly mediated through increased hepatic uptake of amino acids. Epinephrine increases production of the gluconeogenic amino acid alanine by muscle and its uptake by the splanchnic bed. Prolonged changes in either the protein synthetic or degradative processes (or both) leading to loss of lean body mass have been shown to increase morbidity and mortality from several diseases, including cancer and acquired immunodeficiency syndrome (AIDS).

Counterregulatory Hormone Effects

GLUCAGON

Glucagon plays a primary role in energy metabolism. This hormone primarily stimulates hepatic glycogenolysis, as well as gluconeogenesis resulting in an overall increase in hepatic glucose output.

GROWTH HORMONE AND CORTISOL

GH and cortisol facilitate glucose production and limit glucose utilization, but neither of them plays a critical role in the acute counterregulatory response to a hypoglycemic episode. Their effects are not immediate (delayed for approximately 6 hours); thus, they are mostly involved in defense against prolonged hypoglycemia. Cortisol contributes to the regulation of gluconeogenic substrate supply through permissive effects on the lipolytic action of catecholamines and GH in adipose tissue and on the glycogenolytic action of catecholamines in skeletal muscle. In addition, it induces hepatic enzymatic gene expression required for enhanced gluconeogenic rates and exerts permissive effects on the stimulation of gluconeogenesis in the liver by glucagon and epinephrine.

EPINEPHRINE

Epinephrine stimulates hepatic glycogenolysis and hepatic and renal gluconeogenesis, largely by mobilizing gluconeogenic precursors including lactate, alanine, glutamine, and glycerol from adipose and muscle stores. Epinephrine also limits glucose utilization by insulin-sensitive tissues. Epinephrine helps increase hepatic glucose output and together with glucagon acts within minutes to increase plasma glucose concentrations.

The increased activation of the sympathetic nervous system and the associated release of epinephrine and norepinephrine suppress pancreatic insulin release and stimulate glucagon release leading to an increased glucagon to insulin ratio. Thus, stimulation of glycogenolysis and inhibition of glycogen synthesis by glucagon and epinephrine as well as the glucagon-stimulated hepatic gluconeogenesis proceed unopposed.

Neuroendocrine Regulation of Energy Metabolism During Extreme Conditions

COUNTERREGULATION TO HYPOGLYCEMIA

The contribution of the activation of the autonomic nervous system is easier understood when described in the context of acute and severe hypoglycemia. Because of the clear advantages of glycemic control in preventing organ injury in diabetic patients, tight regulation of plasma glucose levels is desired and recommended in this patient population. However, the most prevalent problem associated with tight glycemic control is the development of insulin-induced hypoglycemia. The decrease in plasma glucose concentrations (hypoglycemia) within and below the physiologic postabsorptive concentration range of approximately 70–110 mg/dL (3.9–6.1 mmol/L) triggers the activation of a counterregulatory neuroendocrine response. Acute insulin-induced hypoglycemia increases neuronal activity in the nucleus tractus solitarius and lateral hypothalamic glucosensors, resulting in increased sympathetic activity.

Enhanced sympathetic activity suppresses pancreatic insulin release and stimulates glucagon and epinephrine release, leading to increased hepatic glucose output. The additional release of GH and cortisol also contribute to the increase in hepatic glucose output and the suppression of tissue glucose uptake, partly through an increase in tissue fatty acid oxidation. As plasma glucose levels are restored, peripheral glucose sensors in the portal vein, small intestine, and liver decrease firing. This afferent signal is transmitted to the hypothalamus and to the nucleus solitarius in the medulla through the vagus nerve, conveying information on the prevailing peripheral glucose levels. The hypothalamus integrates these signals and initiates an appropriate response through the inhibition of hepatic and adrenal nerve activity, with consequently decreased release of adrenomedullary catecholamines, removing the inhibition on pancreatic insulin release and thus allowing hyperglycemia to induce pancreatic insulin secretion. Thus, in this system, glucose acts as a feedback signal contributing to integration of the neuroendocrine mechanisms that regulate its homeostasis.

REGULATION OF ENERGY METABOLISM DURING EXERCISE

The neuroendocrine response to exercise is targeted to provide for the increased energy demands of the exercising muscle and includes activation of the sympathetic nervous system, release of GH, activation of the hypothalamic-pituitary-adrenal axis with consequent release of catecholamines and cortisol, suppression of insulin release, and stimulation of glucagon release (Figure 10–2). This neuroendocrine response stimulates lipolysis, and hepatic and muscle glycogenolysis leading to an increase in free fatty acids, gluconeogenic substrate mobilization, and hepatic glucose output (because of an increase in both gluconeogenesis and glycogenolysis). Both hepatic and skeletal muscle glycogenolysis are stimulated by the increase in catecholamine release. However, because muscle lacks glucose-6-phosphatase, the glucose-6-phosphate produced by muscle glycogenolysis is either oxidized in muscle cells or released into the circulation as lactate. The increased lactate delivered to the liver is then used for hepatic gluconeogenesis. Hepatic glycogenolysis predominates during intense exercise, but gluconeogenesis contributes substantially to the increased hepatic glucose output during prolonged exercise as the liver glycogen stores decline and the supply of gluconeogenic precursors increases. As exercise intensity increases from mild to moderate and intense, energy substrate selection switches from lipid to carbohydrate dependence. GH and cortisol contribute only minimally to the exercise-induced increase in liver glucose output.

Skeletal muscle is the main site of oxidation of fatty acids, and endogenous triacylglycerols represent an important source of energy both at rest and during low- and moderate-intensity exercise. During moderate-intensity exercise, lipolysis increases approximately 3-fold, mainly because of an increase in β-adrenergic stimulation, leading to an increased release of glycerol (used as a hepatic gluconeogenic substrate) and fatty acids into the circulation. The increase in adipose tissue and muscle blood flow facilitates the delivery of fatty acids to skeletal muscle for oxidation. In combination, the decrease in insulin and enhanced sympathetic stimulation, result in increased lipolysis and triacylglycerol oxidation; which serves as the main energy substrate for muscle. As the intensity of exercise increases, fat oxidation increases further until exercise intensities reach approximately 65% maximum oxygen consumption (VO_2 max). After this point, the rate of fat oxidation declines, most likely because of reduced fatty acid delivery from adipose tissue to muscle.

The contribution of amino acid oxidation to total energy expenditure is negligible during short-term intense exercise and accounts for 3–6% of the total ATP supplied during prolonged exercise in humans. Although it is not quantitatively important regarding energy supply, the intermediary metabolism of several amino acids, notably glutamate, alanine, and the branched-chain amino acids, influences the availability of tricarboxylic acid cycle intermediates. Sustained dynamic exercise stimulates amino acid oxidation, chiefly of the branched-chain amino acids, and ammonia production in proportion to exercise intensity. If the exercise is intense enough, it causes a net loss of muscle protein (as a result of decreased protein synthesis, increased breakdown, or both); some of the amino acids are oxidized as energy, whereas the rest provide substrates for gluconeogenesis and possibly for acid-base regulation.

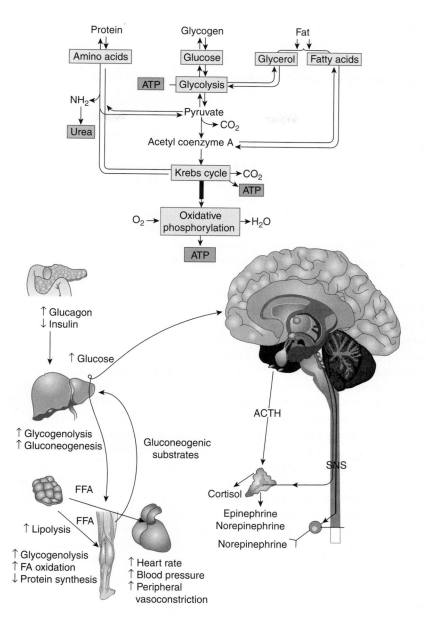

Figure 10–2. Neuroendocrine response to exercise. The principal pathways activated by stress are the hypothalamic-pituitary-adrenal axis and sympathetic nervous system resulting in the increased release of corticotropin-releasing hormone (CRH), arginine vasopressin (AVP), catecholamines, endorphins, and growth hormone (GH). In the periphery, increased production and release of cortisol, glucagon and catecholamines, and suppressed release of insulin favor an overall catabolic response. Stimulation of hepatic glycogenolysis and gluconeogenesis, muscle glycogenolysis, and adipose tissue lipolysis ensure the production and mobilization of energy stores to sustain the enhanced metabolic demands of the individual. Reproductive and growth functions are inhibited, conserving energy to sustain fundamental processes that ensure survival. ACTH, adrenocorticotropic hormone; ATP, adenosine triphosphate; FA, fatty acid; FFA, free fatty acid; SNS, sympathetic nervous system.

Maintenance of Long-Term Energy Balance and Fat Storage

The neuroendocrine mechanisms involved in maintaining energy balance have been described earlier. Furthermore, the hormonal regulation of the 2 principal energy stores in the body—hepatic glycogen and adipose tissue triglycerides—has been outlined. The balanced transition from fed to fasted and the consumption of adequate energy commensurate with the level of physical activity of a given individual ensure that adequate energy reserves are available for short-term increases in metabolic demands, such as those described for exercise. An imbalance in either energy intake or expenditure leads to 1 of 2 extremes: loss of lean body mass or wasting syndrome resulting from an overall catabolic state, or obesity resulting from a combination of excess caloric intake and decreased physical activity. The salient features of these 2 conditions are described below.

CATABOLIC STATE

When the fasted state is prolonged into a state of starvation, or under conditions of increased energy substrate demands, the contributions of the counterregulatory hormones cortisol, epinephrine, norepinephrine, and glucagon become evident, favoring overall catabolic effects. During such conditions, insulin effects are practically abolished. Because of the important anabolic effects of insulin, it follows that the metabolic responses that predominate are those that lead to catabolism of stored energy (glycogenolysis, lipolysis) and of lean tissues (muscle proteolysis), leading to loss of lean body mass, or wasting. It is important to note that energy metabolism can be pushed to a starvation-like state not only by discontinuation of food intake, in the classic sense of starvation, but also during conditions of stress, such as from a surgical intervention, cancer, severe infection, sepsis, burns, and traumatic injury. Under these conditions, additional factors such as inflammatory cytokines (eg, tumor necrosis factor [TNF], interleukins 1 and 6) interact with mediators of the neuroendocrine response. In addition, the production of GH, IGF-1, and the respective binding proteins becomes dysregulated, also contributing to the lack of anabolic processes and dominance of catabolic responses. Overall, the increased release of stress hormones and proinflammatory cytokines and the impairment in the release and action of insulin and growth factors, in association with altered release of androgens, lead to an overall catabolic response that affects the liver, adipose tissue, muscle, and, in extreme circumstances, visceral tissues. The deleterious impact of the loss of lean body mass on survival from disease underscores the relevance of understanding the hormonal mechanisms involved in the regulation of energy metabolism and their importance in the management of the critically ill patient.

OBESITY

Obesity is defined as a significant increase above the ideal weight (the weight that maximizes life expectancy). The increase in body mass index (BMI), an indicator of the adiposity or fatness that accompanies obesity, has become an important health problem for the developed world. Life expectancy is reduced when body mass index is significantly increased above the ideal level. Obesity is

Table 10–2. Classification of overweight according to the World Health Organization

BMI (kg/m²)*	Definition	WHO classification
<18.5	Thin	
18.5–24.9	Healthy or normal	
25.0–29.9	Overweight	Grade 1 overweight
30.0–39.9	Obese	Grade 2 overweight
=40.0	Morbidly obese	Grade 3 overweight

BMI, body mass index; WHO, World Health Organization.
*BMI is defined as mass in kilograms divided by the square of the height in meters.

associated with an increased risk of diabetes, dyslipidemia, hypertension, heart disease, diabetes, and cancer. Approximately 20% of the US population is considered obese, according to the definition of the World Health Organization (Table 10–2).

Body weight and the excess weight gain leading to obesity are determined by interactions among genetic, environmental, and psychosocial factors that affect the physiologic mediators of energy intake and expenditure, several of which pertain to the endocrine system. The altered balance between energy intake and energy expenditure leads to excess weight gain and obesity. Energy expended by the individual can be in the form of work (physical activity) or heat production (thermogenesis), which can be affected by environmental temperature, diet, and the neuroendocrine system (catecholamines and thyroid hormone). The uncoupling of ATP production from mitochondrial respiration dissipates heat and affects the efficiency with which the body utilizes energy substrates. The expression of proteins involved in this process (uncoupling protein-1 expressed in brown adipose tissue and uncoupling protein-3 in skeletal muscle) is modulated by catecholamines, thyroid hormones, and leptin. Studies are currently under way to establish their roles in the regulation of BMR and in the development of obesity.

The role of genetics in the predisposition to obesity has been demonstrated convincingly. Susceptibility genes that increase the risk of developing obesity have been identified, and their relevance has been shown in studies in which pairs of twins were exposed to periods of positive and negative energy balance. The differences in the rate of weight gain, the proportion of weight gained, and the sites of fat deposition showed greater similarity within pairs than between pairs, indicating a close genetic relationship. Although a clear correlation between energy expenditure and weight gain has not been demonstrated, increasing physical activity; which represents 20%–50% of total energy expenditure, has been actively promoted as an approach to prevent obesity and improve insulin responsiveness. Environmental factors are also thought to unmask genetic tendencies toward obesity.

From the standpoint of endocrine physiology, it is important to note that the responsiveness to hormones that regulate lipolysis varies according to the distribution of fat depots. The lipolytic response to norepinephrine is greater in abdominal than in gluteal or femoral adipose tissue in both men and women. The exaggerated release of free fatty acids from abdominal adipocytes directly into the portal system, an increased hepatic gluconeogenesis, and hepatic glucose release, and hyperinsulinemia are hallmarks of patients with upper-body obesity. The endocrine properties of the different fat pads may be more important than the anatomic location of the fat pad. The severity of medical complications is more closely related to body fat distribution; being greater in individuals with upper-body obesity than those with an excess total body fat. Differential fat deposition leading to upper-body or abdominal obesity is reflected in a high waist-hip ratio, an index used for predicting risks associated with fat accumulation. The presence of visceral obesity, insulin resistance, dyslipidemia, and hypertension is collectively termed the **metabolic syndrome** or **syndrome X**.

Excess energy intake in relation to the energy expended by the organism leads to the accumulation of fat. The fat mass itself is determined by the balance between breakdown (lipolysis) and synthesis (lipogenesis) (see Figure 10–1). The sympathetic nervous system is the principal stimulator of lipolysis, leading to a decrease in fat stores, particularly when the energy demands of the individual are increased. When intake exceeds energy utilization, lipogenesis occurs in liver and adipose tissue. Lipogenesis is influenced by diet (increased by carbohydrate-rich diets) and hormones (principally GH, insulin, and leptin) through modification of transcription factors (eg, peroxisome proliferator-activated receptor γ [PPAR-γ]). The main hormones involved in fat storage are insulin (which stimulates lipogenesis), and GH and leptin (which reduce lipogenesis). The transcription factor PPAR, the target for the insulin sensitizer thiazolidinedione drugs (see Chapter 7), affects gene transcription of several enzymes involved in glucose and fat metabolism and is involved in preadipocyte differentiation into mature fat cells. Other hormones involved in the regulation of body fat stores include testosterone, dehydroepiandrosterone, and thyroid hormone.

REGULATION OF ENERGY INTAKE

Regulation of energy intake is mediated by several factors. Central integration of peripheral signals, including those mediated by mechanoreceptors and chemoreceptors, signals the presence and energy density of food in the gastrointestinal tract. Hypothalamic glucose sensors monitor fluctuations in circulating glucose concentrations. Hormones signal the central release of peptides that regulate appetite and satiety. Two hormones that have been identified as crucial in the long-term regulation of energy balance are insulin (see Chapter 7) and **leptin**, the product of the *ob* gene (discussed later). Both hormones are released in proportion to body fat. They are transported into the brain, where they modulate the expression of hypothalamic neuropeptides known to regulate feeding behavior and body weight, resulting in inhibition of food intake and increase in energy expenditure.

Although insulin release is directly correlated to meals; that of leptin does not correlate with food intake but reflects body fat mass.

HYPOTHALAMIC INTEGRATION

The hypothalamus receives innervation from several areas, notably the nucleus tractus solitarius (NTS) and area postrema in the brainstem. These areas relay many neural and hormonal signals from the gastrointestinal tract. Mechanical stretch receptors sense stretch of the stomach and other areas of the intestine. The principal hormone associated with control of satiety is the peptide cholecystokinin (CCK). CCK, is released from the duodenum in response to the presence of lipids or protein in the intestinal lumen (see Figure 10–2). This hormone acts via local sensory receptors in the duodenum sending signals to the brain regarding the intestinal nutritional content. The NTS also relays taste information to the hypothalamus and other centers. Other signals regarding smell, sight, memory of food, and the social context under which it is ingested are also integrated and may also influence energy intake by modulating output from the hypothalamus. Integration of these signals results in the activation of gene expression of mediators implicated in the regulation of satiety and development of obesity. These genes control thermogenesis (uncoupling proteins), hormone synthesis (**ghrelin**, leptin, and CCK and adiponectin), and neurotransmitter (**neuropeptide Y**) availability, as summarized in Table 10–3.

The relative contributions of these mediators to the regulation of caloric intake, energy expenditure, body weight, and fat mass are not completely understood. However, important new discoveries, such as the secretory function of adipose tissue, have provided new insight into potential factors contributing to obesity. Adipose tissue is now classified not just as an energy storage tissue but as an endocrine tissue participating in a complex network regulating energy homeostasis, glucose and lipid metabolism, vascular homeostasis, immune response, and even reproduction. Among the hormones identified that are produced by adipose tissue are leptin, cytokines (TNF-α, interleukin 6), adipsin and acylation-stimulating protein, angiotensinogen, plasminogen activator inhibitor-1, adiponectin, resistin, and steroid hormones (see Table 10–3). Secretion of almost all of these hormones and cytokines is dysregulated as a consequence of both excess and deficiency in the mass of adipose tissue, suggesting that they are involved in the pathophysiology of both obesity and cachexia. Of particular interest are the contributions of the proinflammatory cytokines to the development of insulin resistance in obese individuals and the potential role of leptin as a regulator of fat mass.

TNF produced by adipose tissue has been implicated in producing insulin insensitivity, both indirectly and directly. Indirectly, TNF stimulates stress hormone production. Directly, TNF decreases insulin-induced receptor substrate 1 tyrosine phosphorylation and its association with the downstream signaling mediators (phosphatidylinositol trisphosphate kinase), and it also inhibits PPAR. These pathways and their role in the regulation of intermediary metabolism and regulation of fat mass are currently under intense investigation.

Table 10–3. Mediators implicated in regulation of energy balance

Mediator	Regulation and target effect
Gastrointestinal tract	
Cholecystokinin	Released in the duodenum during a meal. Stimulates the vagus nerve projecting to the NTS and signals within the hypothalamus to induce satiety.
Ghrelin	Produced primarily by the stomach. Levels increase before meals and decrease following a meal. Stimulates growth hormone release, increases food intake. Overall has anti-leptin action. Plasma levels are low in obese patients.
PYY$_{3-36}$	Member of the NPY family, released in the distal small intestine and colon in response to food. Blood levels remain elevated between meals. Reduces food intake.
GLP-1	Peptide produced in the intestinal cells in response to high intestinal luminal glucose concentrations. Amplifies glucose-induced insulin release from the β-cell.
Adipose tissue	
Adiponectin (AdipoQ)	Increases insulin sensitivity and tissue fat oxidation, resulting in reduced circulating fatty acid levels and reduced intramyocellular and liver triglyceride content. Levels decreased in obese patients; plasma levels correlate negatively with triglycerides.
Acylation-stimulating protein	Stimulates triglyceride synthesis in adipocytes, resulting in more rapid postprandial lipid clearance. Stimulates translocation of glucose transporters to the cell surface.
Leptin	Secreted by fat cells in proportion to fat stores. Acts on hypothalamic neurons to decrease food intake. Leptin is necessary for maturation of the reproductive axis.
Resistin	Peptide hormone induced during adipogenesis. It antagonizes insulin action.
Hypothalamus	
NPY	Produced by hypothalamic neurons that express AgRP. Release is under leptin, insulin, and cortisol regulation. Stimulates food intake via the NPY5 receptor.
α-MSH	Product of POMC in hypothalamic neuronal subset under leptin regulation. Decreases food intake through melanocortin-4 receptors in the hypothalamus.
CART	Peptide produced by hypothalamic POMC-expressing neurons stimulated by leptin and amphetamines. Reduces food intake.
AgRP	Released from hypothalamic NPY-expressing neurons. Inhibits neuronal melanocortin-4 receptors and increases food intake.
Orexins (A and B)	Produced by neurons in the lateral hypothalamus perifornical area. Regulated by glucose, leptin, NPY, and POMC neurons. They stimulate food intake.

AdipoQ, adipocyte complement-related protein of 30 kDa; AgRP, agouti-related peptide; CART, cocaine- and amphetamine-regulated transcript; GI, gastrointestinal; GLP-1, glucagon-like Peptide 1; MSH, melanocyte-stimulating hormone; NTS, nucleus tractus solitarius; PYY, polypeptide YY; POMC, proopiomelanocortin.

LEPTIN

Leptin is a peptide hormone produced predominantly in adipose tissue. Leptin is thought to serve as an indicator of energy stores (lipostat), as well as a modulator of energy balance. The specific effects of leptin on fat metabolism are as follows:

- Decrease in fat storage
- Increase in sympathetic-mediated energy expenditure
- Increase in expression of uncoupling proteins
- Decrease in triglyceride content by increasing fatty acid oxidation
- Decrease in activity and expression of esterification and lipogenic enzymes
- Decrease in lipogenic activity of insulin, favoring lipolysis

The release of leptin into the circulation is pulsatile. Plasma concentrations follow a circadian rhythm, and are highest between midnight and early morning and lowest in the early to midafternoon. These changes in leptin plasma concentrations are not influenced by meal ingestion or meal-induced increases in the circulating insulin concentration. The overall effect of leptin is to deplete fat stores and promote leanness in a feedback regulatory system. In this feedback loop, leptin functions as a sensor that monitors the level of energy stores (adipose tissue mass). The signal is received and integrated by hypothalamic neurons, and an effector response, most likely involving modulation of appetite centers and sympathetic nervous system activity, regulates the 2 main determinants of energy balance: intake and expenditure.

The effects of leptin are mediated through the leptin receptor, located throughout the central nervous system and peripheral tissues. Leptin binding to its receptor activates gene transcription on hypothalamic neurons resulting in reduced expression of 2 orexigenic (feeding-inducing) neuropeptides, neuropeptide Y (NPY) and agouti-related peptide (AgRP); and enhanced expression of 2 anorexigenic peptides, α-melanocyte-stimulating (α-MSH) hormone and cocaine- and amphetamine-regulated transcript (CART). Thus, leptin-induced inhibition of food intake results from both the suppression of orexigenic and the induction of anorexigenic neuropeptides (Figure 10–3).

The role of leptin in humans appears to be mostly one of adaptation to low energy intake rather than a brake on overconsumption and obesity. Leptin concentrations decrease during fasting and energy-restricted diets, independent of body fat changes, stimulating an increase in food intake before body energy stores become depleted. Because leptin levels do not increase in response to individual meals, it is not thought to serve as a meal-related satiety signal. Finally, it is notable that obese individuals have high plasma leptin concentrations that do not result in the expected reduction in food intake and increase in energy expenditure, suggesting that obesity may be related to leptin resistance and not leptin deficiency.

Congenital leptin deficiency is a rare autosomal recessive disease resulting from mutations in the leptin gene. Affected individuals are markedly obese mainly

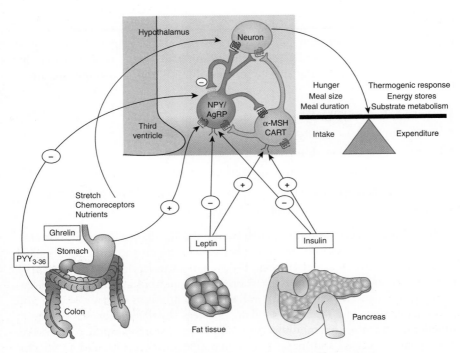

Figure 10–3. Hypothalamic integration of energy intake. The hypothalamus receives innervation from several areas, notably the nucleus tractus solitarius and area postrema in the brainstem, that relay many neural and hormonal signals from the gastrointestinal tract, such as mechanical signals indicating stretch of the stomach and other areas of the intestine, and hormonal signals indicating the presence of food in the gut, such as cholecystokinin. Additional signals regarding smell, sight, memory of food, and the social context under which it is ingested are also integrated and may also influence energy intake by modulating output from the hypothalamus. Hormones also alter hypothalamic gene expression resulting in modulation of energy intake. Leptin and insulin decrease appetite by inhibiting the production of neuropeptide Y (NPY) and agouti-related protein (AgRP), while stimulating melanocortin-producing neurons in the arcuate-nucleus region of the hypothalamus. NPY and AgRP stimulate eating, and melanocortins inhibit eating. Ghrelin stimulates appetite by activating the NPY/AgRP-expressing neurons. PYY_{3-36}, released from the colon, inhibits these neurons and transiently decreases appetite. Integration of these signals results in the activation of gene expression of mediators implicated in the regulation of satiety, control of thermogenesis, and energy expenditure. CART, cocaine- and amphetamine-regulated transcript; α-MSH, α-melanocyte-stimulating; PYY, polypeptide YY.

because of increased food intake (hyperphagia) and have inadequate gonadotropin-releasing hormone (GnRH) release, manifesting in hypogonadotropic hypogonadism characterized by failure to reach puberty, including absence of growth spurt, secondary sex characteristics, and menarche.

Ghrelin is a hormone produced by the enteroendocrine cells of the stomach, and to lesser extent by the placenta, pituitary, and hypothalamus. Circulating levels of ghrelin decrease during meals and are highest in the fasted state. Ghrelin levels are decreased in obese individuals and increased in individuals consuming low-calorie diets, involved in chronic strenuous exercise, and with cancer anorexia and anorexia nervosa. In humans, ghrelin has been shown to be a potent GH secretagogue and appetite stimulant.

ELECTROLYTE BALANCE

Regulation of Sodium Balance

Sodium is the primary electrolyte that regulates extracellular fluid (ECF) levels and osmolarity in the body. Sodium is an essential mineral required for the integrity of multiple organ functions, particularly through the regulation of fluid balance and ultimately the regulation of blood pressure. It is essential for maintaining hydration, water balance, osmotic equilibrium, plasma volume, and acid-base balance and for preserving nerve impulses and muscle contractions. Sodium concentration determines the ECF tonicity, which reflects the balance between sodium and water in the ECF. The osmolarity (the amount of solute per unit volume) of bodily fluids is tightly regulated by balancing the intake and excretion of sodium with those of water. Extreme variation in osmolarity causes cells to shrink or swell, damaging or destroying cellular structure and disrupting normal cellular function.

Regulation of extracellular Na^+ concentration controls the distribution of water between the ECF and intracellular fluid (ICF) and maintains cell volume, ensuring normal physiologic function. Sodium is maintained in the ECF by the action of Na^+/K^+-ATPase, whereas water crosses cell membranes through ubiquitously expressed aquaporins (maintaining ICF and ECF isotonicity). Water balance is maintained by matching the amount of water consumed in food and drink (and generated by metabolism) to the volume of water excreted. Consumption is regulated by central nervous system stimulation of thirst and salt craving, whereas excretion is principally regulated hormonally at the kidney. Additional loss of water (1 L/d) occurs through the skin, lungs, and feces.

The overall *mass* of Na^+ is under aldosterone regulation, whereas the Na^+ *concentration* in plasma is under antidiuretic hormone (ADH) regulation. Thus, low Na^+ concentrations do not necessarily mean that total Na^+ mass is low. In chronic heart failure, osmolarity can be low, yet Na^+ mass can be high because of excess water and Na^+ in the ECF, with greater increases in total body water than in Na^+ mass.

INTAKE, DISTRIBUTION, AND EXCRETION OF SODIUM

Sodium concentrations average 140 mmol/L in plasma and 10 mmol/L intracellularly. The concentration of sodium in gut secretions and sweat is similar to that in the ICF (10–50 mmol/L). Sodium concentrations and intravascular volume are physiologically controlled in parallel. For a given amount of total-body water, intravascular volume is determined by sodium concentrations, which control the distribution between ICF and ECF.

The minimum recommended intake of sodium is 500 mg/d; which is markedly exceeded by the average diet in the United States (average 4–5 g/d). One teaspoon of table salt contains approximately 6 g of sodium chloride (2.3 mg of sodium). Sodium intake is usually considered to be unregulated; however, specific hypothalamic areas are involved in salt appetite, although their physiology is not completely understood.

Sodium balance is maintained primarily through hormonal regulation of renal sodium excretion. Fecal loss is small (0.8–8 mmol/d) even when sodium intake is high. Skin loss is small except under conditions of excessive sweating. Small changes in percentage renal reabsorption of sodium cause a large change in the amount of sodium excreted. The total amount of filtered sodium load (about 25,200 mmol/d) is equal to the glomerular filtration rate (180 L/d) multiplied by plasma sodium concentrations (140 mmol/L). Therefore, to maintain sodium balance on a dietary intake of 150 mmol/d, a total of 25,050 mmol (ie, 99.4% of the filtered load) must be reabsorbed. Approximately 60%–70% of the filtered sodium is reabsorbed in the proximal tubule. An additional 20%–30% of filtered sodium is reabsorbed in the ascending limb of the loop of Henle. Sodium reabsorption in the thick ascending limb is passive, down an electrical gradient set up by the active transport of chloride ions, and is the site of inhibition by loop diuretics. Thus, a significant (80%–95%) obligatory reabsorption of filtered sodium occurs in the renal tubule before reaching the distal tubule, preventing large renal sodium losses. The majority of the remaining sodium (5%–10%) is reabsorbed in the distal tubule and collecting duct. It is here that the finer regulation of sodium excretion through aldosterone occurs, and this is the site of inhibition by the diuretic hydrochlorothiazide (see Chapter 6).

Hormonal Regulation of Sodium and Water Balance

The system that controls total-body water is a negative feedback homeostatic mechanism, of which thirst and ADH are the major effectors. Two stimuli regulate the system: tonicity of the ECF through osmoreceptors, and intravascular volume through stretch or baroreceptors. As discussed in Chapter 3, the system works primarily to maintain intravascular volume and to a lesser extent to maintain tonicity. Thirst is stimulated by an increase in tonicity (1%–2% changes are sufficient to elicit thirst) and by reductions in the ECF volume. Water intake is inhibited by hypotonicity and ECF volume expansion.

Sudden decreases in blood volume are sensed by mechanoreceptors in the left ventricle, carotid sinus, aortic arch, and renal afferent arterioles (Figure 10–4; see Figure 2–7). These mechanoreceptors respond to decreased stretch resulting from decreases in systemic arterial pressure, stroke volume, renal perfusion, or peripheral vascular resistance by triggering an increase in sympathetic outflow from the central nervous system, activation of the renin-angiotensin-aldosterone system, and nonosmotic release of arginine vasopressin (AVP or ADH), as well as stimulation of thirst. Low blood pressure results in decreased renal perfusion pressure

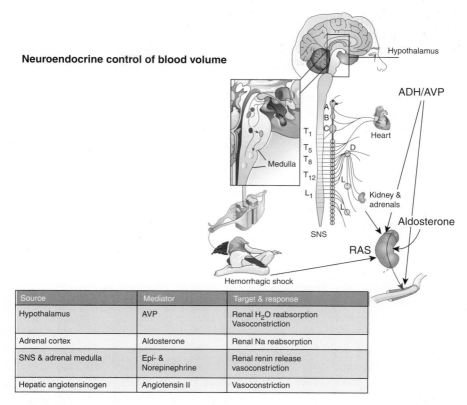

Figure 10–4. Neuroendocrine control of blood volume. Sudden decreases in blood volume are sensed by mechanoreceptors in the left ventricle, carotid sinus, aortic arch, and renal afferent arterioles triggering an increase in sympathetic (SNS) outflow from the central nervous system, activation of the renin-angiotensin-aldosterone (RAS) system, and the nonosmotic release of arginine vasopressin (AVP), as well as the stimulation of thirst. The decrease in renal perfusion pressure and glomerular filtration rates, stimulate the release of renin, the enzyme responsible for angiotensinogen conversion to angiotensin I (later converted by angiotensin-converting enzyme [ACE] to angiotensin II). Angiotensin II, aldosterone, and antidiuretic hormone (ADH) produce vasoconstriction, venoconstriction, and renal retention of Na^+ and water.

and lower glomerular filtration rates, which stimulate the release of renin from juxtaglomerular cells in the afferent and efferent arterioles. Renin is an enzyme synthesized in the juxtaglomerular cells of the kidney that cleaves angiotensinogen (a peptide produced by the liver) to angiotensin I, which is later converted by angiotensin-converting enzyme to angiotensin II. This renin-angiotensin system is part of an extremely powerful feedback system for long-term control of blood pressure and volume homeostasis. Together, angiotensin II, aldosterone, and ADH produce vasoconstriction, and renal retention of Na^+ and water.

Antidiuretic hormone—ADH directly controls water excretion by the kidneys (see Chapter 2). ADH secretion and compensatory thirst are stimulated by hypothalamic osmoreceptors and by decreased stimulation of aortic and carotid stretch receptors. Release of ADH is inhibited by increased stretch of mechano-receptors (stretch receptors) in the atria of the heart. ADH stimulates insertion of aquaporins into the cell membrane, increases water reabsorption in the collecting ducts, and concentrates excreted urine.

Angiotensin II—Angiotensin II elevates blood pressure by several mechanisms, including direct vasoconstriction, potentiation of the activity of the sympathetic nervous system at both the central and peripheral levels, stimulation of aldosterone synthesis and release with consequent sodium reabsorption by the kidney (see Chapter 6), stimulation of ADH release and increased water retention, intra-renal efferent arteriolar constriction (which maintains glomerular filtration rate when renal perfusion is impaired, also known as "glomerular tubular feedback"). Because of the effectiveness of the renin-angiotensin system in regulating blood pressure, blockade of the system with angiotensin-converting enzyme inhibitors offers a powerful therapeutic tool in diseases such as hypertension and congestive heart failure.

Aldosterone—Aldosterone increases sodium reabsorption and potassium excretion in the distal tubule and the collecting duct of the nephron, playing a central role in determining total-body Na^+ mass, and thus long-term blood pressure regulation. Aldosterone release from the adrenals is under positive regulation by Angiotensin II.

Atrial natriuretic peptide (ANP)—ANP is a 28-amino-acid peptide, synthesized primarily in cardiac atrial cells, and released in response to atrial stretch via mechanosensitive ion channels. Release of ANP is increased by volume expansion, immersion in water up to the neck, changing from the standing to the supine position, exercise, and sympathetic stimulation. ANP binds to transmembrane receptors with cytoplasmic domains that are guanylyl cyclases. The effects of ANP are to increase glomerular filtration rate and decrease proximal tubular sodium reabsorption leading to increased natriuresis. Additional effects of ANP include inhibition of renin, aldosterone, and AVP release, and vasodilation.

Integrity of the arterial circulation, as determined by cardiac output and peripheral vascular resistance, is the primary determinant of renal sodium and water excretion in health and disease. Specifically, either a primary decrease in cardiac output or arterial vasodilatation causes arterial underfilling, which results in the activation of neurohumoral reflexes that stimulate sodium and water retention. The renal excretion of sodium and water normally parallels sodium and water intake, so that an increase in plasma and blood volume is associated with increased renal sodium and water excretion. The increase in blood volume results in pressure diuresis and natriuresis (loss of water and sodium), restoring blood volume to normal.

ABNORMALITIES IN SODIUM AND WATER BALANCE

Abnormalities in sodium and water balance can be classified into 4 categories. Excess Na^+ is characterized by expansion of the ECF volume and frequently by low effective circulating blood volume (ie, heart failure, hypoalbuminemia, renal insufficiency). Deficit in Na^+ is characterized by reduced ECF volume. Excess water is caused by either excess intake or enhanced ADH release and is manifested by hyponatremia and hyposmolarity. Water deficit is caused by lack of intake or excess loss (renal and nonrenal) and is manifested by hypernatremia and hyperosmolarity.

Regulation of Potassium Balance

Potassium is the most abundant cation in the body and the main intracellular electrolyte. Most (98%) of the potassium in the body is sequestered within cells. The ratio of extracellular to intracellular potassium (1:10) is the major determinant of resting membrane potential and is maintained by a Na^+/K^+-ATPase. Serum potassium levels range between 3.6 and 5.0 mmol/L. Small losses (1%, or 35 mmol) of total-body potassium content can seriously disturb the delicate balance between intracellular and extracellular potassium and can result in profound physiologic changes. Because only a small percentage of the total-body stores is present in the ECF, hypokalemia (serum levels less than 3.6 mmol/L) is not necessarily synonymous with whole-body potassium deficiency. Manifestations of hypokalemia include generalized muscle weakness, paralytic ileus, and cardiac arrhythmias.

INTAKE, DISTRIBUTION, AND EXCRETION OF POTASSIUM

The minimum daily requirement of potassium is approximately 1600–2000 mg (40–50 mmol or mEq). The daily intake of potassium in the western diet is approximately 80–120 mmol. Only a small fraction (10%) of potassium is excreted through the gastrointestinal tract. The majority is excreted by the kidney, accounting for 90% of daily potassium losses. Thus, the kidney is responsible for long-term potassium homeostasis, as well as for regulating the serum potassium concentration. On a short-term basis, serum potassium is also regulated by the shift of potassium between the ICF and ECF. This short-term regulation of serum potassium is principally controlled by insulin and catecholamines through regulation of the transcellular distribution of potassium. Dietary potassium, which is rapidly absorbed by the gut, increases serum potassium transiently. The release of insulin and catecholamines during a meal quickly shifts the potassium into the cells.

Potassium excretion by the kidney is tightly regulated and is determined primarily by events beyond the early distal tubule, where either reabsorption or secretion of K^+ can occur. The filtered K^+ (approximately 700–800 mmol/d) is largely reabsorbed by proximal nephron segments, including the proximal convoluted tubules and thick loop of Henle. Only approximately 10% of filtered K^+ reaches the distal convoluted tubule. Excretion of K^+ occurs mainly through secretion by distal segments, predominantly the distal convoluted tubule and the collecting duct, and is mediated primarily by apical membrane K^+ channels in the principal cells. Potassium excretion almost always exceeds the amount delivered to the early distal tubule (except under conditions of sustained K^+ depletion), indicating that the rate of secretion is the key determinant of K^+ excretion. The principal site for the regulation of K^+ excretion is the distal tubule, where secretion is indirectly but tightly coupled to sodium reabsorption via the amiloride-sensitive sodium channel; and under regulation by aldosterone. Increased sodium reabsorption increases potassium secretion, whereas decreased sodium reabsorption decreases K^+ secretion. Any condition that decreases the activity of renal K^+ channels results in hyperkalemia (eg, amiloride intake or aldosterone deficiency), whereas increased activity results in hypokalemia (eg, primary aldosteronism or Liddle syndrome; see Chapter 6). Because the kidney is the major regulator of K^+ homeostasis, renal dysfunction results in abnormal levels of serum K^+.

Potassium contributes to regulation of its balance by stimulating aldosterone secretion by the glomerulosa cells of the adrenal cortex (Figure 10–5). This effect is facilitated by angiotensin II released in response to activation of the renin-angiotensin system when renal perfusion pressure is decreased. Aldosterone enhances renal and colonic K^+ secretion, promoting the loss of K^+ in the urine and stool. Sustained hyperkalemia does not occur in individuals with normal renal function despite marked increases in potassium intake because of an adaptive change in distal tubular K^+ secretion, such that intake is matched by rapid and equivalent increases in K^+ excretion. The mechanisms involved in the chronic adaptation to increased levels of K^+ include changes in apical K^+ and Na^+ conductance and in basolateral Na^+/K^+-ATPase pump activity, an increase in apical Na^+ delivery and reabsorption, and an increase in K^+ excretion per nephron to match K^+ intake.

Hormonal Regulation of Potassium Balance

Total-body stores of potassium and its cellular distribution in the body are closely regulated by key hormones.

Aldosterone—Aldosterone is the major regulator of body stores of potassium through its effect on the excretion of potassium by the kidney. Aldosterone increases the synthesis and activity of Na^+/K^+-ATPase in the basolateral membrane of the distal tubule, promoting the exchange of cytosolic Na^+ for K^+. The overall result is an increase in Na^+ reabsorption and an increase in K^+ excretion.

Insulin—Insulin stimulates entry of K^+ into the cell through activation of the electroneutral Na^+/H^+ antiporter, leading to Na^+ influx. The increase in intracellular Na^+ produced by insulin triggers the activation of the electrogenic Na^+/K^+-ATPase, which extrudes Na^+ from the cell in exchange for K^+. The treatment of patients with diabetic ketoacidosis with high insulin doses produces a significant influx of K^+ into the cells that may result in hypokalemia, manifested by changes in the electrocardiogram.

Catecholamines—Catecholamines (β-adrenergic receptor stimulation) increase cellular K^+ uptake by stimulating cell membrane Na^+/K^+-ATPase. Indirectly, catecholamines stimulate glycogenolysis, resulting in an increase in plasma glucose concentrations, release of insulin from the pancreas, and insulin-mediated effects on K^+ redistribution. Stimulation of the α-adrenergic receptor shifts K^+ out of the cell and can also affect K^+ distribution through inhibition of pancreatic insulin release.

Insulin and catecholamines are both stimulated by the ingestion of glucose- and K^+-rich foods, thereby maintaining K^+ homeostasis despite large dietary

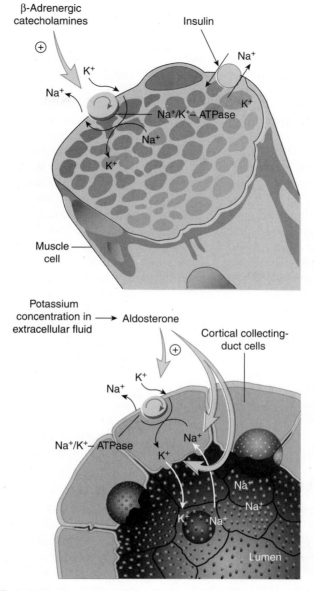

Figure 10–5. An increase in extracellular fluid potassium concentration stimulates the secretion of aldosterone and a decrease inhibits its secretion. Aldosterone promotes potassium excretion through its effects on Na$^+$/K$^+$-adenosine triphosphatase (ATPase) and epithelial sodium and potassium channels in collecting-duct cells. Angiotensin II has a synergistic effect on the stimulation of aldosterone production induced by hyperkalemia. Insulin stimulates entry of K$^+$ into the cell through the activation of the electroneutral Na$^+$/K$^+$ antiporter. The increase in intracellular Na$^+$ produced by insulin triggers the activation of the electrogenic Na$^+$/K$^+$-ATPase, which extrudes Na$^+$ from the cell in exchange for K$^+$. Catecholamines (β-adrenergic receptor stimulation) increase cellular potassium uptake by stimulating cell membrane Na$^+$/K$^+$-ATPase. Stimulation of the α-adrenergic receptor produces a shift of K$^+$ out of the cell. (Modified, with permission, from Gennari F. Current concepts: hypokalemia. *N Engl J Med.* 1998;339:451. Copyright © Massachusetts Medical Society. All rights reserved.)

intake. These hormones are essential in moving K^+ primarily into the intracellular compartment of the liver and striated muscle cells.

Intracellular K^+ homeostasis is also affected by changes in acid-base balance and osmolarity. Sudden changes in plasma osmolarity redistribute water between the ICF and ECF. This movement of water out of a cell creates a solvent drag phenomenon, pulling K^+ out of the cell and therefore increasing serum K^+. Similarly, metabolic acidosis caused by a loss of bicarbonate or a gain in hydrogen ion concentration [H^+] leads to a shift of K^+ across cell membranes and hyperkalemia. However, integrity of renal function and stimulation of aldosterone release rapidly correct this imbalance. These examples do not entail net changes in body K^+. In contrast, in diabetic ketoacidosis, there is a net loss of K^+ from the body because of osmotic diuresis, despite elevations in ECF K^+ concentrations (hyperkalemia), because of insulin deficiency. Following aggressive insulin treatment, hypokalemia becomes apparent. Opposite effects are observed during alkalosis. In metabolic alkalosis, the excess bicarbonate causes H^+ in the ECF to decrease, leading to entry of Na^+ into the cell in exchange for H^+. Na^+ is pumped out of the cell by the Na^+/K^+-ATPase in exchange for K^+ movement into the cell creating a shift of K^+ into the cells.

Low serum K^+ concentration (hypokalemia; less than 3.6 mmol/L) is perhaps the most common electrolyte abnormality encountered in clinical practice. Hypokalemia is almost always the result of K^+ depletion induced by abnormal fluid losses (ie, vomiting, colonic diarrhea, profuse sweating, diuretic use, or nasogastric suction). Patients present with muscle weakness and changes in the electrocardiogram. More rarely, hypokalemia occurs because of an abrupt shift of K^+ from the ECF into cells, frequently as an effect of prescription drugs.

Regulation of Calcium Balance

Serum calcium concentrations are tightly regulated and concentrations are held constant at 1 mmol of ionized calcium or 10 mg/dL of total calcium. Calcium accounts for 1%–2% of adult human body weight, with the majority (99%) found in bones and teeth. Calcium helps maintain the cell membrane electrical potential and is involved in signaling mechanisms, enzymatic activity, coagulation cascade, neurotransmitter release, and intercellular communication. Because of its role in these and other critical functions, its tight regulation is important in preventing diseases such as osteoporosis, renal and heart disease, and hypertension.

The recommended calcium intake varies with age, sex, and reproductive stage. Higher intakes are recommended for children, adolescents, pregnant and lactating mothers, postmenopausal women, and the elderly (1200–1500 mg/d) than for healthy adults up to age 65 years (1000 mg/d). A positive correlation between protein intake and urinary calcium has been established. This relationship may explain the apparently higher calcium requirement of the diet in the developed world as compared with that of underdeveloped countries. The catabolism of dietary protein generates ammonium ion and sulfates from sulfur-containing amino acids, leading to the acidification of plasma. This decrease in pH triggers bone resorption to supply buffers such as citrate and carbonate, with the consequent release of calcium into the circulation, resulting in calciuria.

HORMONAL REGULATION OF CALCIUM BALANCE

Calcium homeostasis is maintained by the complex interaction of several hormones, particularly vitamin D, parathyroid hormone (PTH), and calcitonin (see Chapter 4). Because the major reservoir for calcium is the bone, and this is the pool of calcium that is involved in actively maintaining serum plasma concentrations within a normal range, the factors that influence bone metabolism such as estrogen, growth factors, glucocorticoids, thyroid hormone, and cytokines also contribute significantly to the overall metabolic control of Ca^{2+} stores. However, it is important to note that it is the "free" calcium in serum that is under tight hormonal regulation, principally by PTH.

Parathyroid hormone—PTH activates 25-hydroxyvitamin D-1α-hydroxylase, the enzyme that converts 25-hydroxyvitamin D to the active form of 1,25-dihydroxyvitamin D [1,25(OH)$_2$D]. PTH also stimulates renal reabsorption of calcium.

Vitamin D—1,25(OH)$_2$D increases dietary Ca^{2+} absorption in the small intestine and increases osteoblast activity, resulting in stimulation of osteoclast-mediated resorption. Vitamin D plays an important role in differentiation of the promyelocyte to the osteoclast precursor to mature osteoclast through osteoblast-generated osteoclast differentiation factor (see Chapter 5). These effects of vitamin D on bone resorption coupled with formation as part of the bone-remodeling process result in calcium mobilization by the skeleton into the plasma compartment. Both PTH and vitamin D are required for this system to operate. In the distal renal tubule, PTH and vitamin D act in concert to produce virtually complete reabsorption of the filtered load of calcium. These sources of calcium cause an increase in serum calcium, which, through feedback inhibition at the parathyroid gland, decreases PTH secretion (see Chapter 5).

Calcitonin—Calcitonin counteracts the effects of PTH and vitamin D. It prevents hypercalcemia by directly inhibiting osteoclast activity, thereby reducing calcium mobilization and release from the skeleton.

Hormonal Regulation of Phosphate Balance

Phosphorus in the form of phosphate ($H_2PO_4^-$), accounts for more than 50% of bone mineral mass. Osteoblasts are unique among all other cell types in that they create a mineral trap (calcium-phosphate) in bone matrix after it has been deposited. This trap depletes the ECF around the osteoblast of both calcium and phosphorus, and if the local concentration of phosphorus drops too low, osteoblasts become phosphorus starved. Throughout the body, phosphorus is found as a component of nucleic acids, phospholipids, signaling molecules (inositol 1,4,5-trisphosphate, phosphatidylinositol 4,5-bisphosphate), and cofactors involved in cellular energy metabolism (ATP, guanosine triphosphate), playing numerous vital roles in cell function. Most food products, whether plant or animal, contain relatively abundant quantities of phosphates. Normal balanced diets provide 800–1500 mg of phosphorus per day. The skeleton contains 85% of the body's phosphorus; the rest is distributed in the ECF and ICF (0.5–0.8 g). Total extracellular phosphorus (about 12 mg/dL) is found in an ionized form and a nonionized form (8.5 mg/dL is in the organic form and 3.5 mg/dL is in the inorganic form). The inorganic form may be found ionized or free (50%); complexed with Ca^{2+}, Mg^{2+}, and Na^+ (35%); or bound to protein (15%).

Phosphate homeostasis is maintained by intestinal absorption, renal excretion, balance of phosphate exchange in and out of the cells, and their hormonal regulation. Because of its critical role in energy-requiring physiologic functions, the extracellular phosphate concentration is maintained in a narrow range, principally through regulation of urinary excretion. When renal function is compromised, impaired phosphate excretion by the kidney leads to hyperphosphatemia and the stimulation of PTH release from the parathyroid gland (Figure 10–6).

 Following intestinal absorption from the diet, most phosphate undergoes urinary excretion. Under normal physiologic conditions, urinary phosphate excretion corresponds roughly to phosphate intake and absorption

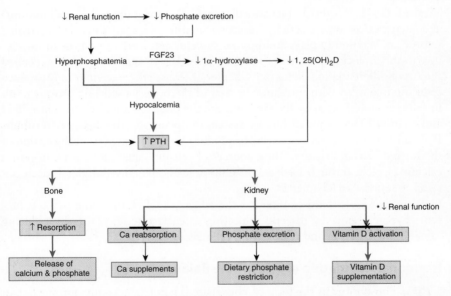

Figure 10–6. Phosphate balance in chronic renal failure. When renal function is compromised, impaired phosphate excretion by the kidney leads to hyperphosphatemia. Hyperphosphatemia stimulates parathyroid hormone (PTH) release from the parathyroid gland and also stimulates release of fibroblast growth factor 23 (FGF23), which in turn suppresses activity of 1α-hydroxylase and vitamin D activation. Decreased $1,25(OH)_2D$ allows for increased PTH release as well. PTH stimulates bone resorption and release of calcium phosphate. Because of the impairment in renal function, PTH is unable to stimulate calcium reabsorption, phosphate excretion, or vitamin D activation. Management of these patients requires supplementation with calcium, control of dietary phosphate intake, and vitamin D supplementation.

from the upper small intestine. Alterations in extracellular phosphate concentrations lead to rapid adjustments in renal excretion and slower and less regulated adjustments in intestinal absorption. Under normal physiologic conditions, approximately 80%–90% of the filtered load of phosphate is reabsorbed primarily in the proximal tubules, with higher rates of reabsorption at early segments. Low dietary phosphate intake can lead to almost 100% reabsorption of filtered phosphate, whereas high dietary phosphate intake decreases proximal tubular reabsorption.

Phosphate excretion by the kidney is stimulated by PTH through the inhibition of brush-border membrane Na^+/PO_4^{2-}cotransport activity. Phosphate reabsorption in the proximal tubule can also be decreased by fibroblast growth factor 23 (FGF23), a peptide produced in osteoblasts and osteocytes. FGF23 suppresses the 1-hydroxylase responsible for synthesis of $1,25(OH)_2D$ and decreases renal phosphate reabsorption through reduction of the expression of the sodium phosphate cotransporters in the kidney and intestine. FGF23 production is stimulated by $1,25(OH)_2D$ and by high phosphate levels. Abnormalities in FGF23 are linked to genetic diseases such as autosomal dominant hypophosphatemic rickets.

Phosphate reabsorption by the kidney is increased by vitamin D and insulin through stimulation of brush-border membrane Na^+/PO_4^{2-}cotransport and inhibition of the phosphaturic action of PTH. Vitamin D also regulates intestinal phosphate absorption by stimulating the brush-border membrane Na^+/PO_4^{2-}cotransport in the upper small intestine. Thus, PTH promotes phosphate excretion, whereas vitamin D and insulin promote phosphate renal reabsorption and intestinal absorption. Vitamin D deficiency leads to increased phosphate renal excretion and decreased intestinal phosphate and Ca^{2+} absorption, resulting in a severe loss of both Ca^{2+} and phosphate from bone (the major site of both of these mineral stores) because of enhanced PTH activity, resulting in loss of bone mineral and osteomalacia. This is in contrast to osteoporosis induced by Ca^{2+} deficiency.

NEUROENDOCRINE REGULATION OF THE STRESS RESPONSE

Alterations in the environment or in the host that require adaptation involve the synchronized interaction of virtually all aspects of neuroendocrine function that have been described. The process of adaptation to a biologic, psychosocial, or environmental insult to the host is referred to as the stress response; in the acute setting, it is also termed the "fight or flight" response. It is now clear that in modern life, this stress response can be chronic, with a significant cost to the health of the individual. This wear and tear of chronic adaptation to daily stressors constitutes the allostatic load of the individual; it is the "pathologic" chronic homeostasis through which we achieve stability at the expense of psychosocial and physical well being.

Chronic activation of the mechanisms that restore homeostasis results in excessive and, in some cases, inadequate responses that ultimately alter the function of virtually all organ systems (eg, hypertension, autoimmune disorders, metabolic

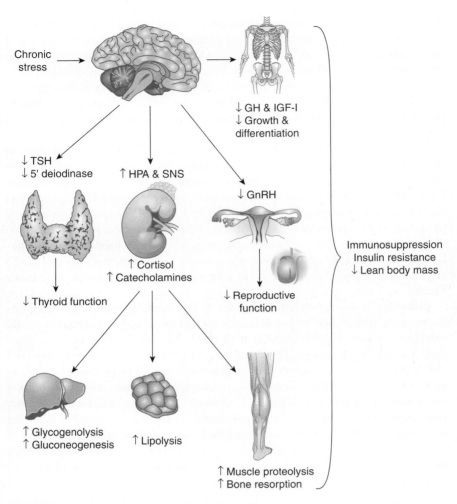

Chronic stress

↓ GH & IGF-I
↓ Growth &
differentiation

↓ TSH
↓ 5' deiodinase

↑ HPA & SNS

↓ GnRH

↓ Thyroid function

↑ Cortisol
↑ Catecholamines

↓ Reproductive
function

Immunosuppression
Insulin resistance
↓ Lean body mass

↑ Glycogenolysis
↑ Gluconeogenesis

↑ Lipolysis

↑ Muscle proteolysis
↑ Bone resorption

Figure 10–7. The chronic activation of the mechanisms that restore homeostasis results alterations in function in virtually all organ systems. The short-term activation of these stress response mechanisms ensures that energy substrates are available to meet the increased metabolic demands of the individual. However, prolonged duration and increased magnitude of their activity leads to erosion of lean body mass and tissue injury. GH, growth hormone; GnRH, gonadotropin-releasing hormone; HPA, hypothalamic-pituitary-adrenal axis; IGF-1, insulin-like growth factor 1; SNS, sympathetic nervous system; TSH, thyroid-stimulating hormone.

syndrome) (Figure 10–7). Many of the effects of this dysregulated state are mediated by chronic activation of the hypothalamic-pituitary-adrenal (HPA) axis and the sympathetic nervous system, producing marked alterations in endocrine function, such as the following:

Inhibition of reproduction function—Enhanced release of corticotropin-releasing hormone (CRH) and β-endorphin suppresses GnRH release directly and indirectly through the release of glucocorticoids. Elevated glucocorticoids suppress the release of GnRH, luteinizing hormone, and follicle-stimulating hormone, and produce gonadotropin resistance at the gonads. This suppression in gonadal function is evident in patients with anorexia nervosa and extreme athletes.

Inhibition of the GH–IGF-1 axis—Chronic activation of the HPA axis suppresses GH release and inhibits the effects of IGF-1 at target tissues.

Suppression of thyroid function—CRH and cortisol suppress the production of thyroid-stimulating hormone and inhibit the activity of peripheral 5′-deiodinase, leading to the euthyroid sick syndrome.

Dysregulation of energy substrate metabolism—An increase in catecholamines stimulates lipolysis and decreases triglyceride synthesis in white adipose tissue. In the liver, increased epinephrine levels stimulate hepatic glycogenolysis and, together with high cortisol levels, increase hepatic glucose output. High cortisol levels resulting from activation of the HPA increase gluconeogenesis, produce insulin resistance in peripheral tissues, inhibit the lipolytic action of GH, and inhibit bone osteoblastic activation (remodeling) by sex steroids. This leads to increases in visceral adiposity and loss of BMD and lean body mass. This aspect of the stress response may be of particular importance in the treatment of diabetic patients during stressful periods such as surgery or infection.

Alterations in the immune response—The significant rise in circulating cortisol levels affects virtually all aspects of the immune response, including cytokine production, leukocyte trafficking and recruitment, and production of chemokines. Overall, glucocorticoids exert an anti-inflammatory response and increase the risk of infections. CRH may have direct proinflammatory effects on cells of the immune system. Activation of the autonomic nervous system also affects the immune response through effects on neutrophil demargination and cytokine production.

Short-term activation of these stress response mechanisms ensures that energy substrates are available to meet the increased metabolic demands of the individual. However, prolonged duration and increased magnitude of these activities lead to erosion of lean body mass and tissue injury. Nevertheless, impaired activation or lack of responsiveness of the HPA and autonomic nervous system can also be deleterious, as in the case of the critically ill patient. Thus, the overall regulation of the neuroendocrine responses that mediate the physiologic functions involved in maintaining and restoring homeostasis is critically important in situations such as illness, trauma, surgery, or fasting.

KEY CONCEPTS

 Energy substrate mobilization, utilization, and storage are under neuroendocrine regulation.

 Hepatic glycogen and adipose tissue triglycerides are the principal sites of energy storage.

 The central nervous system integrates the counterregulatory response to acute decreases in energy substrate availability.

 Regulation of sodium balance determines blood volume and blood pressure control.

 The kidney is responsible for long-term potassium homeostasis and serum potassium concentration.

 Insulin and catecholamines regulate the cellular distribution of potassium.

 Serum calcium levels are tightly regulated through hormone-mediated effects on bone.

 Phosphate is regulated principally through effects on renal excretion.

 STUDY QUESTIONS

10–1. Which of the following neuroendocrine responses contributes to meeting the enhanced energy demands during exercise?

a. Glucagon stimulation of hepatic glycogen synthesis

b. Epinephrine stimulation of hepatic glycogenolysis

c. Norepinephrine-induced stimulation of insulin release

d. Cortisol inhibition of gluconeogenesis

10–2. Which of the following processes takes place immediately after a balanced meal?

a. Suppression of pancreatic insulin release

b. Increased muscle and fat glucose uptake

c. Increased hepatic glycogenolysis

d. Suppressed lipogenesis

10–3. Activation of the renin-angiotensin-aldosterone system during loss of effective intravascular volume results in all of the following except:

   a. Increased renal sodium and fluid retention

   b. Potentiation of the activity of the sympathetic nervous system

   c. Peripheral venodilation

   d. Enhanced ADH release

10–4. Regulation of body K^+ content and distribution can be affected by all of the following except:

   a. Aldosterone-induced increase in K^+ excretion

   b. Insulin stimulation of intracellular K^+ efflux

   c. β-Adrenergic stimulation of cell membrane Na^+/K^+-ATPase

   d. Sudden changes in plasma osmolarity

10–5. Mechanisms involved in the regulation of Pi balance include:

   a. PTH stimulation of Pi excretion

   b. Decreased proximal tubular reabsorption by vitamin D

   c. Insulin suppression of proximal tubular Pi reabsorption

   d. Vitamin D inhibition of intestinal Pi absorption

SUGGESTED READINGS

Ahima RS, Flier JS. Leptin. *Annu Rev Physiol*. 2000;62:413.

Friedman JM. Obesity in the new millennium. *Nature*. 2000;404:632.

Frühbeck G, Gómez-Ambrosi J, Muruzábal FJ, Burell MA. The adipocyte: a model for integration of endocrine and metabolic signaling in energy metabolism regulation. *Am J Physiol Endocrinol Metab*. 2001;280:E827.

Gennari F. Current concepts: hypokalemia. *N Engl J Med*. 1998;339:451.

Habib KE, Gold PW, Chrousos GP. Neuroendocrinology of stress. *Endocrinol Metab Clin North Am*. 2001;30:695.

Havel PJ. Peripheral signals conveying metabolic information to the brain: short-term and long-term regulation of food intake and energy homeostasis. *Exp Biol Med*. 2001;226:963.

Hillebrand JJ, de Wied D, Adan RA. Neuropeptides, food intake and body weight regulation: a hypothalamic focus. *Peptides*. 2002;23:2283.

Kojima M, Kangawa K. Ghrelin: structure and function. *Physiol Rev*. 2005;85:495.

Jequier E. Leptin signaling, adiposity, and energy balance. *Ann N Y Acad Sci*. 2002;967:379.

Kopelman PG. Obesity as a medical problem. *Nature*. 2000;404:635.

Liu Z, Barrett EJ. Human protein metabolism: its measurement and regulation. *Am J Physiol Endocrinol Metab*. 2002;283:E1105.

Margetic S, Gazzola C, Pegg GG, Hill RA. Leptin: a review of its peripheral actions and interactions. *Int J Obes Relat Metab Disord*. 2002;26:1407.

Mora S, Pessin JE. An adipocentric view of signaling and intracellular trafficking. *Diabetes Metab Res Rev*. 2002;18:345.

Tsao TS, Lodish HF, Fruebis J. ACRP30, a new hormone controlling fat and glucose metabolism. *Eur J Pharmacol*. 2002;440:213.

Wilding JPH. Neuropeptides and appetite control. *Diabet Med*. 2002;19:619.

Appendix: Normal Values of Metabolic Parameters and Tests of Endocrine Function

Table A. Plasma and serum values

Hormone	Time/condition of sample	Normal value or range SI (traditional units)
ACTH	8:00 AM	<18 pmol/L (<80 pg/mL)
Aldosterone	8:00 AM	<220 pmol/L (<8 ng/dL)
Potassium		3.5–5.0 mmol/L (3.5–5.0 mEq/L)
Angiotensin II	8:00 AM	10–30 nmol/L (10–30 pg/mL)
Arginine vasopressin	Random fluid intake	1.5–5.6 pmol/L (1.5–6 ng/L)
Plasma osmolarity		285–295 mOsmol/L
Sodium		136–145 mmol/L (136–145 mEq/L)
Cortisol	8:00 AM 4:00 PM	140–690 nmol/L (5–25 µg/dL) 80–330 nmol/L (3–12 µg/dL)
DHEA		7–31 nmol/L (2–9 µg/L)
DHEAS		1.3–6.7 µmol/L (500–2500 µg/L)
17-Hydroxyprogesterone	Women Follicular Luteal Men	0.6–3 nmol/L (0.20–1 µg/L) 1.5–10.6 nmol/L (0.5–3.5 µg/L) 0.2–9 nmol/L (0.06–3 µg/L)
Calcium	Plasma	2.2–2.6 mmol/L (9–10.5 mg/dL)
Phosphorus	Inorganic	1.0–1.4 mmol/L (3–4.5 mg/dL)
Vitamin D		40–160 pmol/L (16–65 pg/mL)
Calcitonin		<50 ng/mL (<50 pg/mL)
Glucagon		50–100 ng/mL (50–100 pg/mL)
Insulin	Overnight fast	43–186 pmol/L (6–26 µU/mL)
Glucose	Overnight fast	4.2–6.4 mmol/L (75–115 mg/dL)
β-OH butyrate		<300 µmol/L (<3 mg/dL)
Lactate	Venous plasma	0.6–1.7 mmol/L (5–15 mg/dL)
Fatty acids	Free	180 mg/L (<18 mg/dL)
Androstenedione	Women Men	3.5–7.0 nmol/L (1–2 ng/mL) 3.0–5.0 nmol/L (0.8–1.3 ng/mL)
Estradiol	Women Men	70–220 pmol/L (20–60 pg/mL) <180 pmol/L (50 pg/mL)

(Continued)

Table A. Plasma and serum values (*continued*)

Hormone	Time/condition of sample	Normal value or range SI (traditional units)
Progesterone	Women Luteal peak Men, prepubescent girls, postmenopausal women	>16 nmol/L (75 ng/mL) <6 nmol/L (<2 ng/mL)
Testosterone	Women Men Prepubertal boys and girls	<3.5 nmol/L (<1 ng/mL) 10–35 nmol/L (3–10 ng/mL) 0.17–0.7 nmol/L (0.05–0.2 ng/mL)
FSH	Women (reproductive age) Ovulatory surge Postmenopausal women Mature men	5–20 IU/L (5–20 mIU/mL) 12–30 IU/L (12–30 mIU/mL) 12–30 IU/L (12–30 mIU/mL) 5–20 IU/L (5–20 mIU/mL)
LH	Women (reproductive age) Ovulatory surge Postmenopausal women Mature men	5–25 IU/L (5–25 mIU/mL) 25–100 IU/L (25–100 mIU/mL) >50 IU/L (>50 mIU/mL) 5–20 IU/L (5–20 mIU/mL)
β-hCG	Men and nonpregnant women	<3 IU/L
Oxytocin	Random Ovulatory peak	1–4 pmol/L (1.25–5 pg/mL) 4–8 pmol/L (5–10 ng/mL)
Prolactin		2–15 µg/L (2–15 ng/mL)
Growth hormone	Post 100 g glucose PO	<5 µg/L (<5 ng/mL)
TSH		0.4–5 mU/L (0.4–5 µU/mL)
Thyroxine (T$_4$)		64–154 nmol/L (5–12 µg/dL)
Triiodothyronine (T$_3$)		1.1–2.9 nmol/L (70–190 ng/dL)
Reverse T$_3$		0.15–0.61 nmol/L (10–40 ng/dL)
Resin T$_3$ uptake		25–35%

ACTH, adrenocorticotropic hormone; DHEA, dehydroepiandrosterone; DHEAS, dehydroepiandrosterone sulfate; FSH, follicle-stimulating hormone; hCG, human chorionic gonadotropin; LH, luteinizing hormone; PO, by mouth; TSH, thyroid-stimulating hormone.

SI: System of International Units.

Conversions:

$$mmol/L = \frac{mg/dL \times 10}{atomic\ weight}$$

$$mg/dL = \frac{mmol/L \times atomic\ weight}{10}$$

Table B. Urinary levels

Hormone or metabolite	Amount excreted
Aldosterone	14–53 nmol/d (5–19 µg/d)
Free cortisol	55–275 nmol/d (20–100 µg/d)
17-Hydroxycorticosteroids	5.5–28 µg/d (2–10 mg/d)
17-Ketosteroids	Men: 24–88 µmol/d (7–25 mg/d)
	Women: 14–52 µmol/d (4–15 mg/d)
Free catecholamines	<590 nmol/d (<100 µg/d)
Epinephrine	<275 nmol/d (<50 µg/d)
Metanephrines	<7 µmol/d (<1.3 mg/d)
Vanillylmandelic acid (VMA)	<40 µmol/d (<8 mg/d)

Answers to Study Questions

CHAPTER 1

1–1. (b)   Hormones bind to specific receptors in their target cells. Lipid-soluble hormones bind to intracellular receptors. Hormone binding to binding proteins increase their half-life. Peptide hormones bind to cell membrane receptors. Thyroid hormones are the only nonsteroid hormones that bind to intracellular receptors. They are transported into the cell.

1–2. (e)   Changes in mineral and nutrient plasma levels (eg, calcium or glucose) affect hormone release. Pituitary tumors can result in either deficient or excessive hormone production. Transatlantic flight can disrupt circadian rhythms affecting hormone release. Strenuous exercise (as in training for the Olympics) is associated with decreased gonadotropin-releasing hormone (GnRH) release.

1–3. (d)   Hormones may inhibit their release through an autocrine mechanism. The substrate a hormone regulates (eg, calcium or glucose) directly regulates release of insulin and parathyroid hormone. Negative feedback regulation can occur at the level of the organ releasing the hormone, at the pituitary or in the hypothalamus. Feedback inhibition may be exerted by nutrients (calcium) and hormones (cortisol).

1–4. (c)   The structure of the hormone dictates location of its receptor. This large glycosylated peptide cannot cross the plasma membrane, so it will bind to a cell membrane receptor. It will likely undergo degradation, so it will not be excreted intact in the urine. Hormones do not directly bind to adenylate cyclase. They bind to receptors that couple with diverse signaling mechanisms.

CHAPTER 2

2–1. (b)   Urinary output is 10 times higher than normal (1.5 L/d). This patient suffered traumatic brain injury that disrupted his hypothalamic-neurohypophysial axis. The large urine volume is the result of decreased arginine vasopressin (AVP) release and decreased water reabsorption (neurogenic diabetes insipidus). Serum sodium and osmolarity will be high because of the excess in water losses.

2–2. (b)   The high volume of diluted urine (low sodium and low osmolality) match the description of the patient's clinical presentation.

2–3. (c) This patient's problem is most likely associated with decreased free-water reabsorption because of lack of arginine vasopressin (AVP)-stimulating aquaporin 2 insertion into the luminal membrane of the collecting duct. Low AVP levels reflect low production and release of AVP. Without adequate AVP-mediated receptor stimulation, there is no reason to expect increased urinary release of cyclic 3′,5′-adenosine monophosphate (cAMP). Nothing suggests that there is increased sodium reabsorption in this individual.

2–4. (c) Throughout pregnancy, uterine changes will make the tissue more responsive to oxytocin-receptor stimulation. This is the result of increased prostaglandin synthesis, decreased β-adrenergic receptor expression, increased gap junction formation, and increased oxytocin receptor expression. These changes are the result of increased estrogen levels during pregnancy.

2–5. (d) This patient presents with low sodium levels and a differential diagnosis of syndrome of inappropriate antidiuretic hormone secretion (SIADH). SIADH is the excessive and inappropriate release of antidiuretic hormone despite a lack of physiologic signal (increased osmolarity or decreased blood volume). This person will have low volume of very concentrated urine.

CHAPTER 3

3–1. (b) This patient presents with visual abnormalities and an enlarged sella turcica suggesting enlarged pituitary gland. It is important to remember the close anatomic relationship of the gland with the optic chiasm. His complaint of decreased libido for the past 6–9 months is suggestive of decreased testosterone, which in turn is the result of excess prolactin production, which suppresses gonadotropin-releasing hormone (GnRH) release. There are no signs of water balance problems. There are no indications of altered glucocorticoid production (no changes in glucose levels) or in growth hormone release (no metabolic or soft tissue growth abnormalities). Increased luteinizing hormone (LH) release would result in increased testosterone production and that would not be associated with decreased libido.

3–2. (c) This is a young woman in her fertile years who manifests visual problems and infertility. This presentation is likely associated with increased prolactin levels. There are no other indications of abnormal endocrine function.

3–3. (b) Laceration of the median eminence would be expected to disrupt hypothalamo-hypophysial portal circulation decreasing the delivery of growth hormone-releasing hormone (GHRH) and as a result insulin-like growth factor 1 (IGF-1). It would be expected that decreased delivery of dopamine to the anterior pituitary would result in an increase in prolactin resulting from removal of inhibitory tone of lactotrophs.

Parathyroid hormone (PTH) is not controlled by the hypothalamus and thus its levels would not be expected to change.

3–4. (c) Growth hormone (GH) will have its most important effects on longitudinal growth during childhood. Intrauterine growth is modestly affected by decreased GH. Similarly, early postnatal weight gain is not dependent on GH action. Hyperglycemia and impaired glucose tolerance, as well as deepening of the voice would be manifestations of excess GH release in adulthood.

3–5. (e) The α-subunit of follicle-stimulating hormone (FSH) is identical to that of thyroid-stimulating hormone (TSH). It is the β subunit that gives the hormone its specificity. Therefore, a recombinant hormone will have the effects attributed to the β subunit of TSH. Thus it would be expected that Na/I symporter activity, thyroglobulin synthesis, and tetraiodothyronine (T_4) release would increase while not affecting luteolysis or ovulation.

CHAPTER 4

4–1. (c) The clinical presentation of this patient is consistent with hyperthyroidism (restlessness, nervousness, insomnia, tachycardia, tremors, and warm moist hands) associated with goiter (enlarged thyroid gland). You expect high triiodothyronine (T_3), low or normal reverse triiodothyronine (rT_3) (less active form of the hormone), and very low thyroid-stimulating hormone (TSH) because of negative feedback inhibition.

4–2. (c) The radioactive iodine scan revealed greater concentration of radioiodine because that is a gland that has all steps in thyroid hormone synthesis fully stimulated. The positive serum titers of thyroid-stimulating immunoglobulin (TSI) confirm that the thyroid-stimulating hormone (TSH) receptor is being constantly stimulated. The TSH receptor is a G-protein-coupled receptor (GPCR), that couples to adenylate cyclase and results in increased cyclic 3′,5′-adenosine monophosphate (cAMP) on stimulation. There should be no change in thyroid-binding protein levels nor a downregulation of the Na/I symporter. The increased thyroid hormone (TH) action is not the result of increased deiodination of tetraiodothyronine (T_4) to triiodothyronine (T_3) in the liver.

4–3. (d) This patient presents in a rural setting complaining of fatigue, constipation, lethargy, and intolerance to cold. All of these are suggestive of low thyroid function. He is on a low salt diet and consumes a predominantly vegetarian diet, with water derived from a local well. All of these are hints at low iodide in the diet. The slowly growing enlarged mass in his neck, taken together with the history are consistent with hypothyroidism caused by decreased dietary iodine and consequently decreased follicular cell iodine concentration.

4–4. (c) The clinical presentation of this patient is consistent with hyperthyroidism (restlessness, nervousness, insomnia, tachycardia, tremors, and warm moist hands). The enlarged thyroid in a female hyperthyroid patient is strongly suggestive of Graves disease. You would expect high triiodothyronine (T_3), low or normal reverse triiodothyronine (rT_3) (rT_3 is increased in chronic illness or nutritional deprivation), suppressed thyroid-stimulating hormone (TSH) (because of negative feedback), and increased titers of circulating thyroid-stimulating immunoglobulin.

CHAPTER 5

5–1. (b) The precipitating factor in this young otherwise healthy patient is dehydration. He has high parathyroid hormone (PTH) levels (probably a problem that had been ongoing). High PTH is associated with increased bone resorption resulting in increased serum calcium (and consequently filtered calcium), which with dehydration, precipitated and formed kidney stones (reason for the pain and the blood in the urine when he passed them). You would expect low serum inorganic phosphate (Pi), because PTH promotes Pi excretion. High PTH would stimulate vitamin D synthesis and thus intestinal calcium absorption. The urinary calcium excretion likely reflects a reabsorption process that has been overwhelmed by the excess calcium filtered. The increase in bone resorption and turnover would be expected to be associated with increased serum alkaline phosphatase.

5–2. (d) This patient has excess production of parathyroid hormone (PTH) that is no longer controlled by high plasma calcium levels. Thus, there is a loss of negative feedback regulation of PTH release. He probably has increased calcitonin release. PTH promotes preosteoclast recruitment and differentiation, not osteoclast apoptosis. The activity of 24 hydroxylase (in the kidney) would be responsive to increased calcium levels, but not that of 25-hydroxylase (in the liver).

5–3. (a) This elderly patient has a history of malignancy with bone metastasis. Bone resorption is expected to be elevated. This explains why her parathyroid hormone (PTH) levels are low (suppressed by high calcium). Phosphate is elevated because it is released during bone resorption with calcium. Alkaline phosphatase levels increase during bone resorption.

5–4. (c) The hypercalcemia of malignancy is caused by increased parathyroid hormone (PTH) related peptide and not PTH itself.

5–5. (d) Most of protein-bound Ca^{2+} is bound to albumin, and this interaction is sensitive to changes in blood pH. Acidosis leads to a decrease in protein binding of Ca^{2+} and an increase in "free" or ionized Ca^{2+} in the plasma. Alkalosis results in increased Ca^{2+} binding and a decrease in ionized Ca^{2+} in the plasma. Hyperventilation leads to respiratory alkalosis and in turn a decrease in ionized calcium. For example, Na^+ channel voltage-gating is dependent on the extracellular Ca^{2+} concentration. Stable Ca^{2+} levels are critical for normal physiologic function. Decreased plasma Ca^{2+} concentrations reduce the voltage threshold for the action potential firing, resulting in neuromuscular hyperexcitability. This can result in numbness and tingling of fingertips, toes, and the perioral region or muscle cramps.

5–6. (c) Medical strategies for the management of osteoporosis include bisphosphonate-mediated apoptosis of osteoclasts, suppression of osteoclast activity by calcitonin, increased osteoblast differentiation by selective estrogen receptor modulators, and enhanced vitamin D–mediated intestinal Ca^{2+} absorption (not secretion).

CHAPTER 6

6–1. (a) This individual has clinical manifestations of excess cortisol that decreases in a dexamethasone suppression test, suggesting the source of cortisol production stimulation is within the hypothalamic-pituitary-adrenal (HPA) axis. Elevated cortisol production indicates that the adrenal cortex is not destroyed. The problem is not congenital. It has been identified at 49 years of age. The production of adrenocorticotropic hormone (ACTH) is unlikely to be in the lung as it responded to the dexamethasone suppression test. The clinical manifestations given are all reflecting increased cortisol and not aldosterone.

6–2. (c) The presentation suggests elevations in cortisol reflected by weight gain, and high glucose levels with all other parameters given within normal range. The increased blood pressure may be caused by increased mineralocorticoid-like activity by excess cortisol. The patient has normal menstrual periods, ruling out prolactinoma as a likely cause. Lung metastatic carcinoma would likely be associated with weight loss and not gain. Excess licorice consumption would be associated with higher serum sodium levels (hers are normal). Graves disease is highly unlikely, as there are no clinical manifestations of excess thyroid function; she is gaining weight and is hyperglycemic.

6–3. (d) The episodic presentation of headaches, associated with high blood pressure and all other parameters within normal ranges suggests increase catecholamine release most likely from a pheochromocytoma. This is also suggested by the adrenal mass that in response to manipulation releases catecholamines (surge in blood pressure during surgery). This patient would have likely had increased free catecholamines or metabolites in the urine.

6–4. (d) In this case, the patient presents with high blood pressure and high sodium and low potassium levels. This suggests increased aldosterone activity and rules out the likelihood of the hypertension being caused by pheochromocytoma. The renin values are low, so aldosterone production is not secondary to the canonical angiotensin II stimulation. The patient is not reported to be on any medications, ruling out iatrogenic Cushing syndrome. Plasma glucose levels are normal, so cortisol is not expected to be increased, ruling out a pituitary adenoma.

21-Hydroxylase deficiency would result in decreased mineralocorticoid activity. An adrenal adenoma making too much aldosterone could explain the patient's clinical presentation.

CHAPTER 7

7–1. (c) Insulin-induced hypoglycemia can be caused by self-administration of insulin (in a suicide attempt) or by the excessive release of insulin from an insulinoma. In the case of an insulinoma, C-peptide is released in a 1:1 ratio with insulin. Measuring C-peptide levels will reflect increased endogenous production of insulin.

7–2. (e) This is a clinical presentation of a hyperglycemic, hyperosmolar, nonketotic coma. This is more frequently seen in type 2 diabetes.

7–3. (b) This is a clinical presentation of hyperglycemia (most likely because the patient is diabetic and has had a recent infection that would have triggered a stress response contributing to the hyperglycemia). The patient is dehydrated and will likely have increased plasma osmolarity because of the hyperglycemia.

7–4. (c) The insulin pump stopped functioning in an individual who is dependent on insulin for glycemic control. The patient is likely to be hyperglycemic because of lack of insulin. Glucagon levels will likely be low because of the hyperglycemia. Without insulin, glycogen breakdown proceeds unopposed. Diabetic ketoacidosis is a more frequent complication in patients with type 1 diabetes. Lack of insulin results in increased circulating levels of free fatty acids and gluconeogenic amino acids. These exceed the liver's capacity for their metabolic utilization, leading to the buildup of ketone bodies in the blood (diabetic ketoacidosis) and their urinary excretion. Diabetic ketoacidosis is precipitated by infections, discontinuation of or inadequate insulin use, new-onset (untreated) diabetes, and other events, such as the stress associated with surgery.

CHAPTER 8

8–1. (c) The presentation of this young male patients with decreased testosterone explains why he has not developed secondary sexual characteristics normal for his age. Increased estradiol production would have led to epiphyseal closure.

8–2. (c) The excessive height and arm length resulting from delayed epiphyseal growth plate closure is caused by decreased estradiol production in bone.

8–3. (b) The small testicular size in someone taking hormone analogs to increase his muscle mass (presumably androgen analogs) would be associated with negative feedback at the hypothalamus and pituitary resulting in decreased follicle-stimulating hormone (FSH) and luteinizing hormone (LH). FSH determines seminiferous tubule growth, and thus testicular size and spermatogenesis.

8–4. (c)   Leptin released from adipose tissue is a permissive factor in initiating puberty. Strenuous exercise regimens or malnutrition leading to decreased fat mass are associated with delayed onset of puberty.

CHAPTER 9

9–1. (d)   Human chorionic gonadotropin (hCG) is the hormone of pregnancy and at 2-months' gestation should be elevated. Progesterone levels will also be increased because of combined production by the corpus luteum and the placenta.

9–2. (a)   Estriol is a reflection of fetal-placental unit health because its synthesis requires precursor synthesis by the mother, and placental and fetal metabolism. Maternal human chorionic gonadotropin (hCG) levels are a useful index of the functional status of the trophoblast (placental health).

9–3. (d)   This clinical presentation of excessive bleeding following delivery associated with other manifestations suggestive of additional hormonal deficiency (fatigue, weight gain) would be consistent with severe decrease in perfusion at the median eminence leading to decreased anterior pituitary function caused by ischemia. Decreased triiodothyronine (T_3) would be the result of a decrease in thyroid-stimulating hormone (TSH) release by the anterior pituitary. It would be expected that luteinizing hormone (LH), follicle-stimulating hormone (FSH) (and consequently estrogen), and adrenocorticotropic hormone (ACTH) would be decreased, prolactin may be low or normal (depending on the extent of cellular damage).

9–4. (d)   Menopausal changes in women result from a decrease in ovarian function, decreased estrogen, and removal of negative feedback resulting in increased luteinizing hormone (LH) and follicle-stimulating hormone (FSH) production and release.

CHAPTER 10

10–1. (b)   The enhanced energy demands during exercise are met by neuroendocrine stimulation of glycogenolysis and sympathetic inhibition of insulin release. Glucagon stimulates gluconeogenesis (not glycogen synthesis), and cortisol facilitates (does not inhibit) gluconeogenesis.

10–2. (b)   Immediately after a balanced meal, insulin release is increased leading to increased glucose transport into adipose tissue and skeletal muscle. The increase in insulin levels suppresses glycogenolysis and stimulates lipogenesis.

10–3. (c) Activation of the renin-angiotensin-aldosterone system during loss of effective intravascular volume results in increased renal sodium and fluid retention through increased Na and water reabsorption, potentiation of the activity of the sympathetic nervous system, venoconstriction (angiotensin-mediated vascular smooth muscle contraction), and increased antidiuretic hormone (ADH) release in response to the decreased blood volume (which is enhanced by angiotensin).

10–4. (d) Regulation of body K^+ content and distribution is affected by aldosterone-induced increase in K^+ excretion in exchange for Na; insulin indirect stimulation of intracellular influx (not efflux) of K^+ through activation of the Na/H antiporter; stimulation of the α-adrenergic receptor producing a shift of K^+ out of the cell; and sudden changes in plasma osmolarity. Sudden changes in plasma osmolarity redistribute water between the intracellular fluid (ICF) and extracellular fluid (ECF). This movement of water out of a cell creates a solvent drag phenomenon, pulling K^+ out of the cell and therefore increasing serum K^+.

10–5. (a) Parathyroid hormone (PTH) is the principal factor in the regulation of inorganic phosphate (Pi) balance, primarily through its renal excretion.

Index

Page numbers followed by *f* and *t* indicate figures and tables, respectively.